Clinical
Psychiatry

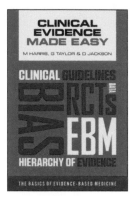
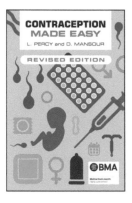
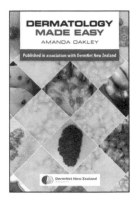
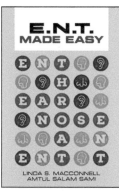
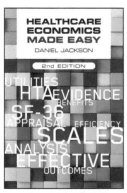
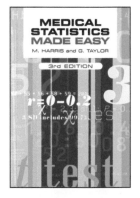
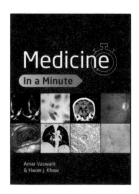
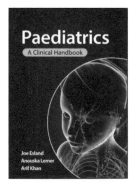
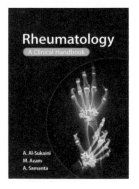
For more details see www.scionpublishing.com

Clinical Psychiatry

A handbook for medical students, residents, and clinicians

Charles DeBattista
Professor of Psychiatry and Behavioral Sciences,
Stanford University School of Medicine, California

Ira D. Glick
Professor Emeritus of Psychiatry and Behavioral Sciences,
Stanford University School of Medicine, California

Based on an original work by:
Mohsin Azam, Mohammed Qureshi, and Daniel Kinnair
Leicester Medical School, Leicester, UK

Scion

This in an updated American edition of *Psychiatry: A Clinical Handbook*, published by Scion Publishing Ltd in 2016 (ISBN 9781907904813)

Scion PublishingLimited

The Old Hayloft, Vantage Business Park, Bloxham Road, Banbury OX16 9UX, UK

www.scionpublishing.com

Important Note from the Publisher

The information contained within this book was obtained by Scion Publishing Ltd from sources believed by us to be reliable. However, while every effort has been made to ensure its accuracy, no responsibility for loss or injury whatsoever occasioned to any person acting or refraining from action as a result of information contained herein can be accepted by the authors or publishers.

Readers are reminded that medicine is a constantly evolving science and while the authors and publishers have ensured that all dosages, applications and practices are based on current indications, there may be specific practices which differ between communities. You should always follow the guidelines laid down by the manufacturers of specific products and the relevant authorities in the country in which you are practicing.

Although every effort has been made to ensure that all owners of copyright material have been acknowledged in this publication, we would be pleased to acknowledge in subsequent reprints or editions any omissions brought to our attention.

Registered names, trademarks, etc. used in this book, even when not marked as such, are not to be considered unprotected by law.

Line artwork by Hilary Strickland Illustration, Bath, UK

Typeset by Medlar Publishing Solutions Pvt Ltd, India

Printed in the UK

Last digit is the print number: 10 9 8 7 6 5 4

Contents

Preface ix

Acknowledgements x

Abbreviations xi

Outline of the book xiii

1   Introduction to psychiatry 1

2   Assessment in psychiatry 7

2.1   Psychiatric history taking 8

2.2   Mental status examination 15

3   Mood disorders 24

3.1   Overview of mood disorders 25

3.2   Depressive disorder 27

3.3   Bipolar affective disorder 35

4   Psychotic disorders 42

4.1   Overview of psychosis 43

4.2   Schizophrenia 45

5   Anxiety disorders 54

5.1   Overview of anxiety disorders 55

5.2   Generalized anxiety disorder 57

5.3   Phobic anxiety disorders 62

5.4   Panic disorder 67

6   Trauma and stressor-related disorders 71

7   Obsessive–compulsive and related disorders 79

8   Somatic symptom disorders 85

9   Feeding and eating disorders 94

9.1   Anorexia nervosa 95

9.2   Bulimia nervosa 102

10 Substance-related and addictive disorders 108
  10.1 Substance misuse 109
  10.2 Alcohol-use disorders 116

11 Personality disorders 125

12 Suicide and self-harm 131
  12.1 Deliberate non-suicidal self-harm 132
  12.2 Suicide and risk assessment 135

13 Neurocognitive disorders 141
  13.1 Delirium 142
  13.2 Dementia 149

14 Child psychiatry 161
  14.1 Autism spectrum disorders 162
  14.2 Attention deficit hyperactivity disorder 169
  14.3 Learning disability 175

15 Management 180
  15.1 Psychotherapies 181
  15.2 Antidepressants 187
  15.3 Antipsychotics 194
  15.4 Mood stabilizers 202
  15.5 Anxiolytics and hypnotics 207
  15.6 Electroconvulsive therapy (ECT) 210
  15.7 Transcranial magnetic stimulation (TMS) 213
  15.8 Vagus nerve stimulation (VNS) 215

16 Mental health law and forensic psychiatry 217
  16.1 Mental health and the law 218
  16.2 Forensic psychiatry 221

17 Common OSCE scenarios 224

18 Board-style questions 240

Glossary of terms 256
Appendix A   Answers to board-style questions 262
Appendix B   Answers to self-assessment questions 269
Appendix C   Figure acknowledgements 277
Index 279

Preface

Psychiatry is a rapidly evolving field. New medications are continually introduced including rapid-acting intravenous and intranasal antidepressants and long-acting antipsychotic injectables that only need to be given 4 times per year. Devices such as transcranial magnetic stimulation are playing a larger role in treatments and empirically based psychosocial treatments including dialectical behavior therapy and cognitive behavior therapy have become standard approaches for treating many mental disorders.

As psychiatry continues to evolve, so do other areas of medicine. The medical student and resident are faced with trying to synthesize a growing body of knowledge in a limited amount of time. This book represents an effort to distill the discipline of psychiatry to its essential elements. We (CD and IG) have spent decades teaching psychiatry to both pre-clinical and clerkship medical students at Stanford University and appreciate the need for efficiency in a reference book. Despite the fact that there are many books directed at medical students, we have found few of them are accessible enough to be consumed in the typical 4–8 week, American psychiatry clerkship. We hope that this book, with its bullet point format, extensive use of figures and tables, and relevant board-type questions can be rapidly reviewed and serve as an important part of preparation for both the National Board of Medical Examiner's (NBME) psychiatry shelf exam, as well as Step 2 and 3 of the US Medical Licensing Examination (USMLE).

In addition to medical students, several other learners will find this book useful. Neurology residents who are taking the American Board of Psychiatry and Neurology (ABPN) specialty board examination in neurology should find the book helpful in their preparation for this exam. Likewise, primary care physicians who increasingly have had to take a larger role in the treatment of mental health problems in their patients because of the shortage of psychiatric specialists, will also find the book helpful. Finally, graduate students in the mental health disciplines including clinical psychology and social work may also benefit from the book.

Charles DeBattista and Ira D. Glick

Acknowledgements

We are grateful to the many medical and graduate students, as well as residents and trainees, we have had the privilege of teaching at the University of California, San Francisco and Stanford University. Robert Heinlein said, "When one teaches, two learn," and we have been the recipients of much valued insights from the students we have taught over many years.

We are also grateful to the authors of the UK version of this book (MA, MQ, and DK) for providing an excellent template on which to build a US version. Finally, we would like to thank Jonathan Ray and the editorial group at Scion Publishing for their assistance in the completion of this text.

Please refer to Appendix C for acknowledgements to the copyright holders of the images provided in this book.

Abbreviations

6-CIT	6-item cognitive impairment test	CT	computed tomography
β-hCG	beta human chorionic gonadotropin	CTO	community treatment order
		CVA	cerebrovascular accident
AA	Alcoholics Anonymous	CXR	chest X-ray
ABCDE	airway, breathing, circulation, disability, exposure/examination	DBT	dialectical behavioral therapy
		DEXA	dual energy X-ray absorptiometry
ABG	arterial blood gas	DLB	dementia with Lewy bodies
ABV	alcohol by volume	DSH	deliberate self-harm
AD	Alzheimer's disease	DSM	The APA classification of mental disorders
add+up	attention deficit disorders uniting parents		
		DVM	diurnal variation in mood
ADDISS	Attention Deficit Disorder Information and Support Service	EAT	eating attitudes test
		ECG	electrocardiogram
ADHD	attention deficit hyperactivity disorder	ECHO	echocardiogram
		ECT	electroconvulsive therapy
ADL	activities of daily living	EDNOS	eating disorder not otherwise specified
AKA	also known as		
ALL	acute lymphocytic leukemia	EEG	electroencephalogram
AMHP	approved mental health professional	EPSE	extrapyramidal side effects
		ER	Emergency Room
AML	acute myloid leukemia	ERP	exposure and response prevention
AMT	Abbreviated Mental Test	FSH	follicle-stimulating hormone
AN	anorexia nervosa	GABA	gamma-aminobutyric acid
APA	American Psychiatric Asssociation	GAD	generalized anxiety disorder
ASD	autism spectrum disorders	GCS	Glasgow Coma Scale
AVPU	alert, voice, pain, unresponsive	GHB	gamma-hydroxybutyrate
AXR	abdominal X-ray	GI	gastrointestinal
BAD	bipolar affective disorder	GP	general practitioner
BD	twice daily (bis die)	GPCOG	General Practitioner Assessment of Cognition
BDNF	brain-derived neurotrophic factor		
		HbA1c	glycated hemoglobin
BN	bulimia nervosa	HPA	hypothalamic–pituitary–adrenal
BNF	British National Formulary	HR	heart rate
BP	blood pressure	ICD	International Classification of Diseases
BZD	benzodiazepines		
CAM	Confusion Assessment Method	ICE	ideas, concerns, and expectations
CAT	cognitive analytic therapy		
CBC	complete blood count	ICP	intra-cranial pressure
CBT	cognitive behavioral therapy	ID	intellectual disability
CCF	congestive cardiac failure	IN	intranasal
CJD	Creutzfeldt–Jakob disease	IPT	interpersonal therapy
CMV	cytomegalovirus	IQ	intelligence quotient
CNS	central nervous system	IV	intravenous
COCP	combined oral contraceptive pill	LD	learning disability
COMT	catechol O-methyltransferase	LFTs	liver function tests
COPD	chronic obstructive pulmonary disease	LH	luteinizing hormone
		MAO	monoamine oxidase
CRP	C-reactive protein	MAOI	monoamine oxidase inhibitor

Abbreviations

MCV	mean cell volume	QDS	four times a day (*quater die sumendum*)
MDMA	methylenedioxymeth-amphetamine	RC	responsible clinician
MDT	multidisciplinary team	RR	respiratory rate
MI	myocardial infarction	SADQ	Severity of Alcohol Dependence Questionnaire
MMPI	Minnesota Multiphasic Personality Inventory	SARI	serotonin antagonist and reuptake inhibitor
MMR	measles, mumps, rubella	SBA	single best answer
MMSE	Mini-Mental State Examination	SNRI	serotonin and norepinephrine reuptake inhibitor
MOCA	Montreal Cognitive Assessment		
MRI	magnetic resonance imaging	SNS	sympathetic nervous system
MSE	mental status examination	SOAD	second opinion appointed doctor
MSU	midstream specimen of urine	SPECT	single-photon emission computerized tomography
N+V	nausea and vomiting		
NERI	norepinephrine reuptake inhibitor	SSRI	selective serotonin reuptake inhibitor
NICE	National Institute for Health and Care Excellence	TASR	Tool for Assessment of Suicide Risk
NKDA	no known drug allergies	TB	tuberculosis
NMDA	*N*-methyl-D-aspartate	TCA	tricyclic antidepressant
NMS	neuroleptic malignant syndrome	TFTs	thyroid function tests
NPIS	National Poisons Information Service	TMS	transcranial magnetic stimulation
NR	nearest relative	ToF	tetralogy of Fallot
OCD	obsessive–compulsive disorder	ToRCH	toxoplasmosis, other (syphilis, varicella-zoster, parvovirus B19), rubella, cytomegalovirus (CMV), and herpes
OD	once daily (*omni die*)		
OSCE	objective structured clinical examination		
OT	occupational therapist	TSQ	trauma screening questionnaire
OTC	over the counter	UTI	urinary tract infection
PANDAS	pediatric autoimmune neuropsy-chiatric disorders associated with streptococcal infections	VaD	vascular dementia
		VBG	venous blood gas
		VDRL	venereal disease research laboratory (test for syphilis)
PCP	primary care physician		
PD	personality disorder	VNS	vagus nerve stimulation
PE	psychoeducation	VSD	ventricular septal defect
PKU	phenylketonuria	WCC	white cell count
PO	oral (*per os*)	WHO	World Health Organization
PRN	when required (*pro re nata*)	Y-BOCS	Yale–Brown obsessive–compulsive scale
PT	prothrombin time		
PTSD	post-traumatic stress disorder		

Outline of the book

Chapter 1: Introduction to psychiatry

- Explains the concept of psychiatry, its relevance in modern-day healthcare and reasons behind studying it. Highlights the book's usefulness for medical students, residents, psychiatric trainees, PCP trainees, and psychiatric nurses.
- Delves briefly into the history of psychiatry as well as key concepts including psychiatric classification systems, the community mental health team (multidisciplinary team) and the bio-psychosocial approach. Furthermore, a mind map illustrates all of the psychiatric disorders covered in this book, which are principally based on the DSM-5 criteria.

Chapter 2: Assessment in psychiatry

- Discusses in depth the two key components of the psychiatric assessment: the psychiatric history and the mental state examination.
- These chapters are packed with hints and tips that can be applied clinically and in OSCEs.

Chapters 3–14: The psychiatric disorders

- A detailed overview of all the psychiatric conditions. A bullet point format is used, with key information in bold, making the valuable points easy to identify.
- For each condition, the following areas will be discussed:
    - **Definition:** A concise definition will be stated for each condition with key words in **bold** to emphasize their importance.
    - **Pathophysiology/Etiology:** Pathophysiology and etiology often overlap and as such we have placed them together in the same section. All psychiatric conditions are multifactorial in their development, and we aim to divide this section into categories for ease of recall, most commonly biological and environmental.
    - **Epidemiology and risk factors:** Up to date sources have been used to highlight the incidence and prevalence of the psychiatric disorders. Risk factors are also listed, where relevant, in order of importance.
    - **Clinical features:** Clinical features are described for all conditions, with helpful use of images, figures and mnemonics where appropriate.
    - **Diagnosis and investigations:** This section covers four valuable sub-sections. Firstly, an area dedicated to history taking includes specific questions articulated to assist you in a clinical situation (often a psychiatric line of questioning is sensitive in nature, with questions needing to be phrased cautiously). Secondly, we delve into the mental status examination (MSE) findings specific to the condition in question. Thirdly, we cite the investigations required to help with diagnosis, with justification offered for all. Finally, we cover the differential diagnoses for the condition (*see below* for associated symbols used in the book).

History taking	Mental status examination	Laboratory studies	Differential diagnosis
Hx	MSE	Ix	DDx

- **Management:** The final section explores the management of the respective conditions. We deploy the use of the bio-psychosocial model in order to divide management strategies into specific strata.
- At the end of each chapter 'self-assessment questions' are provided in the form of short answer questions. These questions are specifically designed to see whether readers have grasped the information provided for each condition and are also an opportunity for students to practice answering exam-style short answer questions.
- Special features include:

OSCE tips	OSCE tip boxes offer helpful hints and tips that will enable you to perform well in OSCE settings.
Key facts	Key fact boxes discuss important points that you are more likely to be tested on in your exams.
DSM-5 Criteria	The clinical features section has a DSM-5 criteria box to list the clinical features and relevant timing of these features required for diagnosing a psychiatric condition.
'MNEMONIC'	We provide invaluable mnemonics throughout the textbook, for various areas we feel that students struggle to recall but are absolutely crucial to know.

Chapter 15: Management

Including key information on:

- **Psychotherapy:** key information including indications, rationale, aim and modes of delivery is provided for the most commonly used psychotherapies, including cognitive behavioral therapy and psychodynamic therapy. Many other forms of simpler and relatively new psychotherapy are also discussed.
- **Pharmacology:** key information (including examples, indications, mechanisms of action, side effects, contraindications, and route and dose) on antidepressants, mood stabilizers, antipsychotics, hypnotics, and anxiolytics is provided. We use **DO** and **DO NOT** boxes to highlight important points to bear in mind when initiating pharmacological agents in psychiatry.
- **Devices:** the indications and side effects of some of the more commonly used devices are discussed including electroconvulsive therapy (ECT), transcranial magnetic stimulation (TMS) and vagus nerve stimulation (VNS).

Chapter 16: Mental health law and forensic psychiatry

- This brief chapter discusses consent, capacity, powers of attorney and psychiatric holds.
- It goes on to discuss the assessment and treatment of offenders with mental health disorders. We also mention the considerations during court proceedings and predictors of violent behavior.

Chapter 17: Common OSCE scenarios

- Being as student friendly as possible we delve into five common OSCE scenarios, likely to appear in exams.
- These should ideally be practiced in a group of three, with a student, simulated patient, and assessor.
- We also provide a detailed point scheme checklist.

Chapter 18: Board-style questions

- A selection of 38 single best answer (SBA) questions are provided that will challenge your knowledge.

Glossary of terms

- Definitions of the key terms and concepts mentioned throughout the course of the book are provided in the glossary. Key words can be looked up swiftly without having to spend time sieving them out!

Appendices

- Answers to the board-style questions are given with detailed explanation and justification of the method for reaching the correct answer.
- Detailed answers are also provided for the self-assessment questions at the end of the section for each psychiatric condition.

Chapter 1

Introduction to psychiatry

What is psychiatry?

- Psychiatry is the branch of medicine that deals with the diagnosis, treatment, and prevention of mental, emotional, and behavioral disorders.
- Subspecialty areas of psychiatry recognized by the American Board of Psychiatry and Neurology include child and adolescent, geriatrics, forensic, addiction, sleep, and consultation–liaison psychiatry. In addition, fellowship training is available in many other areas, including administrative, social and community, research, neuropsychiatry, and interventional psychiatry among others.
- Mental illness is very common. Research suggests that **1 in 4** people will experience a mental health problem over the course of a year. The prevalence of this set of conditions ranks alongside cardiovascular diseases and malignancies.

History of psychiatry

- Mental disorders have always been part of the human condition.
- Mental disorders have been described as early as the Ancient Egyptian Empire. However, it is only since the turn of the twentieth century that psychiatry as we know it today, has begun to take shape. See *Fig. 1.1* for notable events in psychiatry.
- The late 1940s, with the discovery of lithium to stabilize moods, and the early 1950s, with chlorpromazine as the first antipsychotic, ushered in the new era of psychopharmacology.

Why study psychiatry?

- Psychiatric disorders, including depression and anxiety, are common in many areas of medicine, but often overlooked. Therefore it is imperative for all healthcare professionals to have knowledge of the impact of mental health disorders.
- In primary care, roughly **20–25%** of patients seen suffer from a psychiatric disorder, either in isolation or accompanying physical illness.
- Psychiatric illness can also affect physical health. There is a **10–25 year reduction in life expectancy** (premature mortality) for patients with severe psychiatric disorders (*WHO*) (*Fig. 1.2*). Psychiatric disorders are one of the leading causes of disability in the developed world. In addition, co-morbid psychiatric disorders significantly worsen the outcome of many conditions from heart disease to cancer.
- The content in this textbook will provide useful information not only for medical students, but for residents, primary care physicians, and psychiatric nurses. The information in this book will provide you with:
  - a basic understanding of the common psychiatric disorders encountered not only by psychiatrists, but by any healthcare provider.
  - knowledge of how to perform a comprehensive and efficient psychiatric assessment including the psychiatric history and mental state examination.
  - information on how to manage a patient holistically by employing the bio-psychosocial approach.

1550 BC: The Ebers Papyrus, most important medical manuscript from Ancient Egypt, describes disorders such as depression and dementia.

400 BC: Ancient Greek physician Hippocrates hypothesizes that physiological abnormalities cause mental problems.

705 AD: First psychiatric hospital built by Muslims in Baghdad.

1247: Europe's first mental health institution, Bethlem Royal Hospital (then referred to as Bedlam asylum), is established. Unstable patients were commonly chained up.

1808: The word 'psychiatry' was first used by Johann Christian Reil in a 188-page paper.

1845: The Lunacy Act passed in England enhancing status of mentally ill persons to patients.

1893: German psychiatrist Emil Kraepelin clinically defines what would later become known as schizophrenia.

1901: Alois Alzheimer identifies the first case of what became known as Alzheimer's disease.

1917: Sigmund Freud publishes one of his most famous works, *Introduction to Psychoanalysis*, outlining his theory of neuroses.

1930s: Convulsive therapy introduced in the treatment of serious psychiatric disorders.

1948: Lithium bicarbonate's ability to stabilize mood swings cited by Australian psychiatrist John Cade.

1951: First antipsychotic, chlorpromazine, and the prototype tricyclic antidepressant, imipramine, developed.

1960: Aaron Beck develops cognitive therapy.

1980: DSMIII published by the American Psychiatric Association.

1988: Fluoxetine, the first SSRI, is released for treatment of depression.

2005: Vagus nerve stimulation (VNS), the first implantable device for the treatment of depression, approved by the FDA

2008: FDA approves first TMS device for the treatment of depression.

Fig. 1.1: Notable events in the history of psychiatry.

Psychiatric classification

- The two main classification systems for mental disorders are the **ICD-10** and **DSM-5** (produced by the American Psychiatric Association).

NOTE: For the purposes of this textbook, we will be primarily using DSM-5 criteria as this system predominates in the USA.

- We will focus on some of the more common psychiatric disorders highlighted below:

1. **Neurodevelopmental disorders**
2. **Schizophrenia spectrum and other psychotic disorders**
3. **Bipolar and related disorders**
4. **Depressive disorders**
5. **Anxiety disorders**
6. **Obsessive compulsive and related disorders**
7. **Trauma and stressor-related disorders**
8. **Dissociative disorder**
9. **Somatic symptom and related disorders**
10. **Feeding and eating disorders**
11. **Personality disorders**
12. **Neurocognitive disorders**
13. **Substance related and addictive disorders**
14. Gender dysphoria
15. Disruptive, impulsive, conduct disorders
16. Elimination disorders
17. Paraphilic disorders
18. Sleep–wake disorders
19. Sexual dysfunction
20. Other mental disorders

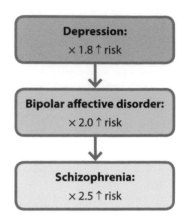

Fig. 1.2: ↑ risk of mortality in the major psychiatric disorders vs. the general population.

Areas of psychiatry

Psychiatry is a broad specialty with many distinct and varying conditions (*Fig. 1.3*).

Psychiatric assessment

Formulating a psychiatric diagnosis is a structured process involving an initial assessment, generating differential diagnoses, and then performing investigations to come to a diagnosis.

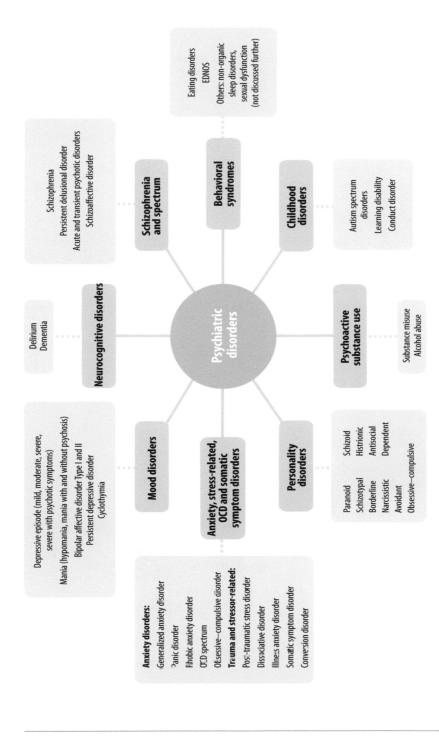

Fig. 1.3: Mind map of all the psychiatric disorders.

Initial assessment

- **Psychiatric history:** see *Section 2.1*.
- **Mental state examination:** see *Section 2.2*.
- **Physical examination:** Certain medical conditions (e.g. anemia, thyroid abnormalities) can present with psychiatric features. If alcohol abuse is suspected, the physical signs which accompany it must be assessed for.

Differential diagnosis

- **Organic:** Due to demonstrable pathology of the brain, e.g. delirium, dementia, and substance-related disorders.
- **Functional:** Any non-organic condition. Have predominantly psychological causes, e.g. psychoses such as schizophrenia or mood disorders such as depression.

Bio-psychosocial approach

- The **bio-psychosocial model**, theorized by the psychiatrist George Engel, is the mainstream ideology of contemporary psychiatry.
- According to the model, health is best understood as a combination of biological, psychological, and social factors as opposed to earlier, purely biological ideas.
- Throughout this book we will utilize the bio-psychosocial approach, particularly in the context of management of psychiatric illness (*Fig. 1.4*).

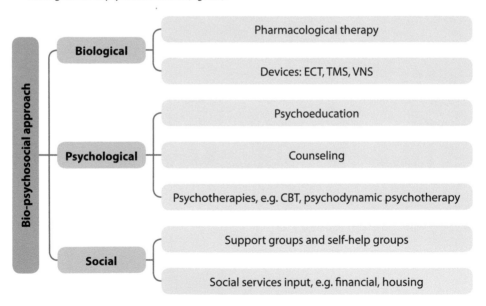

Fig. 1.4: Bio-psychosocial approach to management in psychiatry.

Chapter 2

Assessment in psychiatry

| 2.1 | Psychiatric history taking | 8 |
| 2.2 | Mental status examination | 15 |

2.1 Psychiatric history taking

Introduction to psychiatric history taking

- Taking a psychiatric history is structurally similar to a medical history. The major differences are in the **social** and **developmental history** (also known as the **personal history**), which are covered in more depth, as well as the **past psychiatric history**.
- A thorough psychiatric history takes at least **1 hour**. You may find it helpful to jot down notes as you go along, as this can aid you in being more methodical in your history taking.
- The areas you need to cover in the history are shown in *Fig. 2.1.1*.
- It is not always appropriate to ask all of the questions in every single case presentation. It can sometimes be more prudent to leave gaps to fill in later, particularly if your patient is suspicious, paranoid, or acutely distressed.
- Parts of the history can be found in the old notes, as well as a **collateral history** from an informant.
- As with any history, it is important to begin with open-ended questions and focus in on certain areas with more specific, closed questions. This gives the patient a chance to talk about their experiences and concerns, while allowing you to gain the information you need.
- As with any medical history, at the conclusion you should be able to generate a list of differential diagnoses based on the symptoms you have elicited during the history taking.
- Everyone has their own style of interviewing and there is no single 'correct way'. However, you need to feel comfortable with the style you adopt, so that the sensitive questions are not phrased awkwardly.

Before the interview (the 4 S's)

- **Site:** Ideally the room should be as **comfortable** and soundproof as can be, but this is not always possible on wards or in the emergency department.
- **Safety:** It is important that you and your patient have easy access to the door and, in some cases like prisons, a chaperone or security may be required. Check local added precautions such as panic buttons and alarms.
- **Setting:** It is best to arrange chairs at 90° to each other. If a desk is required to make notes, this should not be directly in between the patient and the interviewer such that it is obstructing. Sit in a relaxed posture. Ensure that there are no interruptions by turning cell phones off and handing pagers to colleagues.

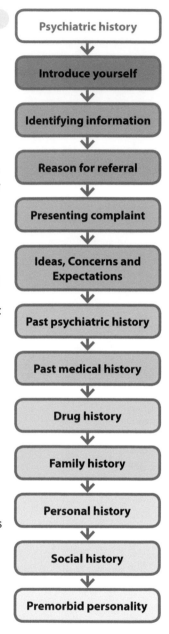

Fig. 2.1.1: Components of the psychiatric history.

- **Study:** Read any referral letter or previous notes to familiarize yourself with the case. Take any appropriate collateral history from a member of staff or family or, best of all, contact the previous mental health provider.

Introduction

- Introduce yourself including your **name** and your **role**.
- Explain the **purpose** of the meeting and how long you have to interview the patient.
- Gain **consent** to take a history.

Identifying information ('NAG MORE')

- **N**ame (full)
- **A**ge
- **G**ender
- **M**arital status and children
- **O**ccupation (present and past)
- **R**eligious and **E**thnic background

NOTE: Some of this information may be gathered during the history, or from the medical notes. We would avoid covering all of this in a conversation with the patient before asking about the presenting complaint.

Reason for referral or admission

- WHEN was the patient admitted (date and time)?
- WHY was the patient admitted?
- WHO was involved in the patient's admission, e.g. PCP, ER, police, social worker?
- Is the patient in hospital voluntarily or detained under a psychiatric commitment

Presenting complaint

- Start with an **open-ended question**, for example 'How can we help you?' or 'What brought you to the hospital?'
- Onset: 'When did you realize things have changed?'
- Severity: 'How has this affected your life?'
- Duration: 'How long has this been going on for?'
- Progression: 'Have you had any fluctuations in the way you have been feeling?'
- Precipitating events/Aggravating and relieving factors: 'Has anything occurred in your life recently which could explain how you are feeling?'
- Associated symptoms: Always screen for depression, psychosis, and suicidal ideation.

OSCE tips 1: Controlling the consultation

If the patient has:
- **Anxiety** → Reassure and normalize their symptoms.
- **Mania** → Try focusing them on the purpose of the interview, explain that you are interrupting to re-direct them and will come back to what they are saying later.
- **Confusion** (delirium or dementia) → Try to orientate the patient to time and place.
- **Psychosis** → Be empathetic and non-judgemental and acknowledge non-verbal cues (e.g. responses to hallucinations).

OSCE tips 2: Screening for other psychiatric disorders (*Table 2.1.1*)

In any psychiatric history, it is important to screen for the main psychiatric problems (e.g. depression and psychosis) even if the patient comes in with a different presenting complaint. Keep it as brief as possible, asking about the main symptoms, e.g. for depression ask about the core symptoms (lowered mood and anhedonia) and for psychosis ask about the presence of delusions and hallucinations.

Table 2.1.1: Specific presenting complaints and how to phrase questions accordingly

Depression	
Low mood	'Have you noticed any changes in your mood recently?'
Anhedonia	'Do you still enjoy the things that you used to enjoy?', 'Is there anything that you enjoy or that consistently makes you happy now?'
Anergia	'How would you describe your energy levels?', 'On a scale of 1 to 10 with 1 being extremely tired and 10 being full of energy, where would you place yourself?'
Psychosis	
Delusions	'Do you worry that other people are spying on you or may be trying to hurt you?', 'Do you feel safe or are you in any danger?' (**persecutory delusion**)
Hallucinations	Make sure you signpost: 'I want to ask you about experiences which people sometimes have, but find difficult to talk about. These are questions I ask everyone.' 'Do you ever see (**visual**) or hear (**auditory**) things that other people seem unable to see or hear?'
Auditory hallucinations	'Are the voices/people talking about you (**third person**) or directly to you (**second person**), are they commenting on what you are doing (third person – **running commentary**) or are they telling you to do certain things? If so, what are they telling you?'
Anxiety	
Generalized anxiety	'Would you say you were a worrier?', 'Do you feel particularly anxious or on edge?', 'How much time do you spend worrying in a day?', 'Do you feel irritable often?', 'Do you find that you are unable to relax?'
Panic attacks	'Do you ever feel so overcome by anxiety that you feel like you are going to die or go crazy?', 'How long do attacks last?', 'Is there anything which triggers these episodes?'
Phobias	'Do you have any fears that you or others may consider to be irrational?', 'Do you have any thoughts that you would consider obsessive?'
Obsessions	'Do any thoughts or worries keep coming back to your mind even though you try to push them away?'

Ideas, concerns, and expectations (ICE)

ICE is a crucial part of the history. Eliciting health beliefs and concerns in a sincere and fluent manner will enable you to build a strong rapport with the patient.

- **Ideas:** 'Do you have any thoughts as to what could be making you feel this way?'
- **Concerns:** 'Is there anything that is particularly concerning or worrying you at the moment?'
- **Expectations:** 'Do you have any thoughts as to the best way in which you feel we can help you?'

> **OSCE tips 3:** Watch out for non-verbal cues!
>
> Picking up on **non-verbal cues** is essential when taking a psychiatric history. Although the mental state examination is specifically targeted towards this, your examination essentially starts as soon as you see the patient. For instance, patients with depression often have poor eye contact and are motorically slow while a psychotic patient may be responding to auditory hallucinations and be internally preoccupied.

Past psychiatric history

- Have there been any similar problems to the presenting complaint, in the past? Previous or ongoing **psychiatric diagnoses** – 'Do you have any psychiatric illness that you are aware of?'
- **Dates** and **duration** of previous episodes of mental illness.
- Whether or not a **psychiatric commitment** was ever implemented.
- Details of previous **hospitalization** and **treatment** including medications, psychotherapy and electroconvulsive therapy. Ask about **response to treatment** and about **side effects**.

Past medical history and drug history

- Ask about any current or previous **medical illnesses** or any past **surgical procedures:** 'Is there anything that you are currently seeing the doctor for?'
- Ask particularly about **head injuries** and **previous cranial surgery**, **neurological conditions** (e.g. epilepsy), and **endocrine abnormalities** (e.g. thyroid disease).

> **OSCE tips 4:** Be careful not to offend patients
>
> A psychiatric history contains extremely sensitive questions and it is important not to cause offense to the patient as this can make the consultation counterproductive. There are tools designed to aid you with this:
> 1. **Signposting** → 'It is important to ask you the following which we ask everyone…'
> 2. **Normalizing** → 'Some people can feel this way…has this happened to you?'
> 3. **Acknowledge embarrassment** → 'I know this is a sensitive topic…'
>
> **This will help establish and build a good rapport with the patient.**

- Find out about **medication** the patient is using (both prescription and over-the-counter). Also, ask specifically about previous use of **psychotropic medication**, and whether the reported medication helped symptoms or caused side effects.
- Enquire about **allergies**, including the **nature** of any allergy (e.g. rash, anaphylaxis).

Family history

- Presence of **psychiatric illness in family members:** 'Has anyone in your family ever suffered from problems like you're having now?'
- **Quality of family relationships:** Collect information about parents, siblings and other significant relatives. 'How do you get on with your family?', 'Are there any recent significant events that have occurred in the family?'
- Brief **medical history of family:** 'Are there any medical conditions which run in the family?'
- It can be very useful to draw a **genogram** to represent information appropriately.

Personal history (Table 2.1.2)

- The **personal history** is crucial in identifying **predisposing factors** to the patient's psychiatric illnesses (*Fig. 2.1.2*).

Table 2.1.2: Personal history	
Early childhood	• **Prenatal and intrapartum complications:** 'When your mother had you, are you aware of any complications during the pregnancy or at birth?' • **Developmental milestones:** 'As far as you are aware, did you walk and talk at the right ages, or were you a slow developer?' • **Childhood illness:** 'Were you frequently unwell as a child, or often in hospital as a baby?' • **Childhood psychiatric illness:** 'As a young child do you feel that you were unusually aggressive or struggled with social interaction?' • **Family dynamics:** 'Were your parents married when they had you?', 'Were you planned?', 'Do you have any siblings or step-siblings?' • **Home atmosphere:** 'What is your earliest memory?', 'Was it a happy one?' • **Childhood abuse:** 'Have you ever been abused in childhood, such as sexual abuse, psychological or physical abuse, or neglect?'
Education	• 'Did you attend mainstream or special education schools?' • 'Did you enjoy school? If not, why?' • 'Were you ever bullied at school?' • 'Were you ever told that you had behavioral problems during school?' • 'Did you finish school?' • 'Did you attend higher education and what qualifications have you achieved?'
Employment	• **Chronological list of jobs:** 'Where have worked so far (in order)?' • **Duration of work:** 'How long did you work for in each job?' • **Redundancy or personal choice:** 'Why did you move on from a particular job?' • **Work environment:** 'How would you describe your relationship with your boss and co-workers?'

Table 2.1.2: Personal history *(continued)*

Relationships	• **Sexual orientation:** 'How would you describe your sexuality? Are you heterosexual, homosexual, or bisexual?' • **Chronological account of major relationships:** 'Would you be able to give me an account of the major relationships you've had in your life?' • **Current relationship:** 'Are you currently in a relationship?' • **Children:** 'Do you have any children from current or previous relationships?', 'Who do the children live with?', 'Could you describe your relationship with your children?'
Forensic history	• 'Have you ever been charged with, or convicted of, any offenses?' • If the answer to the above is yes, 'What sentence did you receive?' • 'Do you have any outstanding charges or convictions at present?'

NOTE: In the case of **women** the interviewer should ask about menstrual patterns and previous miscarriages, stillbirths, or terminations.

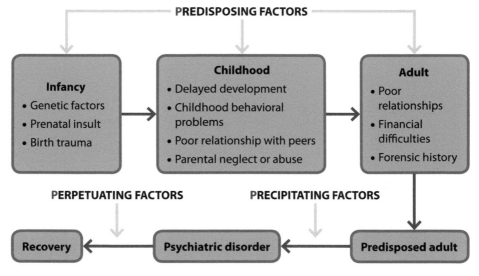

Fig. 2.1.2: Etiological factors in psychiatric illness can be divided into the three Ps (**P**redisposing, **P**recipitating and **P**erpetuating factors). The predisposing factors highlight the importance of taking a personal history.

Social history

- This includes current **accommodation** (state of housing, heating, living conditions), **social support** (friends and family), **financial circumstances** (any debts or benefits) and **hobbies** or **leisure activities**.

Alcohol and substance misuse

- The **CAGE questionnaire** is a useful tool to screen for **alcohol dependence** → if two or more positive, see if they meet criteria for alcohol use disorder (see *Section 10.2*, Alcohol-use disorders).

- How much **alcohol** in a day (units consumed) and type of alcohol.
- Use of **illicit drugs:** 'Have you ever used any recreational drugs?'
- Record **drug names**, **routes** of administration and **years/frequency** of use: 'How much do you spend on this in a week?'
- **Smoking** status: Calculate the **pack-year** smoking history
  (Number of cigarettes smoked per day × duration of smoking in years) ÷ 20

NOTE: The 20 in this equation is the number of cigarettes in a pack.

Premorbid personality

- The **premorbid personality** is an assessment of the patient's personality and character *before* the onset of mental illness.
- 'How would people have described you before?', 'Would they describe you differently now?'
- It is almost always useful to gain a **collateral history** from a family member or friend about premorbid personality in order to corroborate the patient's account.

Summary

- Succinctly **summarize** your understanding of what the patient has told you.
- Provide an opportunity for the patient to ask **questions**.

OSCE tips 5: Psychiatric history summarized

1. **Introductory information:** Age, sex, occupation, ethnic background, marital status.
2. **Reason for referral:** When was the patient admitted, why was the patient admitted and by whom?
3. **Presenting complaint** and **history of presenting complaint:** Onset, severity, duration, precipitating events, associated symptoms.
4. **Past psychiatric history:** Nature, date and duration of previous mental disorders, names of doctors and hospitals, outcomes, history of self-harm, attempted suicide and risk to others.
5. **Past medical history** and **drug history:** Co-morbid physical illness, past and childhood illnesses, surgery, medications (dose, route, side effects) including over-the-counter. Allergies, including type of reaction.
6. **Family history:** Anyone in family suffering from or previously suffered from a mental disorder, alcohol or drug dependency, self-harm or attempted suicide?
7. **Social history:** Self-care, family and social support, finances, smoking, alcohol, illicit drugs.
8. **Personal history:** Early childhood, education, employment, relationships, forensic history.
9. **Premorbid personality:** Personality and character *before* the onset of mental illness.

OSCE tips 6: An example of presenting your psychiatric history

This is Mr X, a 35-year-old man who presents with a 3-month history of low mood, anhedonia and lack of energy, along with biological symptoms of weight loss, reduced libido, and early morning wakening. There are no psychotic features and there is no current suicidal ideation. He has no previous psychiatric history and no past history of self-harm or suicidal acts, and is otherwise medically fit on no regular medication and with no significant family history. There is no history of significant alcohol or substance misuse. In conclusion, Mr X is likely to be suffering from a severe mood disorder and I would like to commence with my mental status examination to further explore Mr X's current mental state, to explore his risk further and to further support my conclusions from the history.

Mental status examination

Introduction

- The mental status examination (MSE) is a systematic appraisal of the appearance, behavior, mental functioning, and overall demeanor of a person. In other words, it reflects a person's psychological functioning at a given point in time.

- The MSE is usually put into a time frame (e.g. the preceding 2 weeks).

- The history and MSE will lead to the formation of differential diagnoses.

- Most of us inherently perform many aspects of the MSE every time we interact with, or observe others.

> **OSCE tips 1:** A useful mnemonic for the MSE: 'ASEPTIC'
>
> Appearance and behavior
> Speech
> Emotion (mood)
> Perception
> Thoughts
> Insight
> Cognition

- Observations of the mental state are important in determining a person's capacity to function, and whether psychiatric follow-up is required.

- Judgements about mental state should always consider the developmental level of the patient and age-appropriateness of the noted behavior.

- If there is any indication of current suicidal or homicidal ideation, then the person must be urgently referred for assessment by a qualified mental health clinician.

- An MSE includes the following eight areas: **appearance**, **behavior**, **speech**, **mood**, **thought**, **perception**, **cognition**, and **insight**.

Appearance and behavior

- **Physical state:** What age does the patient appear? Ethnic origin? Do they appear physically unwell? Are they sweating? Are they unkempt? What is their weight? Any extrapyramidal side effects from antipsychotics? Posture (hunched in depression or upright in anxiety)?

- **Clothing and accessories:** Flamboyant, bright clothing in mania. Dirty, stained, or torn clothing in depression, schizophrenia, substance misuse, and dementia.

- **Personal hygiene:** Self-neglect in substance misuse, depression, schizophrenia.

- **Eye contact:** Inappropriate eye contact (staring in parkinsonism), averting gaze (depression).

- **Facial expression:** Tearful (depression), overly happy (mania).

- **Body language:** Relaxed, tense, or withdrawn. Comment on how the body language might have changed during the consultation.

- **Motor activity and abnormal movements:** Psychomotor retardation (slowing of movements) in depression. Agitation may be seen in manic states, or when distressed. Examples of abnormal movements include tardive dyskinesia and acute dystonia (typical antipsychotics), tremor (anxiety disorders or lithium toxicity), catatonia (schizophrenia), tics (Tourette's syndrome).

- **Level of arousal:** Calm or agitated (delirium, mania).

- **Ability to build rapport:** Can be affected by factors relating to the patient and by how the interviewer manages the conversation.

- **Disinhibition:** e.g. in fronto-temporal dementia, hypomania, mania.

Speech

- **Rate:** Rapid and pressured (mania), mumbling and slow (depression, dementia).
- **Rhythm:** Normal, flattened, or ↑ intonation (the pattern of pitch changes in connected speech).
- **Volume:** Loud (mania), normal, quiet (depression).
- **Content:** Excessive punning (mania), clang association (ideas that are related only by similar or rhyming sounds rather than actual meaning), monosyllabic (a vocabulary composed primarily of monosyllables), spontaneous speech or only in answer to questions.
- **Quantity:** Increased (mania), normal or decreased, i.e. poverty of speech (dementia, depression, schizophrenia).
- **Tone:** Monotonous (depression) or tremulous (anxiety).
- **Dysarthria** (disorder in articulating speech) and **dysphasia** (disorder in language).

Mood and affect (Fig. 2.2.1)

- **Mood** refers to a patient's **sustained, subjective, experienced emotion over a period of time**.

- **Affect** is assessed by observing a patient's **posture, facial expression, emotional reactivity**, and **speech**.

- It can be useful to conceptualize the relationship between emotional affect and mood as being similar to that between the weather **(affect)** and the season **(mood)**. **Affect** refers to immediate expressions of emotion, e.g. smiling at a joke, while **mood** refers to emotional experience over a more prolonged period. Affect is often described as '**reactive**' if no abnormalities are present.

- The patient's mood should be observed throughout the interview with both verbal and non-verbal cues. **Mood** is assessed:

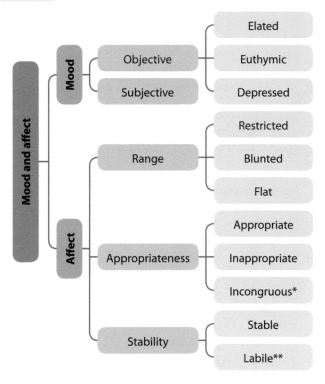

Fig. 2.2.1: Describing mood and affect.
***Incongruous affect:** e.g. schizophrenic patient who reports feeling suicidal with a happy facial expression. ****Labile mood:** refers to a fluctuating mood state, e.g. that in mania (from elated to euthymic) or delirium.

1. **Objectively** (your impression of their mood): euthymic, elated, or depressed.

2. **Subjectively** (the patient's report of their own mood): 'How are you feeling in yourself?', 'How has your mood been lately?'

NOTE: It can be helpful to ask the patient to rate their mood on a scale from 1 to 10 where 1 is 'as low as the patient has ever felt', and 10 is 'as good as the patient has ever felt.'

Thought

One of the first things to do is to assess the patient's way of thinking. Normal human thought has three characteristics: thought content, thought form, and thought stream (*Fig. 2.2.2*).

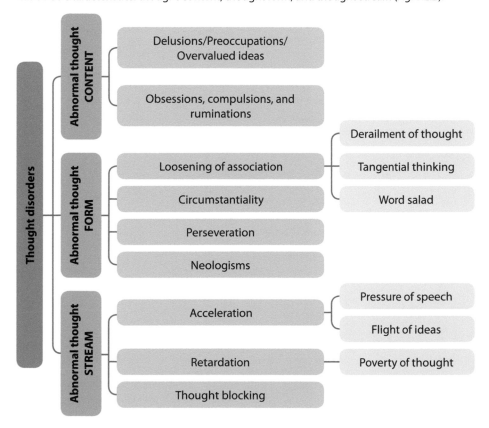

Fig. 2.2.2: Thought divided into abnormalities of thought content, form, and stream.

Thought content (*what is being thought about*)

- **Delusions: Fixed false beliefs**, which are **firmly held despite evidence to the contrary** and go **against** the individual's normal **social** and **cultural belief system**. 'Do you have any personal beliefs that others find strange?' See *Fig. 2.2.3* for classification of delusions.

- **Obsessional thoughts: Distressing thoughts** that enter the mind **despite the patient's effort to resist them**. This is a feature of obsessive–compulsive disorder. 'Do certain ideas or images keep entering your mind, even when you try to keep them out?'

- **Preoccupations/overvalued ideas: Strongly held beliefs** which are particularly important in four disorders: depressive, anxiety, eating, and sexual. **Preoccupations** differ from obsessions in that they can be put out of the mind with effort, whereas obsessions repeatedly enter the patient's mind despite their attempted resistance.

Classifying delusions			
In terms of **CAUSE**	In association with **MOOD**	In terms of **PLAUSIBILITY**	In terms of **CONTENT**
Primary vs. secondary	Mood congruent vs. mood incongruent	Bizarre vs. non-bizarre	See *Table 2.2.1*

Fig. 2.2.3: There are several ways of classifying delusions. In terms of cause: **primary** is unconnected to previous ideas or events whereas **secondary delusions** arise from, and are understandable in the context of, previous ideas or events. **Bizarre delusions** are completely impossible and not in keeping with reality. In **mood congruent delusions**, the content is appropriate to the patient's mood and vice versa in mood incongruent.

Table 2.2.1: Types of delusions in terms of content	
Type of delusion	**Definition (a fixed, false belief that…)**
Grandiose	…one has special powers, is talented, wealthy, or important. Grandiose delusions may be religious in nature, e.g. one is chosen by God.
Persecutory	…other people are conspiring against them in order to inflict harm or destroy their reputation.
Reference	…random events, objects or the behavior of others, have a special significance to oneself.
Guilt	…one has done something sinful or shameful.
Hypochondriacal	…one has a medical illness, despite sound medical evidence to the contrary.
de Clérambault's syndrome (erotomania)	…an exalted person is in love with them. A form of paranoid delusion that is amorous in nature – usually seen in women.
Othello syndrome (morbid jealousy)	…the patient's spouse or sexual partner is being unfaithful, without having any actual proof to support their claim.
Capgras' syndrome	…a familiar person or place has been replaced with an exact duplicate – a delusion of misidentification.
Nihilistic (includes Cotard's syndrome)	…they are worthless or dying. In severe cases they claim that everything is non-existent including themselves (*Cotard's syndrome*).
Infestation	…one is infested by small organisms.

Table 2.2.1: Types of delusions in terms of content *(continued)*	
Type of delusion	**Definition**
Folie à deux	A syndrome in which a delusional belief is shared between two people. This is very rare but can occasionally be seen. Often the two people are from the same family.
Delusional memory (rare primary delusion)	Where a delusional belief is based upon the recall of memory or false memory for a past experience. For example, a man recalls seeing a woman giggling at him in a restaurant a couple of weeks ago and now realizes that this person knew he was infested by small organisms.

Thought form (*in what manner, or shape, is the thought brought about*)

Formal thought disorder refers to abnormalities of the way thoughts are linked together:

- Loosening of association: Refers to the loss of the normal structure of thinking. This occurs mainly in schizophrenia. There are three types: (1) **Derailment of thought** (Knight's move thinking): Discourse consisting of a sequence of unrelated or only remotely related ideas. (2) **Tangential thinking:** The person diverts from the original train of thought but never returns to it. It is more indicative of psychopathology as opposed to circumstantiality (*see below*). (3) **Word salad:** Refers to speech that is reduced to a senseless repetition of sounds and phrases.
- Circumstantiality: **Thinking proceeds slowly** with many **unnecessary details** and **digressions**, before **returning to the original point**. This is seen in obsessional personalities and learning disability (LD).
- Neologisms: Are **words and phrases devised by the patient** or a new meaning to an already known word. May be seen in schizophrenia and autism.
- Perseveration: Uncontrollable and inappropriate repetition of a particular response, such as a word, phrase, or gesture. This most often occurs in dementia.

Stream or flow (*the amount and speed of thinking*)

- Acceleration: Accelerated thoughts can manifest as: (1) **Pressured thought**, and (2) **Flight of ideas** – language that may be difficult to understand when it switches quickly from one loosely connected idea to another. These often occur in manic illness.
- Retardation: Slow speed of thinking which occurs in depressive illnesses.
- Thought blocking: Refers to the sudden cessation of flow of thoughts. The previous idea may then be taken up again or replaced by another thought. This mainly occurs in schizophrenia.

Schneider's first rank symptoms (*Table 2.2.2*)

- Screen for schizophrenia by asking about Schneider's first rank symptoms: **Delusional perception**, **third person auditory hallucinations**, **thought interference** (thought insertion, withdrawal, and broadcast), and **passivity phenomenon**.

Table 2.2.2: Schneider's first rank symptoms	
Delusional perception	A true perception, to which a patient attributes a false meaning. For example, a perfectly normal event such as the sun going down may be interpreted by the patient as meaning that they are chosen by God.
Third person auditory hallucination	See *Table 2.2.3* and *OSCE tips 2*.
Thought interference	1. **Thought insertion:** 'Does it feel like your thoughts are your own?' In thought insertion the patient experiences thoughts inside their mind that they identify as not belonging to them, and that have been put there by an external agency. 2. **Thought withdrawal:** 'Does it feel as though your own thoughts are being taken away from you?' 3. **Thought broadcast:** 'Does it feel as though your thoughts are being heard out loud?'
Passivity phenomenon	'Do you ever feel that your mood or actions are being controlled by someone or something else?'

Thoughts of suicide and self-harm

- Ask about **suicidal ideation:** 'Do you think life is worth living?', 'Have things ever got so bad that you have thought of taking your own life?', 'Have you made any plans to end your life?'
- Ask about **self-harm**, **self-neglect**, **exploitation of others**, and possible **violent** or **homicidal thoughts**. 'Have you had desires to hurt others? If so, in what way?'

Perception

- Determine whether there are any hallucinations. A hallucination is a **perception** in the **absence** of an **external stimulus**. It is a common feature of psychosis.
- Hallucinations may be **visual, auditory, olfactory, gustatory**, or **somatic** (*Table 2.2.3*). **Auditory hallucinations** are the **most common** in mental health disorders.
- Hallucinations may be confused with the following:
  1. **Pseudohallucination:** Would include the experience of hearing voices inside your head. They are not true external hallucinations.
  2. **Illusion:** A false mental image produced by misinterpretation of an external stimulus (*Fig. 2.2.4*). Often occurs in normal people.
  3. **Depersonalization:** Feeling of detachment from the normal sense of self. 'Do you ever feel unreal or that a part of your body is unreal?'
  4. **Derealization:** Feeling of unreality in which the environment and people are experienced as unreal. The patient has got insight and realizes that these experiences are originating from their own mind. 'Do you ever feel that the things around you are unreal?', 'Have you ever had the feeling that things around you are like a stage set?'

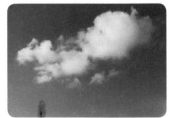

Fig. 2.2.4: Illusion of a sleeping baby formed by the clouds.

Table 2.2.3: Screening for hallucinations		
Type of hallucination	**Definition**	**How to phrase question** **NOTE:** Prior to asking these questions open with an introductory point, e.g. 'Sometimes when people are distressed they can hear or see things that other people cannot…'
Visual	Seeing things in the absence of an external stimulus, e.g. seeing a unicorn or leprechaun.	'Can you see certain things that others cannot?', 'Do you sometimes see something but when you try to touch it you cannot feel it there?'
Auditory	Hearing sounds or voices in the absence of an external stimulus: **Second person** – voice(s) directly addressing the patient; **Third person** – voices talking amongst themselves, or about the patient; **Running commentary** – voice(s) giving account of what the patient is doing.	'Can you hear things that others cannot?', 'Do the voices sound like normal voices?', 'Can you give me examples of what the voices say?', 'If so, how many voices are there?', 'Do you recognize these voices?', 'When do you hear the voices?', 'Do they speak to you, or about you?', 'Do they comment on what you do?', 'Do the voices tell you to do things?', 'Do you reply to the voices?'
Olfactory	Smelling things in the absence of external stimuli. It is usually an unpleasant smell.	'Have you noticed any unusual smells that you cannot account for and there is nothing to explain them?'
Gustatory	Tasting things in the absence of external stimuli.	'Can you taste things for which there is no explanation?'
Somatic	Abnormal bodily sensations in the absence of external stimuli, e.g. the feeling of insects crawling up the patient's skin.	'Have you noticed any unusual sensations in your body?'

OSCE tips 2: Finding the cause of the hallucination

- **Visual hallucinations** are more characteristic of an organic brain disease or substance misuse (they are rarer in schizophrenia, where auditory hallucinations in the second or third person are more common).
- **Second person auditory hallucinations**, particularly derogatory in nature, are seen in a number of conditions including schizophrenia, severe depression with psychosis, and mania with psychosis.
- **Third person auditory hallucinations**, particularly running commentary, are typical of schizophrenia (one of Schneider's first rank symptoms). You do not see third person auditory hallucinations in other psychotic conditions.

Cognition

- **Cognition** consists of **consciousness**, **orientation**, **attention** (ability to focus on the matter at hand), **concentration** (ability to sustain focus), and **memory** (short-term and long-term).
- **Assess general observations:** Are they able to concentrate and make conversation or do they appear confused?
- **Orientation to time**, **place**, **and person**: 'Do you know where we are?', 'Do you remember who I am?', 'Do you know roughly what time it is to the nearest hour?'
- Tools such as the Mini-Mental State Examination **(MMSE)** or the Montreal Cognitive Assessment **(MOCA)** can be helpful in testing memory, attention, language, and visuospatial skills (see *Section 13.2*, Dementia).
- **Impaired cognition** is the core feature of organic disorders such as **dementia** and **delirium**.

Insight

- **Insight** is the **extent to which the patient understands the nature of the problem** and if they are in agreement with treatment. Insight can be **intact** (accept that they have mental disorder and are thus willing to accept treatment), **partial** (accept that they may have a mental disorder but decline medication, or may deny mental disorder and accept medication), or **non-existent** (categorically deny any mental disorder).
  - 'Do you believe that you have a mental health issue such as depression?'
  - 'If so, would you take medication for it, or let us help you in alternative ways?'
  - 'If we were to give you some medication to help you, would you take it?'

OSCE tips 3: MSE summarized

1. **Appearance** and **behavior:** Physical state, clothing and accessories, eye contact, facial expression, body language, motor activity, ability to build a rapport.
2. **Speech:** Rate, rhythm, tone, volume, quantity, content.
3. **Mood** and **affect:** Subjective mood (patient's own words), objective mood (euthymic, elated, depressed). Affect (flat, blunted, restricted, appropriate, inappropriate, stable, labile, incongruous).
4. **Thought:** Delusions? Obsessions? Suicidal ideation? Thought interference? Passivity phenomenon? Formal thought disorder?
5. **Perceptions:** Visual, auditory, somatic, gustatory, olfactory hallucinations.
6. **Cognition:** Orientation to time, place and person, memory (MMSE if time permits), concentration and attention.
7. **Insight:** Full, partial, none.

OSCE tips 4: Presenting a mental state examination – an example

I performed a mental state examination on Mr X, aged 35 who is currently unemployed. I immediately noted that he appeared **unkempt** as I entered the room. Throughout the examination I noticed he looked **tearful** and had a **downward gaze**, but he was able to build a rapport with me. His speech seemed **soft and slow in nature** with **poverty of speech**. **Subjectively** he describes his mood as **low** and **objectively** he appears **depressed**. His affect appears to be reactive as he became more tearful when speaking about distressing events. He does not have formal thought disorder and no disorder of thought stream, or thought interference. There were no delusions currently present when asked. It is vital to note, however, that he did have **suicidal ideation** but had no active suicide plans. His wife and kids are protective factors for him. He also suffers from **second person auditory hallucinations** which were **derogatory** in nature. There are no abnormal perceptions in any other modalities. He is oriented to time, place, and person though his cognition has not been formally tested. His **insight is intact** as he feels that he is suffering from depression and feels he requires medication for this. In conclusion, I think that Mr X is suffering from **severe major depressive episode with psychotic features and suicidal ideation** and should be referred either informally (if possible) or on a formal basis (if he refuses) for further assessment and appropriate inpatient treatment.

Chapter 3

Mood disorders

3.1	Overview of mood disorders	25
3.2	Depressive disorder	27
3.3	Bipolar affective disorder	35

3.1 Overview of mood disorders

Definitions

- **Mood:** Refers to a patient's temporary emotional state of mind and is elicited from the patient in their own words. Common clinical descriptors of mood include euthymic (normal), dysphoric (low), hyperthymic (high), as well as common patient descriptors such as depressed, anxious, irritable, and angry.
- **Affect:** Refers to the outward display of an emotional state. Affect can be described in range (restricted, full, blunted, flat), appropriateness to speech or circumstances and, as with mood, type: depressed, tearful, irritable, angry, labile, elevated, etc. The assessment of mood and affect are described in *Section 2.2, Mental status examination*.
- Mood states such as transient depression are a normal part of human experience. It is only when a mood state causes significant and persistent distress or disability that it is considered as a mood disorder.

Types of mood disorders

Mood disorders are usually grouped as follows:

- Manic episode
- Bipolar affective disorder
- Major depressive episode
- Recurrent depressive disorder
- Persistent mood disorder
- Other mood disorder, or unspecified mood disorder.

See also *Figs. 3.1.1* and *3.1.2*.

Mood disorders can be **primary** or **secondary**:

1. **Primary mood disorder:** a mood disorder that does not result from another medical or psychiatric condition. Broadly speaking, a primary mood disorder is either **unipolar** (**depressive disorder, dysthmia, persistent depressive disorder**) or **bipolar** (**bipolar affective disorder, cyclothymia**).
2. **Secondary mood disorder:** a mood disorder that results from another medical or psychiatric condition.

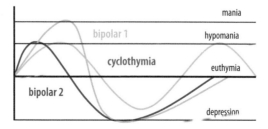

Fig. 3.1.1: Relationship of bipolar 1, bipolar 2 and cyclothymia to mood.

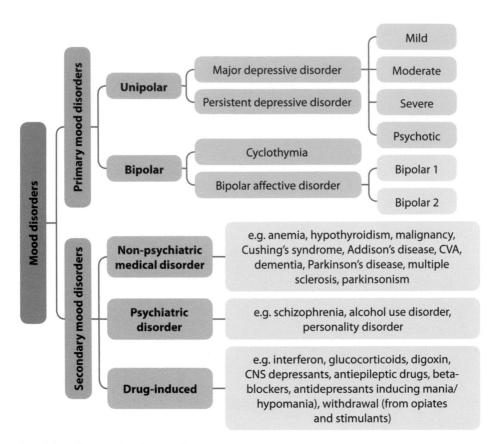

Fig. 3.1.2: Classification of mood disorders.

3.2 Depressive disorder

Depressive disorder

Definition

Depressive disorder is a **mood disorder** characterized by a persistent **low mood and/or a loss of pleasure** and is accompanied by a number of **emotional, cognitive**, and **vegetative symptoms**.

Pathophysiology/Etiology

- Depression is a highly complex **multifactorial disorder** influenced by a number of **bio-psychosocial factors** (see *Table 3.2.1*).
- **Monozygotic twin studies** show the heritability of depression as **40–50%**, and multiple genes are involved.
- The **monoamine hypothesis** states that a deficiency of **monoamine levels or activities (norepinephrine, serotonin, and dopamine)** are associated with depression; this is supported by the fact that antidepressants which increase the concentration of these neurotransmitters in the synaptic cleft, improve the clinical features of depression.

Table 3.2.1: Etiological factors in depressive disorder		
	Biological	**Psychological**	**Social**
Predisposing	• Female gender (2:1) • Postpartum period • Genetics: 40–50% monozygotic concordance rates, family history • Neurochemical: ↓ serotonin, ↓ norepinephrine, ↓ dopamine • Endocrine: ↑ activity of HPA axis • Physical co-morbidities • Past history of depression	• Personality type • Failure of effective stress control mechanisms • Poor coping strategies • Other mental health co-morbidities (e.g. dementia)	• Stressful life events • Loss • Lack of social support
Precipitating	• Poor compliance with medication • Corticosteroids	• Acute stressful life events (e.g. personal injury, loss of loved one, bankruptcy)	• Unemployment • Poverty • Divorce
Perpetuating	• Chronic health problems (e.g. diabetes, COPD, and chronic pain syndromes)	• Poor insight • Negative thoughts about self, the world and the future (Beck's triad)	• Alcohol and substance misuse • Poor social support • ↓ Social status

DSM-5 Criteria for major depressive episode

A. Five (or more) of the following symptoms have been present during the same 2-week period and represent a change from previous functioning; at least one of the symptoms is either (1) depressed mood or (2) loss of interest or pleasure.
   NOTE: Do not include symptoms that are clearly attributable to another medical condition.
   1. Depressed mood most of the day, nearly every day, as indicated by either subjective report (e.g. feels sad, empty, or hopeless) or observation made by others (e.g. appears tearful). (**Note:** In children and adolescents, can be irritable mood.)
   2. Markedly diminished interest or pleasure in all, or almost all, activities most of the day, nearly every day (as indicated by either subjective account or observation).
   3. Significant weight loss when not dieting or weight gain (e.g. a change of more than 5% of body weight in a month), or decrease or increase in appetite nearly every day. (**Note:** In children, consider failure to make expected weight gain.)
   4. Insomnia or hypersomnia nearly every day.
   5. Psychomotor agitation or retardation nearly every day (observable by others; not merely subjective feelings of restlessness or being slowed down).
   6. Fatigue or loss of energy nearly every day.
   7. Feelings of worthlessness or excessive or inappropriate guilt (which may be delusional) nearly every day (not merely self-reproach or guilt about being sick).
   8. Diminished ability to think or concentrate, or indecisiveness, nearly every day (either by subjective account or as observed by others).
   9. Recurrent thoughts of death (not just fear of dying), recurrent suicidal ideation without a specific plan, or a suicide attempt or a specific plan for committing suicide.
B. The symptoms cause clinically significant distress or impairment in social, occupational, or other important areas of functioning.
C. The episode is not attributable to the physiological effects of a substance or another medical condition.
NOTE: Criteria A–C constitute a major depressive episode. Major depressive episodes are common in bipolar I disorder but are not required for a diagnosis of bipolar I disorder.
NOTE: Responses to a significant loss (e.g. bereavement, financial ruin, losses from a natural disaster, a serious medical illness or disability) may include feelings of intense sadness, rumination about the loss, insomnia, poor appetite, and weight loss noted in Criterion A, which may resemble a depressive episode. Although such symptoms may be understandable or considered appropriate to the loss, the presence of a major depressive episode in addition to the normal response to a significant loss should also be carefully considered. This decision inevitably requires the exercise of clinical judgment based on the individual's history and the cultural norms for the expression of distress in the context of loss.
D. The occurrence of the major depressive episode is not better explained by schizoaffective disorder, schizophrenia, schizophreniform disorder, delusional disorder, or other specified and unspecified schizophrenia spectrum and other psychotic disorders.
E. There has never been a manic episode or a hypomanic episode.
NOTE: This exclusion does not apply if all of the manic-like or hypomanic-like episodes are substance-induced or are attributable to the physiological effects of another medical condition.

- Abnormalities of the **hypothalamic–pituitary–adrenal (HPA) and thyroid axis** have been linked to depression. Severe depression is characterized by a relative hypercortisolemia and a change in the diurnal secretion of cortisol. In addition, depression is associated with a blunted TSH response to TRH, and loss of nocturnal TSH rise, among other abnormalities.
- The neurotrophic hypothesis postulates that diminished neuroplasticity in the hippocampus underlies depression.
- Psychosocial factors such as **personality type**, **stressful life events**, and **failure of effective stress control mechanisms** increase the likelihood of developing depression.

Epidemiology and risk factors (see Table 3.2.1)

- Depressive disorders are among the leading causes of disability worldwide. Globally **>350 million** people suffer from depression.
- In the US, 6–7% of the population experience an episode of depression in any given year.
- Onset can occur at any age with a median around 32 years.

OSCE tips 1: Risk factor mnemonic – 'FF, AA, PP, SS': - Female/Family history - Alcohol/Adverse events - Past depression/Physical co-morbidities - ↓ Social support/↓ Socioeconomic status	**OSCE tips 2:** A useful mnemonic for the main symptoms of depression – 'DEAD SWAMP': - Depressed mood - Energy loss (anergia) - Anhedonia - Death thoughts (suicide) - Sleep disturbance - Worthlessness or guilt - Appetite or weight change - Mentation (concentration) reduced - Psychomotor retardation

Clinical features

- The symptoms of a depressive disorder can be divided into **core**, **cognitive**, and **biological** (see Table 3.2.2).

Table 3.2.2: Clinical features of depressive disorder

Core symptoms	
Anhedonia	Lack of interest in things which were previously enjoyable to the patient.
Low mood	Present for at least 2 weeks.
Lack of energy	Also known as anergia.
Cognitive symptoms	
Lack of concentration	Diminished ability to think or concentrate, nearly every day.
Negative thoughts	See Fig. 3.2.1.

Table 3.2.2: Clinical features of depressive disorder *(continued)*	
Excessive guilt	Feelings of worthlessness or excessive or inappropriate guilt, nearly every day.
Suicidal ideation	Recurrent thoughts of death, recurrent suicidal ideation without a specific plan.
Biological/vegetative symptoms	
Fatigue	Loss of energy almost every day
Sleep disturbance	Insomnia (early morning awakening most common). Hypersomnia is atypical subtype.
Loss of libido	Reduced sexual drive.
Biological symptoms	
Psychomotor retardation	Refers to slow speech as well as slow movement.
Weight loss and loss of appetite	Significant weight loss when not dieting, or decrease in appetite nearly every day. Weight gain and increased appetite may occur in atypical depression.
Psychotic symptoms	
Hallucinations	These are usually second person auditory hallucinations. Less common than delusions.
Delusions	These are usually paranoid but may be hypochondriacal, somatic, guilt, nihilistic, or persecutory in nature.

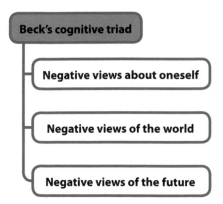

Fig. 3.2.1: Beck's cognitive triad represents three types of negative thought. The triad involves negative thoughts about: the self (i.e. the patient feels worthless), the world/environment (i.e. the world is unfair), and the future (i.e. the future is hopeless).

Diagnosis and investigations

Hx

- **Explore the core symptoms:** 'How has your mood been recently?' **(low mood)**, 'Do you still enjoy the things that you used to?' **(anhedonia)**

- **Explore the cognitive symptoms:** 'Are you able to concentrate on activities, for example, reading and remembering what you read, following the plot of a TV program?' **(lack of concentration)**, 'Are you having difficulty making decisions?' **(indecisiveness)**, 'Are you hopeful for the future?' **(negative thoughts)**, 'Do you feel life is worth living?', 'Have you had any thoughts of ending your own life?' **(suicidal)***

- **Explore the biological symptoms:** 'Do you find your mood worse during certain times of the day?' **(DVM)**, 'What time did you used to wake up before you felt low in mood?', 'What time do you wake up now?' **(EMW)**, 'Do you feel that your thoughts or movements are slower (usually observed)?' **(psychomotor retardation)**, 'When people feel down, sometimes their sexual drive also goes down, has this happened to you?' **(loss of libido)**

*If the patient suggests that they are actively suicidal, you must carry out a full risk assessment (see Suicide and risk assessment, *Section 12.2*).

OSCE tips 3: DO NOT forget to rule out important differential diagnoses!

Remember to always consider other important differential diagnoses even when the symptoms described are very typical of depression. Always ask yourself, 'Is there another psychiatric condition to consider?' e.g. bipolar affective disorder (i.e. did the patient ever have a hypomanic or manic episode?). 'Have I ruled out non-psychiatric medical illnesses that can present with depression?' e.g. hypothyroid, Cushing's, Parkinson's, etc. Also always ask about suicidal thoughts!

MSE		
Appearance	Signs of self-neglect, thin, unkempt, depressed facial expression, tearful.	
Behavior	Poor eye contact, tearful, psychomotor retardation, slow movements, slow responses, may sometimes present with psychomotor agitation.	
Speech	May be slow, non-spontaneous, reduced volume and tone.	
Mood	Low, sad, etc. (subjectively) and affect: restricted, tearful (objectively).	
Thought	Pessimistic, guilty, worthless, helpless, suicidal, delusions (if psychotic).	
Perception	Second person auditory hallucinations (often derogatory).	
Cognition	Impaired concentration.	
Insight	Usually good.	

> **Ix** Laboratory studies are used to exclude organic causes for depression. They are not mandatory and should be used according to clinical judgement:
>
> - **Screening questionnaires:** e.g. **PHQ-9**, **MADRS**, and **Beck depression inventory**.
> - **Blood tests: CBC** (e.g. to check for anaemia), **TFTs** (e.g. to test for hypothyroidism), **electrolytes**, **BUN/Cr**, **LFTs**, **calcium levels** (biochemical abnormalities may cause physical symptoms which can mimic some depressive symptoms), **glucose** (hyperglycemia can cause anergia).
> - **Imaging: MRI** or **CT scan** may be required where presentation or examination is atypical or where there are features suspicious of an intracranial lesion e.g. unexplained headache or personality change.

> **DDx** - **Other mood disorders:** Bipolar affective disorder, other depressive disorders (see *Key facts 1*).
> - **Secondary to physical condition** e.g. hypothyroidism (see Overview of mood disorders, *Section 3.1*).
> - **Secondary to psychoactive substance abuse.**
> - **Secondary to other psychiatric disorders:** Psychotic disorders, anxiety disorders, adjustment disorder, personality disorder, eating disorders, dementia.
> - **Normal bereavement.**

Key facts 1: Other depressive subtypes and time specifiers

Time specifiers
- **Seasonal affective disorder:** Characterized by depressive episodes recurring annually at the same time each year, usually during the fall or winter months.
- **Postpartum depression:** Affects approximately 10% of women. Most cases start within a month and typically peak at 3 months. Clinical features are similar to depression seen in other circumstances.

Depressive subtypes
- **Melancholic depression:** Persistent severe depressed mood (no mood reactivity), severe vegetative symptoms, prominent diurnal variation (worse symptoms in the morning with improvement late in the day).
- **Atypical depression:** This typically occurs with mild–moderate depression with reversal of symptoms, e.g. overeating, weight gain, and hypersomnia. There is a relationship between atypical depression and seasonal affective disorder.
- **Psychotic major depression:** Psychotic symptoms, primarily delusions (paranoid, somatic, nihilistic, guilt, etc.) in the context of a depressive episode.
- **Persistent depressive disorder:** Depressive state for at least 2 years, which does not meet the criteria for a mild, moderate, or severe depressive disorder and is not the result of a partially treated depressive illness.
- **Baby blues:** Seen in around 60–70% of women, typically 3–7 days following birth, and is more common in primiparae. Mothers are anxious, tearful, and irritable. Reassurance and support is all that is required.

Management

- The broad treatment of depression is highlighted using the **bio-psychosocial approach** (*Fig. 3.2.2*).
- The management of depression depends on the **severity** of the depression.

Management of mild depression

- **Watchful waiting:** Should be considered and reassess the patient again in **2 weeks**.
- **Antidepressants: Not** recommended as a first-line therapy for mild depression unless: (1) depression has **lasted a long time**; (2) **past history** of **moderate–severe** depression; (3) **failure of other interventions**; (4) or the depression **complicates the care of other physical health problems**.
- **Self-help programs:** Patient works through a **self-help manual** with a healthcare professional providing support and checking progress.
- **Computerized cognitive behavioral therapy (CBT):** Based on **conventional CBT**, involves a **computer program** educating them about depression and challenging negative thoughts.

Biological
• **Antidepressants**
• **Adjuvants** e.g. antipsychotics, lithium, thyroid hormone, etc.
• **TMS, ECT, VNS**

Psychological
• **Psychotherapies** (See *Key facts 2*)
• **Self-help programs**
• **Physical activity**

Social
• **Social support groups**

Fig. 3.2.2: Bio-psychosocial approach to depression.

- **Physical activity program:** Exercise has been shown to benefit mental health. **Group exercise class** under the supervision of a qualified trainer may be recommended.
- **Psychotherapies** (see *Key facts 2*): If the options above fail, psychotherapies can be tried.

Management of moderate–severe depression

- **Suicide risk assessment:** Should be performed on all patients. A psychiatric hold may be necessary.
- **Psychiatry referral:** Indicated if: (1) **suicide risk** is **high**; (2) depression is **severe**; (3) **recurrent** depression; (4) or **unresponsive** to **initial treatment**; (5) **psychotic symptoms** present.
- **Antidepressants: First-line** antidepressants are **selective serotonin reuptake inhibitors** (SSRIs) e.g. citalopram, serotonin noradrenaline reuptake inhibitors (SNRIs), e.g. duloxetine, bupropion, mirtazapine, and vortioxetine. Second and third line agents include **tricyclic antidepressants (TCAs)** and **monoamine oxidase inhibitors**. Should be **continued for 6–12 months** after resolution of symptoms for first depressive episode, 2 years after resolution but may require chronic treatment in patients with a history of two or more serious episodes.
- **Adjuvants:** Antidepressants may be **augmented** with **lithium, antipsychotics, thyroid hormone**, and other agents.
- **Psychotherapy:** Refer for **CBT** and **interpersonal therapy (IPT)**
- **Social support:** Engaging with activities in the community that the individual is avoiding or attending social support groups with others.

- **ECT:** Indications specific to depression include: (1) acute treatment of **severe depression** which is **life-threatening**; (2) **rapid response required**; (3) **depression** with **psychotic features**; (4) **severe psychomotor retardation** or **catatonia**, (5) or **failure of other treatments**.
- **Transcranial magnetic stimulation (TMS):** Indications include medication-resistant or intolerant patients who are less seriously ill than those requiring ECT (see *Chapter 15* on management).
- **Vagus nerve stimulation (VNS):** Patients with recurrent or chronic depression unresponsive to other strategies (see *Chapter 15* on management).

Key facts 2: Psychotherapies used to manage depression (see *Section 15.1*, Psychotherapies)

- **CBT:** Depression causes negative thoughts, which can lead to negative behaviors. CBT allows people to identify and tackle negative thoughts; conducted in groups or individually.
- **IPT:** Helps to identify and solve relationship problems, whether it is with family, partners or friends.
- **Behavioral activation:** Encourages depressed patients to develop more positive behavior or activities that they would usually avoid.
- **Counseling:** Enables patients to explore their problems and symptoms. Counselors offer support and guide patients to help themselves for a particular focus, e.g. bereavement or relationship counseling.
- **Psychodynamic therapy:** Aim is to explore and understand the dynamics and difficulties of a patient's life, which may have begun in childhood.

Self-assessment

A 45-year-old woman presents with a one-month history of low mood, lack of energy, and weight loss, in the setting of a recent divorce. She explains an inability to keep her concentration focused on work and expresses feelings of worthlessness and hopelessness. You suspect depression.

1. Besides low mood, what is the other core symptom of major depression?
2. What are the physical symptoms of depression?
3. Which non-psychiatric medical cause of depression must you rule out and what blood test must be ordered to test this?
4. You determine the patient to be suffering from severe depression. What is the first-line pharmacological treatment of moderate–severe depression? Give an example of a drug that falls in this group.
5. Give three indications for the use of ECT in the management of depression.

Answers to self-assessment questions are to be found in *Appendix B*.

Bipolar affective disorder

Definition

Bipolar affective disorder (previously known as 'manic depressive illness') is a **chronic episodic mood disorder**, characterized by at least one episode of **mania** (or **hypomania**) and usually occurs with depressive episodes. Either one can occur first but the term bipolar also includes those who at the time of diagnosis have suffered only manic episodes, as most patients with mania will eventually develop depression.

Pathophysiology/Etiology

- The cause of bipolar affective disorder (BAD) involves both **biological** and **environmental** factors (*Fig. 3.3.1*).
- The **monoamine hypothesis** is applicable to elevated mood just as it is to depressed mood. It states that elevated mood is a result of **increased central monoamines (norepinephrine** and **serotonin)**.
- **Dysfunction of the HPA axis** (abnormal secretion of cortisol, as found in unipolar depression) and dysfunction of the hypothalamic–pituitary–thyroid axis may contribute to BAD.
- BAD shows **strong heritability** with **monozygotic twin studies** showing a **50–85%** concordance rate. The lifetime risk of developing BAD for 1st degree relatives of a BAD patient is **5–10%, compared to 1% in the general population**.
- **Stressful** or **significant life events** may precipitate the onset of a first manic episode. Subsequent episodes may occur spontaneously.

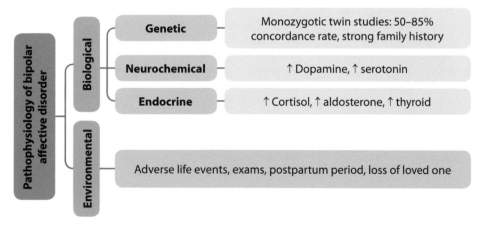

Fig. 3.3.1: Outline of the biological and environmental factors associated with BAD.

Epidemiology and risk factors (*Table 3.3.1*)

- The lifetime risk of developing BAD is **1–3%**.
- The mean age of onset is **19** years of age.
- The male to female affected ratio is **1:1** for bipolar 1 disorder. Bipolar 2 disorder is more common in females.

Table 3.3.1: Risk factors for bipolar affective disorder (**A**ggressive **S**penders)

Age – in early 20s	**S**trong family Hx
Anxiety disorders	**S**ubstance misuse
After depression	**S**tressful life events

Clinical features

- The symptoms of BAD include those of mania or depression. Manic symptoms are listed in *Table 3.3.2* and the symptoms of depression have been discussed in *Section 3.2*, Depressive disorder.
- The severity of mania can be divided into: (1) **hypomania**; (2) **mania without psychosis**; (3) and **mania with psychosis** depending on the severity of symptoms (*Fig. 3.3.2*).
- Different types of bipolar disorder have been recognized according to DSM-5 (*Table 3.3.3*).

Table 3.3.2: Symptoms of mania 'I DIG FASTER'	
Irritability	**Activity/Appetite increased**
Distractibility/Disinhibited (sexual, social, spending)	**Sleep decreased**
Insight impaired/Increased libido	**Talkative** – pressure of speech
Grandiose delusions	**Elevated mood/Energy increased**
Flight of ideas	**Reduced concentration/Reckless** behavior and spending

Hypomania	Mania without psychosis	Mania with psychosis
• **Mildly elevated mood** or **irritable mood** present for **≥4 days**. Symptoms of mania, where present, are to a **lesser extent** than true mania. Considerable interference with work and social life but **not severe disruption**. **Partial insight** may be preserved.	• As with hypomania but to a **greater extent**. Symptoms present for **>1 week**, with **complete disruption** of work and social activities. May have **grandiose ideas** and excessive spending could lead to debts. There may be **sexual disinhibition**, and reduced sleep may lead to **exhaustion**.	• **Severely elevated** or **suspicious mood** with the addition of psychotic features such as **grandiose** or **persecutory delusions** and **auditory hallucinations** that are mood congruent. Patient may show signs of **aggression**.

Fig. 3.3.2: Summary of manic mood disorders that contribute to bipolar affective disorder.

Table 3.3.3: Classification of bipolar affective disorder		
Bipolar I	**Bipolar II**	**Rapid cycling**
Involves periods of severe mood episodes from mania to depression.	Milder form of mood elevation, involving hypomania that alternates with periods of severe depression.	More than four mood swings in a 12-month period with no intervening asymptomatic periods. Poor prognosis.

DSM-5 Criteria for mania and hypomania

Mania

A. A distinct period of abnormally and persistently elevated, expansive, or irritable mood and abnormally and persistently increased goal-directed activity or energy, lasting at least 1 week and present most of the day, nearly every day (or any duration if hospitalization is necessary).

B. During the period of mood disturbance and increased energy or activity, three (or more) of the following symptoms (four if the mood is only irritable) are present to a significant degree and represent a noticeable change from usual behavior:
   1. Inflated self-esteem or grandiosity.
   2. Decreased need for sleep (e.g. feels rested after only 3 hours of sleep).
   3. More talkative than usual or pressure to keep talking.
   4. Flight of ideas or subjective experience that thoughts are racing.
   5. Distractibility (i.e. attention too easily drawn to unimportant or irrelevant external stimuli), as reported or observed.
   6. Increase in goal-directed activity (either socially, at work or school, or sexually) or psychomotor agitation (i.e. purposeless, non-goal-directed activity).
   7. Excessive involvement in activities that have a high potential for painful consequences (e.g. engaging in unrestrained buying sprees, sexual indiscretions, or foolish business investments).

C. The mood disturbance is sufficiently severe to cause marked impairment in social or occupational functioning or to necessitate hospitalization to prevent harm to self or others, or there are psychotic features.

D. The episode is not attributable to the physiological effects of a substance (e.g. a drug of abuse, a medication, or other treatment) or to another medical condition.

NOTE: A full manic episode that emerges during antidepressant treatment (e.g. medication, electroconvulsive therapy) but persists at a fully syndromal level beyond the physiological effect of that treatment is sufficient evidence for a manic episode and, therefore, a bipolar I diagnosis.

NOTE: Criteria A–D constitute a manic episode. At least one lifetime manic episode is required for the diagnosis of bipolar I disorder.

Hypomania

Hypomania criteria are the same as for mania, but are less severe (not severe enough to require hospitalization and do not include psychotic symptoms) and can last as little as 4 days instead of 7 days.

Reprinted with permission from the *Diagnostic and Statistical Manual of Mental Disorders*, 5th Edition, (© 2013). American Psychiatric Association.

Diagnosis and investigations

Hx
- 'How would you describe your mood?' (**elevated, depressed, or irritable mood**).
- 'Have you ever felt on top of the world?' (**elevated mood**).
- 'Do you feel that you have so much energy that those around you can't keep up?' (↑ **energy**).
- 'Are you able to concentrate on reading or following a conversation?' (↓ **concentration**).
- 'Do you find yourself needing less sleep but not getting tired?' (↓ **sleep and** ↑ **energy levels**).
- 'Do you find that your thoughts are flowing more easily or faster?' (**racing thoughts**).

Hx
- 'Have you had any new interests or exciting ideas lately?' **(delusions/overvalued ideas)**.
- 'Do you have any special abilities that are unique to you?' **(grandiose delusions)**.
- 'Are you afraid that someone is trying to harm you?' **(persecutory delusions)**.
- Also ask about **family history** of bipolar affective disorder and **substance misuse**.
- **Pressure of speech** and **flight of ideas** can be assessed from the conversation.

OSCE tips 1: Remember to always screen for mania/hypomania in a depressed patient!

- A patient may present with the classic symptoms of depression but may actually be suffering from bipolar.
- They may not initially reveal to you that they have previously had a manic episode(s) so it is very important that you specifically ask whether they have had previous instances where their mood has been significantly elevated. Also ask about previous periods of disinhibition.
- Ask about a family history of bipolar disorder, a history of post-partum depression, early onset depression, and psychotic depression, because all are associated with bipolar disorder. Also ask about substance abuse.
- Be vigilant. Do not fall into the trap of diagnosing depressive disorder immediately and prescribe an antidepressant as this may destabilize a patient in the bipolar spectrum.

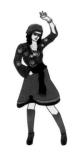

Fig. 3.3.3: Individual with inappropriate bright clothing in keeping with possible mania.

MSE

Appearance	Flamboyant/unusual combination of clothing (see *Fig. 3.3.3*), heavy makeup, and jewelry. Personal neglect when condition is severe.	
Behavior	Overfamiliar, disinhibited (flirtatious, aggressive), increased psychomotor activity, distractible, restless.	
Speech	Loud, ↑ rate and quantity, pressure of speech, uninterruptible, puns and rhymes, neologisms.	
Mood	Elated, euphoric, and/or irritable.	
Thought	Optimistic, pressured thought, flight of ideas, loosening of association, circumstantiality, tangentiality, overvalued ideas, grandiose/persecutory delusions.	
Perception	Usually no hallucinations. Mood-congruent auditory hallucinations may occur.	
Cognition	Attention and concentration often impaired. Fully oriented.	
Insight	Generally very poor.	

OSCE tips 2: The challenge of history taking in a manic patient

- Eliciting a thorough history from a manic patient is a true test of your communication skills as the task is made difficult by their irritability (80% of manic patients), distractibility and disinhibition.
- Be polite but firm in your approach. Flight of ideas, circumstantiality and tangentiality may cause patients to veer off topic, so the key is to gently redirect the patient back to the asked question.
- Any OSCE station will be time-limited so you will need to take control of the interview to ensure that you ask appropriate questions in order to make a clear diagnosis.

Ix

- **Self-rating scales:** e.g. Mood Disorder Questionnaire.
- **Blood tests: CBC** (routine), **TFTs** (both hyper-/hypothyroidism are differentials), **BUN/Cr** (baseline renal function with view to starting lithium), **LFTs** (baseline hepatic function with view to starting mood stabilizers), **glucose**, **calcium** (biochemical disturbances can cause mood symptoms).
- **Urine drug test: Illicit drugs** can cause manic symptoms. Drug and alcohol abuse occurs in 60% of bipolar patients.
- **CT/MRI head** (optional): to rule out space-occupying lesions (can cause manic symptoms such as disinhibition).

DDx

- **Mood disorders:** hypomania, mania, mixed episode, cyclothymia.
- **Psychotic disorders:** schizophrenia, schizoaffective disorder.
- **Secondary to medical condition:** hyper-/hypothyroidism, Cushing's disease, cerebral tumor (e.g. frontal lobe lesion with disinhibition), stroke.
- **Drug related:** illicit drug ingestion (e.g. amphetamines, cocaine), acute drug withdrawal, side effect of corticosteroid use.
- **Personality disorders:** histrionic, emotionally unstable.

Management

- Full **risk assessment** is vital including suicidal ideation and risk to self (e.g. financial ruin from overspending). This will determine the urgency of referral to specialist mental health services.
- Remember to **ask about driving**. Accidents are more common in patients who are manic, hypomanic, or severely depressed.
- A psychiatric hold may be needed if the patient is violent or a risk to self. **Hospitalization** may be required if there is: (1) **reckless behavior** causing **risk to patient or others**; (2) significant **psychotic symptoms**; (3) **impaired judgement**; (4) or **psychomotor agitation**.

OSCE tips 3: A useful mnemonic for the management of bipolar affective disorder: **'CALMER'**

- Consider hospitalization/CBT
- Antipsychotics (Atypical)
- Lorazepam
- Mood stabilizers (e.g. lithium)
- Electroconvulsive therapy
- Risk assessment

- The pharmacological management of bipolar affective disorder is shown in *Table 3.3.4*. Also see *Section 15.4*, Mood stabilizers.
- For **bipolar depression**, offer a **high-intensity psychological intervention** (e.g. **CBT**).
- **ECT** is not first-line, but it can be used when antipsychotic drugs are ineffective and the patient is so severely disturbed that further medication or awaiting natural recovery is not feasible.
- Patients who present with an acute episode should be followed-up **once a week initially** and then **2–4 weekly** for the first few months.
- The **bio-psychosocial approach** to BAD is shown in *Fig. 3.3.4*.

Biological
• **Mood stabilizers, antipsychotics**
• **ECT:** for severe uncontrolled mania or depression

Psychological
• **Psychoeducation**
• **CBT** for depression

Social
• **Social support groups**
• **Self-help groups**
• **Encourage calming activities**

Fig. 3.3.4: Bio-psychosocial approach to the management of BAD.

Table 3.3.4: Pharmacological management of BAD	
Acute manic episode/mixed episode	**Bipolar depressive episode**
• First-line: **an antipsychotic** such as **olanzapine**, **risperidone**, or **quetiapine** (**haloperidol** is also effective). They have a rapid onset of action compared to mood stabilizers and are therefore used in severe mania. If the first antipsychotic is not effective or poorly tolerated then a second is usually offered. • **Mood stabilizers** lithium or valproate should be added as second-line treatment (see Mood stabilizers, *Section 15.4*). • **Benzodiazepines** may further be required to aid sleep and reduce agitation. • **Rapid tranquilization** may be required with **haloperidol** and/or **lorazepam**.	• **Atypical antipsychotics** are effective in bipolar depression. Options include **olanzapine** (combined with **fluoxetine**), or **quetiapine**, lurasidone, or cariprazine. • **Mood stabilizers** such as lithium or lamotrigine may be effective. • **Antidepressants** alone are usually avoided – if used, they should be used with care in BAD, even if depression is the main feature, as they have the potential to induce mania. They should be prescribed in conjunction with the cover of anti-manic medication.
Long-term management of bipolar affective disorder	
• **Lithium**, **valproate**, or **lamotrigine** can be used to prevent relapses (maintenance prescription). • 2nd generation (atypical) antipsychotics can also be used as a maintenance prescription and are frequently combined with mood stabilizers (see *Chapter 15* on management) if one class of drugs is not sufficient to prevent relapse.	

Key facts: The use of lithium as prophylaxis

- Lithium is the standard **long-term therapy** in bipolar affective disorder. It minimizes the risk of relapse and improves quality of life.
- Before lithium treatment is started **BUN/CR** (lithium has renal excretion), **TFTs**, **pregnancy status**, and baseline **ECG** should be checked. Lithium has a **narrow therapeutic window** and so drug levels should be closely monitored and patients should be informed of potential side effects and toxicity.
- **Side effects** include: polydipsia, polyuria, *fine* tremor, weight gain, edema, hypothyroidism, impaired renal function, memory problems, and teratogenicity (Ebstein anomaly) (in 1st trimester).
- Signs of **toxicity (1.5–2.0 mmol/L)**: N+V, *coarse* tremor, ataxia, muscle weakness, apathy.
- Signs of **severe toxicity (>2.0 mmol/L)**: nystagmus, dysarthria, hyperreflexia, oliguria, hypotension, convulsions, and coma.
- Due to its side effect profile and risk of toxicity lithium requires dose monitoring:
  - **Lithium levels – 12 hours** following first dose, then **weekly** until **therapeutic level (0.6–1.2 mmol/L)** has been stable for **4 weeks**. Once stable check every **3 months**.
  - **BUN/CR** – every **6 months**; **TFTs** – every **12 months**.
- A combination of **lithium and sodium valproate** is first-line treatment for **rapid cycling**.

Self-assessment

A 21-year-old female presents with low mood and anhedonia. She is unemployed and lives with her mother following her father's death in a tragic car accident when she was a young girl. You suspect depression and start her on citalopram. A week later her distressed mother comes to see you as she suspects her daughter has not told you the full story. She mentions that there are periods when her daughter seems full of herself, talks constantly without pausing and acts recklessly (e.g. overspending resulting in the family being in debt). She is also concerned about her daughter's alcohol consumption.

1. What is the most likely diagnosis? *(1 point)*
2. Give six differential diagnoses. *(3 points)*
3. Based on the DSM-5 criteria, give three of the possible symptoms required to confirm an episode of mania. *(3 points)*
4. What is the difference between hypomania and mania? *(2 points)*
5. Name two mood stabilizers that could be offered to a patient with an acute manic episode. What needs to be taken into consideration for a woman this age? *(4 points)*

Answers to self-assessment questions are to be found in *Appendix B*.

Chapter 4

Psychotic disorders

4.1   Overview of psychosis   43
4.2   Schizophrenia   45

Overview of psychosis

- **Psychosis** is defined as a mental state in which **a patient cannot distinguish between what is real and what is not**. It typically presents with:

  1. **Delusions:** A **fixed false belief**, which is **firmly held** despite evidence to the contrary and goes against the individual's **normal social and cultural belief system**. See MSE, *Section 2.2* for classification and types of delusions.

  2. **Hallucinations:** A **perception** in the **absence** of an **external stimulus**. It is a common feature of psychosis. See MSE, *Section 2.2* for types of hallucinations.

  3. **Thought disorder:** An impairment in the ability to form thoughts from logically connected ideas. See MSE, *Section 2.2*.

- Psychotic disorders are commonly grouped as follows: schizophrenia, schizophreniform disorder, delusional disorder, brief psychotic disorder, substance-induced psychotic disorder, schizoaffective disorder, catatonia, and other schizophrenia spectrum disorder. They are relatively common, with **schizophrenia** being the **most common**.

- The **incidence** of schizophrenia is **about 1% worldwide**.

- There are a variety of conditions that can present with **psychosis**, like bipolar disorder (*Fig. 4.1.1*).

- **Non-organic** causes of psychosis other than schizophrenia are covered in *Table 4.1.1*.

Causes of psychosis

Causes of psychosis	
Non-organic causes	**Organic causes**
Schizophrenia Schizoaffective disorder Brief psychotic episode Mood disorders with psychosis Delusional disorder Catatonia	Drug-induced psychosis* Iatrogenic (medication)** Complex partial epilepsy Delirium Dementia Huntington's disease Systemic lupus erythematosus Syphilis Endocrine disturbance, e.g. Cushing's syndrome Metabolic disorders including vitamin B_{12} deficiency and porphyria

Fig. 4.1.1: Organic and non-organic causes of psychosis.
*Alcohol, cocaine, amphetamine, methamphetamine, methylenedioxy-methamphetamine (MDMA), mephedrone, cannabis, LSD, psilocybins (e.g. magic mushrooms), ketamine; **levodopa, methyldopa, steroids, antimalarials.

Table 4.1.1: Other causes of psychosis

Brief psychotic disorder	A psychotic episode presenting very similarly to schizophrenia but lasting **<1 month** and so not meeting the criteria for schizophrenia.
Schizoaffective disorder	Characterized by symptoms of both **schizophrenia and a mood disorder** (depression or mania) in the **same episode of illness**. The mood symptoms should meet the criteria for either a depressive illness or a manic/hypomanic episode together with one or two typical symptoms of schizophrenia. This disorder is very rare.
Delusional disorder	The development of a **single or set of delusions** for a period of at least **3 months** in which the delusion is the only, or the most prominent, symptom with other areas of thinking and functioning well preserved, unlike in schizophrenia. The content of the delusion is often **persecutory**, **grandiose**, or **hypochondriacal** in nature. The onset and content of the delusion are often related to the patient's life situation. Symptoms often respond well to antipsychotics.
Induced delusional disorder (Folie à deux)	Induced delusional disorder, also known as 'shared paranoid disorder', is an uncommon disorder characterized by the presence of similar delusions in two or more individuals. **Folie imposée** is where a dominant person ('primary') initially forms a delusional belief during a psychotic episode and imposes it on another person(s) ('secondary'). **Folie simultanée** is when two people considered to suffer independently from psychosis, influence the content of each other's delusions so that they become identical or very similar.
Mood disorders with psychosis	Psychosis occurs **secondary to depression or mania**. On the other hand, schizophrenia usually develops spontaneously.
Postpartum psychosis	The **acute onset** of a **manic** or depressive **episode** shortly after childbirth (usually develops **in the first 2 weeks** following birth). It affects approximately **0.9–2.6%** of women.

Schizophrenia

Definition

Schizophrenia is the most common **psychotic condition**, characterized by two (or more) of the following, each present for a significant portion of time during a one-month period (or less if successfully treated); at least one of these must be:

1. delusions

2. hallucinations

3. disorganized speech plus

4. grossly disorganized or catatonic behavior, and

5. negative symptoms (i.e. diminished emotional expression or avolition).

This disorder leads to major functional impairment and it occurs in the absence of organic disease, previous alcohol or drug-related disorders and is not secondary to sustained elevation or depression of mood.

Pathophysiology/Etiology (see Table 4.2.1)

- The etiology of schizophrenia involves both **biological** and **environmental factors**.
- There is an increased likelihood of schizophrenia in those with a **positive family history**, and **monozygotic twin studies** show a **48%** concordance rate.
- The **dopamine hypothesis** states that schizophrenia is secondary to **over-activity** of **mesolimbic dopamine pathways** in the brain. This is supported by conventional antipsychotics which work by blocking dopamine (D2) receptors, and by drugs that potentiate the pathway (e.g. anti-parkinsonian drugs and amphetamines) causing psychotic symptoms.
- Factors that interfere with early neurodevelopment such as **obstetric complications**, **fetal injury**, and **low birth weight** lead to abnormalities expressed in the mature brain.
- **Adverse life events** and **psychological stress** increase the likelihood of developing schizophrenia.
- **Expressed emotion** is the theory that those with relatives that are 'over' involved or that make hostile or excessive critical comments are more likely to relapse.
- The **stress–vulnerability model** predicts that schizophrenia occurs due to environmental factors interacting with a genetic predisposition (or brain injury). Patients have different vulnerabilities and so different individuals need to be exposed to different levels of environmental factors to become psychotic.

Epidemiology and risk factors (see *Table 4.2.1*)

Table 4.2.1: Etiological factors in schizophrenia

	Biological	Psychological	Social
Predisposing	• **Genetic:** Monozygotic twin studies – 48% concordance • **Neurochemical:** ↑ dopamine, ↓ glutamate, ↓ serotonin, ↓ GABA • **Neurodevelopmental:** Intrauterine infection, premature birth, fetal brain injury, and obstetric complications • Age 15–35 • Extremes of parental age: ≤20 years or ≥35 years	• **Family history:** The closer the family relationship to an affected relative, the higher the risk	• **Substance misuse** • **Low socioeconomic status** • **Migrants:** Higher incidence in migrant populations (e.g. African-Caribbean), but not in offspring born in the new location • Living in an urban area – although this could be as a result of urban drift into cities. • Birth in late winter/early spring season (controversial)
Precipitating	• **Using phencyclidine or using psychostimulants**	• Adverse life events • Poor coping style	• Adverse life events
Perpetuating	• Substance misuse • Poor compliance to medication	• Adverse life events	• ↓ Social support • Expressed emotion

- Schizophrenia affects approximately **24 million** people worldwide. The incidence of schizophrenia is estimated to be **1 per 100** people.
- Peak age of onset is **15–35 years**.
- **Males** and **females** are **equally** affected but a systematic review showed men aged <45 years had twice the rate of schizophrenia as women.

Clinical features

- The symptoms of schizophrenia can be referred to as positive (thought or feelings added to a patient's experience) when there is the appearance of hallucinations and delusions. This is in contrast to **negative** symptoms (an absence or deficiency) which refers to loss of function. The clinical features of schizophrenia depend upon the type of schizophrenia, with **paranoid schizophrenia** being the most common.

Positive symptoms (**D**elusions **H**eld **F**irmly **T**hink **P**sychosis)

- **Delusions:** A delusion is a **fixed false belief**, which is **firmly held** despite evidence to the contrary and goes **against** the individual's **normal social** and **cultural belief system**. Usually **persecutory**, **grandiose**, **nihilistic**, or **religious** in nature. **Ideas of reference** are thoughts in which a patient infers that common events refer to them directly (e.g. personal messages from television and newspapers).

- **Hallucinations:** A hallucination is a **perception** in the **absence** of an **external stimulus**. They are usually **third person auditory hallucinations** which may be of running commentary nature.

- **Formal thought disorder:** Abnormalities of the way thoughts are linked together. See *Section 2.2*, MSE.

Key facts 1: Schneider's first rank symptoms

Schneider's first-rank symptoms of schizophrenia are symptoms which, if one or more are present, are strongly suggestive of schizophrenia:

- **Delusional perception:** A new delusion that forms in response to a real perception without any logical sense, e.g. 'the traffic light turned red so I am the chosen one.'
- **Third person auditory hallucinations:** usually a running commentary.
- **Thought interference:** thought insertion, withdrawal, or broadcast.
- **Passivity phenomenon.**

- **Thought interference:** This could either be the feelings that thoughts are being inserted (**thought insertion**), removed (**thought withdrawal**), or heard out loud by others (**thought broadcast**).

- **Passivity phenomenon: Actions**, **feelings**, or **emotions** being controlled by an external force.

Negative symptoms (the **A** factor)

- **Avolition (↓ motivation):** Reduced ability (or inability) to initiate and persist in goal-directed behavior.
- **Asocial behavior:** Loss of drive for any social engagements.
- **Anhedonia:** Lack of pleasure in activities that were previously enjoyable to the patient.
- **Alogia (poverty of speech):** A quantitative and qualitative decrease in speech.
- **Affect blunted:** Diminished or absent capacity to express feelings.
- **Attention (cognitive) deficits:** May experience problems with attention, language, memory, and executive function.

NOTE: The onset of clinical features may be preceded by a **prodrome** where the patient becomes **reserved**, **anxious**, **suspicious**, and **irritable** with a disturbance in normal everyday functioning.

DSM-5 Criteria for schizophrenia

A. Two (or more) of the following, each present for a significant portion of time during a 1-month period (or less if successfully treated). At least one of these must be (1), (2), or (3):
1. Delusions.
2. Hallucinations.
3. Disorganized speech (e.g. frequent derailment or incoherence).
4. Grossly disorganized or catatonic behavior.
5. Negative symptoms (i.e. diminished emotional expression or avolition).
B. For a significant portion of the time since the onset of the disturbance, level of functioning in one or more areas, such as work, interpersonal relations, or self-care, is markedly below the level achieved prior to the onset (or when the onset is in childhood or adolescence, there is failure to achieve expected level of interpersonal, academic, or occupational functioning).
C. Continuous signs of disturbance persist for at least 6 months. This 6-month period must include at least 1 month of symptoms (or less if successfully treated) that meet Criterion A (i.e. active-phase symptoms) and may include periods of prodromal or residual symptoms.

DSM-5 Criteria for schizophrenia *(continued)*

During these prodromal or residual periods, the signs of the disturbance may be manifested by only negative symptoms or by two or more symptoms listed in Criterion A present in an attenuated form (e.g. odd beliefs, unusual perceptual experiences).

D. Schizoaffective disorder and depressive or bipolar disorder with psychotic features have been ruled out because either 1) no major depressive or manic episodes have occurred concurrently with the active-phase symptoms, or 2) if mood episodes have occurred during active-phase symptoms, they have been present for a minority of the total duration of the active and residual periods of the illness.

E. The disturbance is not attributable to the physiological effects of a substance (e.g. a drug of abuse, a medication) or another medical condition.

F. If there is a history of autism spectrum disorder or a communication disorder of childhood onset, the additional diagnosis of schizophrenia is made only if prominent delusions or hallucinations, in addition to the other required symptoms of schizophrenia, are also present for at least 1 month (or less if successfully treated).

Specify if:

The following course specifiers are only to be used after a 1-year duration of the disorder and if they are not in contradiction to the diagnostic course criteria.

First episode, currently in acute episode: First manifestation of the disorder meeting the defining diagnostic symptom and time criteria. An *acute episode* is a time period in which the symptom criteria are fulfilled.

First episode, currently in partial remission: *Partial remission* is a period of time during which an improvement after a previous episode is maintained and in which the defining criteria of the disorder are only partially fulfilled.

First episode, currently in full remission: *Full remission* is a period of time after a previous episode during which no disorder-specific symptoms are present.

Multiple episodes, currently in acute episode: Multiple episodes may be determined after a minimum of two episodes (i.e. after a first episode, a remission and a minimum of one relapse).

Multiple episodes, currently in partial remission.

Multiple episodes, currently in full remission.

Continuous: Symptoms fulfilling the diagnostic symptom criteria of the disorder are remaining for the majority of the illness course, with subthreshold symptom periods being very brief relative to the overall course.

Unspecified.

Specify if:

With catatonia (refer to the criteria for catatonia associated with another mental disorder, pp. 119–120, for definition).

Coding note: Use additional code 293.89 (F06.1) catatonia associated with schizophrenia to indicate the presence of the comorbid catatonia.

Specify current severity:

Severity is rated by a quantitative assessment of the primary symptoms of psychosis, including delusions, hallucinations, disorganized speech, abnormal psychomotor behavior, and negative symptoms. Each of these symptoms may be rated for its current severity (most severe in the last 7 days) on a 5-point scale ranging from 0 (not present) to 4 (present and severe). (See Clinician-Rated Dimensions of Psychosis Symptom Severity in the chapter "Assessment Measures.")

NOTE: Diagnosis of schizophrenia can be made without using this severity specifier.

OSCE tips: History taking from psychotic patients

- The most common OSCE scenario will be a patient with paranoid schizophrenia displaying positive and perhaps negative symptoms. The other types of schizophrenia are much less common.
- History taking will require you to be familiar with, and look comfortable and confident, asking questions to elicit psychotic symptoms. For the patient their psychotic experiences are real, and you need to demonstrate an empathetic and supportive approach to history taking and MSE.
- Remember to consider the other differentials, both organic and psychiatric, including mood disorders, and drug-induced psychosis.
- A good social history focusing on day to day activities and interests may help you to elicit negative symptoms of schizophrenia.
- You need to sensitively ask questions about insight and risk, as this will determine your management.

Diagnosis and investigations

Hx
- 'Have you ever had the experience of hearing noises or voices talking when there is nobody around and nothing else to explain it?' **(auditory hallucinations)**
- 'How many voices are there?' **(type of auditory hallucination)**
- 'Do these voices speak directly to you or about you?' **(second or third person auditory hallucination, respectively)**
- 'Do these voices ever make comments about what you're doing?' **(third person auditory hallucinations – running commentary)**
- 'Are you afraid that someone else is trying to harm you?' **(persecutory delusion)**
- 'Have you noticed that people are doing or saying things that have a special meaning to you?' 'When you watch television or read the newspaper do you ever worry that there are messages specifically for you?' **(delusions of reference)**
- 'Do you have any special powers or abilities?' **(grandiose delusions)**
- 'Have you ever felt that thoughts are being taken out of your mind?' **(thought withdrawal)**
- 'Have you ever experienced thoughts inside your head that are not yours and have been put there by someone else?' **(thought insertion)**
- 'Have you ever felt under the control of an outside force?' **(passivity phenomenon)**

MSE	**Appearance**	Can be normal **(positive)**, or inappropriate with poor self-care **(negative)**.
	Behavior	Preoccupied, restless, noisy, or suspicious **(positive)**. A few show sudden, unexpected changes in behavior. Withdrawn, poor eye contact, and apathy **(negative)**.
	Speech	May reflect underlying thought disorder (loosening of associations, pressured and distractible speech), interruptions to flow of thought (thought blocking), and poverty of speech **(negative)**.
	Mood	Incongruity of affect or mood changes such as depression, anxiety, or irritability. Flattened affect **(negative)**.
	Thought	Delusions (e.g. persecutory, delusions of control, delusions of reference), thought insertion/withdrawal/broadcast, formal thought disorder (loosening of associations, word salad, concrete thinking, circumstantiality/tangentiality) **(all positive)**.
	Perception	Hallucinations (especially third person auditory in nature) **(positive)**.
	Cognition	Normal orientation. Attention and concentration often impaired **(positive)**. May be evidence of premorbid cognitive impairment. Specific cognitive deficits **(negative)**.
	Insight	Generally poor.

Ix
- **Blood tests: CBC** (anemia, infection), **TFTs** (thyroid dysfunction can present with psychosis), **glucose** or **HbA1c** (as atypical antipsychotics can cause metabolic syndrome), **serum calcium** (hypercalcemia can present with psychosis), **electrolytes, BUN/Cr** and **LFTs** (assess renal and liver function before giving antipsychotics), **cholesterol** (as atypical antipsychotics cause metabolic syndrome), **vitamin B$_{12}$ and folate** (deficiencies can cause psychosis).
- **Urine drug test: Illicit drugs** can cause and exacerbate psychosis.
- **ECG:** Antipsychotics cause **prolonged QT interval**, but this is rare.
- **CT scan:** To rule out organic causes such as **space-occupying lesions**.
- **EEG:** To rule out **temporal lobe epilepsy** as possible cause of **psychosis**.

DDx See *Fig. 4.1.1*, Overview of psychosis.

Management

- **Risk assessment** is vital and the use of a **psychiatric hold** may be required for those who refuse informal admission.
- The care of the schizophrenic patient is a joint effort between primary and secondary care and a combination of inpatient and outpatient care. Involvement of the psychiatric consultant,

community psychiatric nurses, PCPs, social workers, carers and voluntary organizations is essential. A **care program approach** may be used (see *Chapter 1*, Introduction to psychiatry).

- It is essential to assess social circumstances and involve family where possible.
- The principal management of schizophrenia is outlined using the **bio-psychosocial model** (see *Table 4.2.2*).

Key facts 2: Poor prognostic factors for schizophrenia

Factors associated with poor prognosis:

- **Strong family history.**
- **Gradual onset.**
- **↓ IQ.**
- **Premorbid history of social withdrawal.**
- **No obvious precipitant.**

Table 4.2.2: Bio-psychosocial approach to the management of schizophrenia

Biological	
Antipsychotics (see *Fig. 4.2.1* and *Section 15.3*, Antipsychotics)	• Antipsychotics can be broadly divided into **1st** and **2nd generation**. • **2nd generation** antipsychotics are **first-line**, e.g. risperidone and olanzapine. • **Long-acting** formulations should be considered if the patient prefers or there is a problem with non-compliance. • **Clozapine** is the most effective antipsychotic and used for **treatment-resistant schizophrenia** (failure to respond to two other antipsychotics).
ECT	• May be appropriate in patients who are **resistant to pharmacological agents**. Effective for **catatonic schizophrenia**.
Psychological	
CBT	• CBT or supportive therapy are both strongly recommended. **Reduces residual symptoms**.
Family intervention	• Particularly useful for families of patients with schizophrenia who have persisting symptoms. **Psychoeducation** helps families **reduce high levels of expressed emotion** which reduces relapse rates.
Art therapy	• Useful for the alleviation of **negative symptoms** in young people.
Social skills training	• Uses a **behavioral approach** to help patients improve **interpersonal**, **self-care**, and **coping** skills needed in everyday life.
Support groups	• National support groups such as **NAMI** can help facilitate successful rehabilitation back into the community.
Peer support	• Delivered by a **peer support worker** who has recovered from psychosis or schizophrenia and remains stable.
Supported employment programs	• As the patient recovers from the acute episode, part or full time employment or return to school may be indicated.

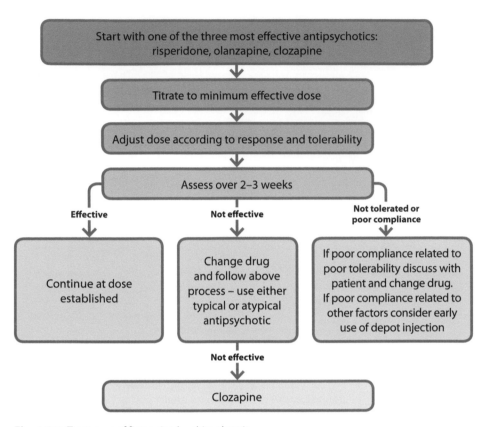

Fig. 4.2.1: Treatment of first-episode schizophrenia.

Self-assessment

A 22-year-old unmarried man presents to the clinic with his mother. He spends most of his time at home and refuses to go out at night alone. He states he saw lightning and is now convinced that the FBI is after him and that FBI agents gather information about his whereabouts. He believes that they are trying to control his thoughts and movement. He also hears them outside his house talking about how they will murder him. He appears suspicious, avoids eye contact, and his answers to questions are delayed, during which he appears internally preoccupied.

1. What is the most likely diagnosis? Name five differential diagnoses. *(3 points)*

2. Which of Schneider's first rank symptoms is this patient suffering from? *(3 points)*

3. What are the negative symptoms of schizophrenia? *(4 points)*

4. What investigations would you perform on this patient and why? *(4 points)*

5. Name an atypical antipsychotic that could be given to this patient. Name four side effects of this medication. *(5 points)*

6. Name some potential psychosocial interventions for this patient. *(4 points)*

Answers to self-assessment questions are to be found in *Appendix B*.

Clinical pearl

Schizophrenia is a lifetime illness, probably of genetic etiology, and as such, improving symptoms and functions is key to help over the course of the illness. Treatment requires a combination of:
1. antipsychotic medication and supportive psychotherapy for the patient
2. ongoing work with the family/significant other or case workers using psychoeducation consistently over the course of the illness
3. long-term rehabilitation and support.

Patients improve with adequate therapy and worsen critically without it, just like untreated diabetes mellitus.

Chapter 5

Anxiety disorders

5.1	Overview of anxiety disorders	55
5.2	Generalized anxiety disorder	57
5.3	Phobic anxiety disorders	62
5.4	Panic disorder	67

5.1 Overview of anxiety disorders

Definitions and epidemiology

- **Anxiety** is an **unpleasant emotional state** involving **subjective fear** and **somatic symptoms**.
- Every human experiences anxiety, but if these anxieties become **excessive** or **disabling** they are described as an illness.
- The **Yerkes–Dodson law** states that anxiety can actually be beneficial up to a **plateau of optimal functioning**. Beyond this level of anxiety however, performance deteriorates (*Fig. 5.1.1*).
- Anxiety disorders are commonly grouped as follows: **phobic anxiety disorders**, such as agoraphobia (with or without panic disorder), social phobia, specific phobia; and **other anxiety disorders**, such as panic disorder, generalized anxiety disorder, separation anxiety, and substance-induced anxiety.
- Anxiety disorders are **common** in primary and secondary care, with associated physical symptoms usually the cause of presentation, as opposed to psychological symptoms.
- The most common anxiety disorders, in order of **prevalence**, are **specific phobia, social anxiety, generalized anxiety disorder, and panic disorder**.
- The one year **prevalence** of anxiety disorders is approximately **14%**.

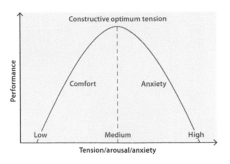

Fig. 5.1.1: Yerkes–Dodson curve.

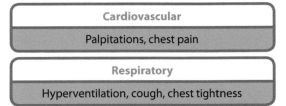

Psychological
Anticipatory fear of impending doom, worrying thoughts, exaggerated startle response, restlessness, poor concentration and attention, irritability, depersonalization and derealization

Cardiovascular
Palpitations, chest pain

Respiratory
Hyperventilation, cough, chest tightness

Gastrointestinal
Abdominal pain ('butterflies'), loose stools, nausea and vomiting, dysphagia, dry mouth

Genitourinary
↑ Frequency of micturition, failure of erection, menstrual discomfort

Neuromuscular
Tremor, myalgia, headache, paresthesia, tinnitus

Fig. 5.1.2: Common symptoms of anxiety.

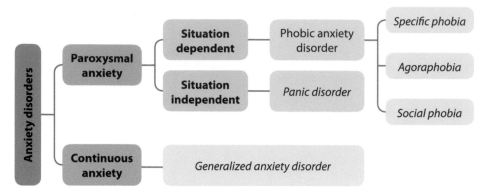

Fig. 5.1.3: The anxiety disorders.

1. **Generalized (free floating) anxiety: Present most of the time** and not associated with specific objects or situations. **Excessive or inappropriate worry** about **normal life events**. Typically **longer duration** (months or even years).

2. **Episodic (paroxysmal) anxiety:** Has an **abrupt onset** and occurs in **discrete episodes**. The episode of anxiety is **severe** with **strong autonomic symptoms**, but usually **short-lived** (typically less than one hour). Can occur in response to specific threats.

Conditions associated with anxiety

• There are many conditions associated with anxiety which can be divided into **medical** (**non-psychiatric**), **substance-related**, and **psychiatric** (see *Table 5.1.1*).

• These are all potential **differential diagnoses** for a patient presenting with features of anxiety.

NOTE: Any **chronic condition** (e.g. COPD, CCF) may cause anxiety and depressive symptoms.

Table 5.1.1: Conditions associated with anxiety	
Medical	Hyperthyroidism, hypoglycemia, anemia, pheochromocytoma, Cushing's disease, chronic obstructive pulmonary disease (COPD), congestive cardiac failure (CCF), malignancies
Substance-related	• Intoxication: e.g. alcohol, cannabis, caffeine • Withdrawal: e.g. alcohol, benzodiazepine, caffeine • Side effects: e.g. thyroxine, steroids, epinephrine
Psychiatric	Eating disorders, somatic symptom disorders, depression, schizophrenia, OCD, post-traumatic stress disorder, adjustment disorder, anxious (avoidant) personality disorder

5.2 Generalized anxiety disorder

Definition

Generalized anxiety disorder (GAD) is a syndrome of **ongoing, uncontrollable, widespread worry** about many events or thoughts that the **patient recognizes** as **excessive** and **inappropriate**. Symptoms must be present on **most days** for at least **6 months** duration.

Pathophysiology/Etiology

- The etiology of GAD can be divided into **biological** and **environmental** causes (*Fig. 5.2.1*). Biological causes can further be split into **genetic** and **neurophysiological**.

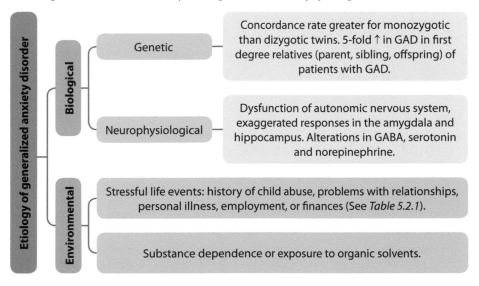

Fig. 5.2.1: Outline of the biological and environmental factors associated with GAD.

Epidemiology and risk factors (*Table 5.2.1*)

- GAD has a prevalence of **2–4%** in the general population.
- It is **more common in** females at a ratio of **2:1**.

Table 5.2.1:	Risk factors for GAD
Predisposing	• Genetics, childhood upbringing, personality type, and demands for high achievement. Being divorced. Living alone or as a single parent. Low socioeconomic status.
Precipitating	• Stressful life events such as domestic violence, unemployment, relationship problems, and personal illness (e.g. chronic pain, arthritis, COPD).
Maintaining	• Continuing stressful events, marital status, living alone, and ways of thinking which perpetuate anxiety (e.g. 'What will happen if others notice that I am anxious?').

Clinical features

- Clinical features of GAD can be divided into the areas shown in *Fig. 5.2.2*.
- **Common features** of presentation *specific* to GAD are listed below ('**WATCHERS**'):
  - **Worry** (excessive, uncontrollable)
  - **Autonomic hyperactivity** (sweating, ↑ pupil size, ↑ HR)
  - **Tension in muscles/Tremor**
  - **Concentration difficulty/Chronic aches**
  - **Headache/Hyperventilation**
  - **Energy loss**
  - **Restlessness**
  - **Startled easily/Sleep disturbance** (difficulty getting to sleep then intermittent awakening and nightmares).

DSM-5 Criteria for GAD

A. Excessive anxiety and worry (apprehensive expectation), occurring more days than not for at least 6 months, about a number of events or activities (such as work or school performance).

B. The individual finds it difficult to control the worry.

C. The anxiety and worry are associated with three (or more) of the following six symptoms (with at least some symptoms having been present for more days than not for the past 6 months):
Note: Only one item is required in children.
  1. Restlessness or feeling keyed up or on edge.
  2. Being easily fatigued.
  3. Difficulty concentrating or mind going blank.
  4. Irritability.
  5. Muscle tension.
  6. Sleep disturbance (difficulty falling or staying asleep, or restless, or unsatisfying sleep).

D. The anxiety, worry, or physical symptoms cause clinically significant distress or impairment in social, occupational, or other important areas of functioning.

E. The disturbance is not attributable to the physiological effects of a substance (e.g. a drug of abuse, a medication) or another medical condition (e.g. hyperthyroidism).

F. The disturbance is not better explained by another mental disorder (e.g. anxiety or worry about having panic attacks in panic disorder, negative evaluation in social anxiety disorder [social phobia], contamination or other obsessions in obsessive–compulsive disorder, separation from attachment figures in separation anxiety disorder, reminders of traumatic events in posttraumatic stress disorder, gaining weight in anorexia nervosa, physical complaints in somatic symptom disorder, perceived appearance flaws in body dysmorphic disorder, having a serious illness in illness anxiety disorder, or the content of delusional beliefs in schizophrenia or delusional disorder).

See *Fig. 5.2.2*.

Diagnosis and investigations

Hx
- 'Talk me through a normal day in your life.' **(open question to identify anxiety)**
- 'Do you ever feel worried with your current state of affairs?', 'Do you worry excessively about minor things on most days of the week?', 'Would you say you are an anxious person?', 'Recently, have you been feeling anxious or on edge?' **(generalized worry)**
- 'Have you noticed any problems with your memory or concentration?' **(↓ concentration)**
- 'Do you ever lie awake at night worrying, or intermittently wake from sleep?', 'Do you ever have unpleasant dreams or nightmares?' **(sleep disturbance)**
- Ask about **somatic symptoms**, e.g. 'Do you ever feel the sensation of your heart beating abnormally fast or pounding on your chest?'

MSE		
Appearance and behavior	Face looks worried with brow furrowed. Restless with tremor. Fidgety. Sweaty when you shake their hand. Hyperventilating. Lip biting. Pallor. Tense posture.	
Speech	Trembling. Slow rate.	
Mood	Anxious.	
Thought	Repetitive worrying thoughts. Thoughts may concern personal health, safety of others, or excessive worry about everyday events, e.g. relationships, finances.	
Perception	No hallucinations.	
Cognition	May complain of poor memory and reduced attention/concentration	
Insight	May or may not have insight.	

NOTE: Observations may reveal a raised heart rate, respiratory rate and blood pressure.

Somatic symptoms
- Difficulty breathing
- Feeling of choking
- Chest pain or discomfort
- Nausea
- Abdominal distress or pain
- Loose motions.

Psychological symptoms
- Feeling dizzy or lightheaded
- Fear of dying
- Fear of losing control
- Derealization and depersonalization.

General symptoms
- Hot flushes or cold chills
- Numbness or tingling
- Headache.

Symptoms of tension
- Muscle tension, aches, or pains
- Restlessness
- Feeling on edge
- Difficulty swallowing
- Sensation of lump in throat.

Non-specific symptoms
- Being startled
- Concentration difficulty and mind blanks
- Persistent irritability
- Sleep problems.

Fig. 5.2.2: Potential symptoms of GAD (DSM-5).

| Ix | • **Blood tests: CBC** (for infection/anemia), **TFTs** (hyperthyroidism), **glucose** (hypoglycemia).
• **ECG:** may show sinus tachycardia.
• **Questionnaires:** GAD-2, GAD-7, Beck's Anxiety Inventory, Hospital Anxiety and Depression Scale. |

| DDx | • **Other anxiety disorders:** panic disorder, specific phobias, OCD, PTSD.
• **Depression.**
• **Hypomania/mania.**
• **ADHD.**
• **Personality disorder** (e.g. avoidant PD, dependent PD). | • **Excessive caffeine. Stimulant, cocaine abuse.**
• **Withdrawal from drugs:** alcohol, benzodiazepines, barbiturates.
• **Organic:** anemia, hyperthyroidism, pheochromocytoma, hypoglycemia (see *Table 5.1.1* in Overview of anxiety disorders, for comprehensive list). |

OSCE tips: Screening for other conditions

In an OSCE, it is very important to screen for depression and substance misuse in patients who you suspect have generalized anxiety disorder, as these conditions are strongly associated.

Management

- The management of generalized anxiety disorder is based on the bio-psychosocial model:
  - Biological: The **first-line drug** treatment of choice is an **SSRI** which has anxiolytic effects. If this does not help, an **SNRI** (e.g. venlafaxine or duloxetine) can be offered. If both of these are ineffective or not tolerated, **pregabalin** or **gabapentin** may be used. Medication should be continued for at least a year. **Benzodiazepines** should not be offered except as **short-term measures** during crises, as they can cause dependence.
  - Psychological: **Psychoeducational groups** are a *low intensity* form of psychological intervention. *Higher intensity* includes **cognitive behavioral therapy** and **applied relaxation** (practicing techniques that lead to muscular or bodily relaxation, which can be applied in situations that trigger anxiety and worry).
  - Social: Include **self-help methods** (such as writing down worrying thoughts and analyzing them objectively) and **support groups. Exercise** should be encouraged and may benefit.
- **Co-morbid depression** or **substance misuse** should be treated (See *OSCE tips*).
- A **stepped care model** can help to determine the most effective interventions for patients with GAD (*Fig. 5.2.3*).

Step 1: Identification and assessment. Psychoeducation about GAD and active monitoring.

Step 2: Low intensity psychological interventions (individual non-facilitated self-help; individual guided self-help; psychoeducational group-based therapy).

Step 3: Higher intensity interventions: CBT or drug therapy.

Step 4: Psychiatric referral, e.g. multi-agency teams. Combination of drug and psychological therapies.

Fig. 5.2.3: Stepped care model for the management of GAD.

Self-assessment

A 35-year-old female presents to you complaining of long-standing tiredness. At first glance, she appears pale, worried, and shaky. On questioning you discover she has been finding it difficult to get to sleep for the past year and when she does eventually get to sleep she is awoken by nightmares. Her mouth is constantly dry despite drinking plenty of water and she frequently gets chest tightness and feels sick. She is worried that this is all impacting on her job as a teacher. You suspect generalized anxiety disorder.

1. How long do symptoms need to be present for in order for this diagnosis to be made? *(1 point)*
2. Suggest three laboratory studies to rule out co-morbid medical conditions. *(3 points)*
3. Other than dry mouth and chest pain, give six somatic symptoms of this disorder. *(3 points)*
4. What is the first-line pharmacotherapy for this condition? *(1 point)*
5. Give two psychosocial forms of management for this condition. *(2 points)*

Answers to self-assessment questions are to be found in *Appendix B*.

Phobic anxiety disorders

Definition

- **Phobia:** is an **intense, irrational** fear of an **object, situation, place,** or **person** that is recognized as **excessive** (out of proportion to the threat) or **unreasonable**.
- **Agoraphobia:** Agoraphobia literally means a 'fear of the marketplace'. It is a fear of **public spaces** or fear of entering a public space from which **immediate escape would be difficult** in the event of a panic attack.
- **Social phobia (social anxiety disorder):** A fear of **social situations** which may lead to **humiliation, criticism,** or **embarrassment**.
- **Specific (isolated) phobia:** A fear restricted to a **specific object or situation** (excluding agoraphobia and social phobia).

Pathophysiology/Etiology *(Table 5.3.1)*

Table 5.3.1: Etiology of phobias	
Agoraphobia	Maintained by avoidance which prevents deconditioning and sets up a vicious cycle of anxiety.
Social phobia	Uncertain etiology. Usually begins in late adolescence, an age at which people are concerned about the impression they make on others.
Specific phobia	Conditioning event in early life, i.e. a frightening experience. Possibly a role for learned behavior, e.g. from parents *(Fig. 5.3.1)*.

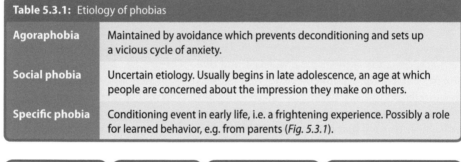

Animals	Nature/forces	Blood/injection/injury	Situational
• Spiders (arachno-) • Insects (entomo-) • Dogs (cyno-) • Birds (ornitho-)	• Thunder (astra-) • Storms (lilapso-) • Water (aqua-)	• Sight of blood (hemo-) • Physical injury or illness (traumato-) • Needles/injection (needle-)	• Closed spaces (claustro-) • Heights (acro-) or flying • Darkness (nycto-) • Hospitals (nosocome-)

Fig. 5.3.1: Some common specific phobias. Prefixes refer to the name of the phobia.

Epidemiology (*Table 5.3.2*) and risk factors (*Table 5.3.3*)

Table 5.3.2: Epidemiology of phobic anxiety disorders

Phobic anxiety disorder	1 year prevalence	Age of onset	♂:♀ ratio
Agoraphobia (affects up to 1/3 of those with panic disorder)	0.4%	Early adulthood (25–30 years of age)	2:1
Social phobia	1.2%	Usually adolescence	1:1
Specific phobia	3.5%	Usually childhood but can develop later in life	1:1

Table 5.3.3: Risk factors for phobias

Aversive experiences (prior experiences with specific objects or situations)
Stress and negative life events
Other anxiety disorders
Mood disorders
Substance use disorders
Family history

Clinical features

- Biological: **Tachycardia** is the usual **autonomic response**, however in phobias of blood, injection, and injury, a **vasovagal response** (bradycardia) is produced, commonly leading to fainting (**syncope**). For a complete list of biological symptoms see GAD, *Section 5.2*.

- Psychological: Include unpleasant **anticipatory anxiety**, **inability to relax**, urge to **avoid** the feared situation, and, at extremes, a **fear of dying**.

- Agoraphobia is strongly linked to panic disorder. Indeed the *DSM-5* divides agoraphobia into: agoraphobia *with* panic disorder and agoraphobia *without* panic disorder.

DSM-5 Criteria for agoraphobia

A. Marked fear or anxiety about two (or more) of the following five situations:
   1. Using public transportation such as automobiles, buses, trains, ships, or planes.
   2. Being in open spaces such as parking lots, marketplaces, or bridges.
   3. Being in enclosed places such as shops, theaters, or cinemas.
   4. Standing in line or being in a crowd.
   5. Being outside of the home alone.
B. The individual fears or avoids these situations because of the thoughts that escape might be difficult or help might not be available in the event of developing panic-like symptoms or other incapacitating or embarrassing symptoms such as fear of falling in the elderly or fear of incontinence.
C. The agoraphobic situations almost always provoke fear or anxiety.
D. The agoraphobic situations are actively avoided, require the presence of a companion, or are endured with intense fear or anxiety.
E. The fear or anxiety is out of proportion to the actual danger posed by the agoraphobic situations and to the sociocultural context.

DSM-5 Criteria for agoraphobia *(continued)*

F. The fear, anxiety, or avoidance is persistent, typically lasting for six months or more.
G. The fear, anxiety, or avoidance causes clinically significant distress or impairment in social, occupational, or other important areas of functioning.
H. If another medical condition such as inflammatory bowel disease or Parkinson's disease is present, the fear, anxiety, or avoidance is clearly excessive.
I. The fear, anxiety, or avoidance is not better explained by the symptoms of another mental disorder, for example, the symptoms are not confined to specific phobia, situational type; do not involve only social situations as in social anxiety disorder; and are not related exclusively to obsessions as in obsessive-compulsive disorder, perceived effects of flaws in physical appearance as in body dysmorphic disorder, reminders of traumatic events as in post-traumatic stress disorder, or fear of separation as in separation anxiety disorder.

NOTE: Agoraphobia is diagnosed irrespective of the presence of panic disorder. If an individual's presentation meets criteria for panic disorder and agoraphobia, both diagnoses should be assigned.

Reprinted with permission from the *Diagnostic and Statistical Manual of Mental Disorders*, 5th Edition, (©2013). American Psychiatric Association.

DSM-5 Criteria for social anxiety disorder (social phobia)

A. Marked fear or anxiety about one or more social situations in which the individual is exposed to possible scrutiny by others. Examples include social interactions (e.g. having a conversation, meeting unfamiliar people), being observed (e.g. eating or drinking), and performing in front of others (e.g. giving a speech).
   NOTE: In children, the anxiety must occur in peer settings and not just during interactions with adults.
B. The individual fears that he or she will act in a way or show anxiety symptoms that will be negatively evaluated (i.e. will be humiliating or embarrassing; will lead to rejection or offend others).
C. The social situations almost always provoke fear or anxiety.
   NOTE: In children, the fear or anxiety may be expressed by crying, tantrums, freezing, clinging, shrinking, or failing to speak in social situations.
D. The social situations are avoided or endured with intense fear or anxiety.
E. The fear or anxiety is out of proportion to the actual threat posed by the social situation and to the sociocultural context.
F. The fear, anxiety, or avoidance is persistent, typically lasting for 6 months or more.
G. The fear, anxiety, or avoidance causes clinically significant distress or impairment in social, occupational, or other important areas of functioning.
H. The fear, anxiety, or avoidance is not attributable to the physiological effects of a substance (e.g. a drug of abuse, a medication) or another medical condition.
I. The fear, anxiety, or avoidance is not better explained by the symptoms of another mental disorder, such as panic disorder, body dysmorphic disorder, or autism spectrum disorder.
J. If another medical condition (e.g. Parkinson's disease, obesity, disfigurement from burns or injury) is present, the fear, anxiety, or avoidance is clearly unrelated or is excessive.

Specify if:
   Performance only: If the fear is restricted to speaking or performing in public.

Reprinted with permission from the *Diagnostic and Statistical Manual of Mental Disorders*, 5th Edition, (©2013). American Psychiatric Association.

Diagnosis and investigations

Hx
- 'What situations cause you anxiety or embarrassment?' **(specific phobia)**
- 'Do you get symptoms in situations from which escape would be difficult?', 'Do you get symptoms in places or situations where help may not be available?', 'Do you get symptoms while being in a crowd or traveling on public transport?' **(agoraphobia)**
- 'Do you ever worry about what people think of you? Does this worry ever lead to you avoiding certain situations?' **(social phobia)**
- 'Do you avoid any situation because you know you will feel panicky?' **(anticipatory anxiety)**

OSCE tips: Features that distinguish phobic anxiety disorders from GAD (**SS, AA, AA**)

Even if a patient is calm when you speak to them, you should screen for phobias as they are **restricting conditions** due to **avoidance of the feared stimulus. Three features** separate phobic anxiety from GAD.
1. Anxiety occurs in **Specific Situations**:
   - *Agoraphobia* – Public transport, supermarkets (especially waiting in line), movie theaters, empty streets.
   - *Social phobia* – Social gatherings, parties, public speaking, meetings, classrooms, eating in public.
2. There is **Anticipatory Anxiety** when there is a prospect of encountering the feared situation.
3. There is **Attempted Avoidance** of circumstances that precipitate anxiety.

MSE		
Appearance & Behavior	Restless and wanting to escape. Pale, sweaty, hyperventilating. May lose consciousness (blood or injection phobia).	
Speech	May be trembling or they may become speechless.	
Mood	Anxious.	
Thought	Unpleasant feelings towards threat. Fear of situation. Desire to escape. Fear of dying.	
Insight	Poor when feared stimulus present. Good when separated from stimulus.	

NOTE: MSE will be largely normal unless exposed to the stimulus for phobia.

Ix
As symptoms occur in a defined situation, diagnosis is usually straightforward with minimal need for investigations. **Questionnaires** include the Social Phobia Inventory and Liebowitz Social Anxiety Scale.

DDx
- **Psychiatric:** Panic disorder, PTSD, anxious personality disorder, somatic symptom disorders, adjustment disorder, depression, schizophrenia (may avoid socializing because of paranoid delusions).
- **Organic:** See *Table 5.1.1* in *Section 5.1*, Overview of anxiety disorders.

Management

General points

- Try to establish a **good rapport** with the patient. Remember, particularly with social phobia, it may have been very challenging for the patient to attend appointments.
- Advise **avoidance of anxiety-inducing substances**, e.g. caffeine.
- Screen for significant co-morbidities such as **substance use, depression**, and **personality disorders**.
- **Refer to a mental health specialist** if there is a risk of **self-harm, suicide, self-neglect**, or **significant co-morbidity**.

Management of the three phobic anxiety disorders (Table 5.3.4)

Table 5.3.4: Management of agoraphobia, social anxiety and specific phobia	
Agoraphobia	• **CBT** is the psychological intervention of choice. The behavioral component includes graduated exposure and desensitization. **Graduated exposure** techniques such as walking increased distances from home day by day, can be used. • **SSRIs** are the first-line pharmacological agent.
Social phobia	• **CBT** (individual or group) specifically designed for social phobia. **Graduated exposure** to feared situations is included both within treatment sessions and as homework. • **Pharmacological interventions** include **SSRIs** (escitalopram or sertraline), **SNRIs** (venlafaxine), or if no response to these, a **MAOI** (transdermal selegiline).
Specific phobia	• The mainstay of treatment is **exposure** either using self-help methods or more formally through **CBT**. • **Benzodiazepines** may be used as anxiolytics in the short term (due to risk of dependence), for instance if a patient needs an urgent CT scan and they are claustrophobic.

Self-assessment

A 35-year-old man experiences intense worry a few weeks before scheduled airline travel. However, he is required to fly several times every year with his work. He developed this 3 years ago following an extremely turbulent flight. He has recurring, vivid images of himself dying in a blazing crash while flying. He is hyperaware of any sound and unexpected movements of the plane. Over the last few months, he has been drinking excessive amounts of alcohol in an attempt to control his symptoms.

1. What type of phobia does this man have? *(1 point)*
2. Give common examples of other types of this phobia. *(2 points)*
3. What are the two other types of phobia and how would you differentiate between them? *(3 points)*
4. How could this patient be managed? *(3 points)*
5. What three features separate phobic anxiety disorders from GAD? *(3 points)*

Answers to self-assessment questions are to be found in *Appendix B.*

Panic disorder

Definition

Panic disorder is characterized by **recurrent**, **episodic**, **severe** panic attacks, which are **unpredictable** and **not restricted** to any particular situation or circumstance.

Pathophysiology/Etiology (Table 5.4.1)

Table 5.4.1: Etiology of panic disorder	
Biological	**Genetics:** Along with OCD, it is one of the most heritable anxiety disorders. **Neurochemical:** Post-synaptic hypersensitivity to serotonin and epinephrine. **Sympathetic nervous system** (SNS): Fear or worry stimulates the SNS → ↑cardiac output which can lead to further anxiety.
Cognitive	Misinterpretation of somatic symptoms (e.g. fear that palpitations will lead to a heart attack).
Environmental	Presence of life stressors can lead to panic disorder.

Epidemiology and risk factors (Table 5.4.2)

- Panic disorder has a prevalence of **2.7%** in the general population.
- It is **three times** more common in ♀.
- The usual age of onset is **late adolescence** but it can occur at any time.

Table 5.4.2: Risk factors for panic disorder		
Family history	Major life events	Age (20–30)
Recent trauma	Females	Other mental disorders
White ethnicity	Asthma	Cigarette smoking
Medication (e.g. CNS drug withdrawal)		

Clinical features (see DSM-5 criteria)

- Panic symptoms usually **peak within 10 minutes** and **rarely persist beyond an hour**.

OSCE tips: A useful mnemonic for some of the key features of panic disorder is 'PANICS Disorder'

Palpitations, Abdominal distress, Numbness/Nausea, Intense fear of death, Choking feeling/Chest pain, Sweating/Shaking/Shortness of breath, Depersonalization/Derealization.

DSM-5 Criteria for panic disorder

A. Recurrent unexpected panic attacks. A panic attack is an abrupt surge of intense fear or intense discomfort that reaches a peak within minutes, and during which time four (or more) of the following symptoms occur:

NOTE: The abrupt surge can occur from a calm state or an anxious state.

1. Palpitations, pounding heart, or accelerated heart rate.
2. Sweating.
3. Trembling or shaking.
4. Sensations of shortness of breath or smothering.
5. Feelings of choking.
6. Chest pain or discomfort.
7. Nausea or abdominal distress.
8. Feeling dizzy, unsteady, light-headed, or faint.
9. Chills or heat sensations.
10. Paresthesias (numbness or tingling sensations).
11. Derealization (feelings of unreality) or depersonalization (being detached from oneself).
12. Fear of losing control or "going crazy."
13. Fear of dying.

NOTE: Culture-specific symptoms (e.g. tinnitus, neck soreness, headache, uncontrollable screaming or crying) may be seen. Such symptoms should not count as one of the four required symptoms.

B. At least one of the attacks has been followed by 1 month (or more) of one or both of the following:
1. Persistent concern or worry about additional panic attacks or their consequences (e.g. losing control, having a heart attack, "going crazy").
2. A significant maladaptive change in behavior related to the attacks (e.g. behaviors designed to avoid having panic attacks, such as avoidance of exercise or unfamiliar situations).
C. The disturbance is not attributable to the physiological effects of a substance (e.g. a drug of abuse, a medication) or another medical condition (e.g. hyperthyroidism, cardiopulmonary disorders).
D. The disturbance is not better explained by another mental disorder (e.g. the panic attacks do not occur only in response to feared social situations, as in social anxiety disorder; in response to circumscribed phobic objects or situations, as in specific phobia; in response to obsessions, as in obsessive-compulsive disorder; in response to reminders of traumatic events, as in post-traumatic stress disorder; or in response to separation from attachment figures, as in separation anxiety disorder).

Reprinted with permission from the *Diagnostic and Statistical Manual of Mental Disorders*, 5th Edition, (©2013). American Psychiatric Association.

Diagnosis and investigations

Hx
- 'Are you nervous all the time or are there periods where you are anxiety-free?' **(episodic)**
- 'Can you predict when these attacks will come on?' **(spontaneous)**
- 'Have you ever been so frightened that you felt you might die or go crazy?' **(intense fear and anxiety)**
- 'Are you worried about your health or any other specific things?' **(major life stressors)**

MSE The MSE findings in panic disorder (if the patient is having a panic attack when seen, which may not be the case) will be largely the same as in GAD (see *Section 5.2*). However, features of **appearance and behavior** may be more intense such as hyperventilation, diaphoresis and restlessness.

Ix As for generalized anxiety disorder (see *Section 5.2*).

DDx
- **Psychiatric:** Other anxiety disorders (e.g. generalized anxiety disorder, phobic anxiety disorder), PTSD, anorexia nervosa, dissociative disorder, bipolar affective disorder, depression, adjustment disorder.
- **Organic:** Pheochromocytoma, hyperthyroidism, hypoglycemia, carcinoid syndrome, arrhythmias, alcohol/substance withdrawal (see *Table 5.1.1* in *Section 5.1*, Overview of anxiety disorders).

Key facts 1: Comparing GAD, panic disorder, and phobic anxiety

	GAD	**Panic disorder**	**Phobic anxiety**
Age of onset	*Variable:* adolescence to late adulthood	Late adolescence to early adulthood	Childhood to late adolescence
When does it occur?	Persistent	Episodic	Situational
Associated behavior	Agitation	Escape	Avoidance
Cognition	Constant worry	Fear of symptoms	Fear of situation
Associations	Depression	Depression, agoraphobia, substance misuse	Substance misuse

Management

- **SSRIs** are **first-line** but if they are not suitable, or there is no improvement after **12 weeks**, then an SNRI such as duloxetine may be considered. **TCA**, e.g. **imipramine** or **clomipramine** would be second line agents. *Benzodiazepines may be given short term (1–6 weeks) with an antidepressant and tapered after the antidepressant begins working.*
- **CBT** is the psychological intervention of choice, focusing on recognition of panic triggers.
- **Self-help methods** include **workbooks** (giving written information on panic disorder and how to overcome it), **support groups**, and **encouraging exercise** to promote good health (exercise introduced gradually as it can precipitate panic in some patients).
- A **stepped care approach** may be recommended (*Fig. 5.4.1*).

Step 1: Recognition and diagnosis	Step 2: Treatment in primary care	Step 3: Review and consideration of alternative treatments	Step 4: Review and referral to specialist mental health services	Step 5: Care in specialist mental health services
Making the diagnosis and identifying common co-morbidities such as depression and substance misuse.	Includes recommendations for psychological therapies, medications, and self-help strategies.	Describes reassessment and consideration of alternative treatments if initial therapy has failed.	States that if two interventions have been offered and there is no improvement in symptoms then referral should be made to specialists.	Discusses reassessment in secondary care, of the patient's social circumstances and environment, and advises shared decisions to be made.

Fig. 5.4.1: Stepped care model for management of panic disorder.

Self-assessment

A 38-year-old man presents to the ER for the second time in 3 weeks with sudden onset shortness of breath, chest pain, palpitations, dizziness, and sweating. He tells the doctor he is afraid of having a heart attack and fears he is going to die whenever it happens. He has stopped driving and has started avoiding crowded areas for fear of inducing further attacks. His past medical history is unremarkable. Cardiac investigations, including ECG and troponin, during both admissions were normal.

1. What is this man describing? *(1 point)*
2. Name three organic disorders that may present similarly. *(3 points)*
3. What are the differences between GAD, panic disorder, and phobic anxiety disorders? *(3 points)*
4. What is the first-line management for this condition? *(1 point)*

Answers to self-assessment questions are to be found in *Appendix B*.

Chapter 6

Trauma and stressor-related disorders

Definitions

There are several conditions associated with reactions to stressful events:

- **Post-traumatic stress disorder (PTSD):** Is an **intense**, **prolonged**, **delayed** reaction following exposure to an **exceptionally traumatic event**. This chapter will focus on PTSD.

- **Acute stress disorder:** An abnormal reaction to **sudden stressful events** (see *Key facts 1*, later in chapter).

- **Adjustment disorder:** Normal adjustment refers to psychological reactions involved in adapting to new circumstances. Adjustment disorder is when there is **significant distress** (greater than expected), accompanied by an **impairment in social functioning** (see *Key facts 1*, later in chapter).

Pathophysiology/Etiology

- The most important component of etiology is exposure to a **traumatic event** in which the individual was **involved directly** or as a **witness** (see *Table 6.1*).

- Not all individuals who experience the same traumatic experience go on to develop PTSD, thus suggesting a pre-existing **vulnerability**. Twin studies of Vietnam War veterans suggest that part of the vulnerability may be **genetic** (see *Table 6.2*).

- **Cognitive theories** suggest that failure to process emotionally charged events causes memories to persist in an unprocessed form which can intrude into conscious awareness.

Epidemiology and risk factors

- Approximately **5%** of adults in the USA suffer from PTSD.

- **20–30%** of individuals experiencing a traumatic event may go on to develop PTSD.

- It can affect people of all ages, but is **more common in** ♀ (♀:♂ ratio is **2:1**).

Table 6.1: Traumatic events

Severe assault (e.g. physical or sexual abuse, robbery, mugging).

Major natural disaster (e.g. earthquakes, floods).

Serious road traffic accident.

Observer/survivor of civilian disaster (e.g. acts of terrorism, the Holocaust).

Involvement in wars (e.g. World War II, Vietnam War).

Freak occurrences (e.g. near drowning when on holiday).

Physical torture.

Prisoner of war or **hostage situation**.

Hearing about **unexpected injury** or **violent death** of a **family member** or **friend**.

Table 6.2: Risk factors for PTSD

Exposure to a major traumatic event	• Professions at risk (armed forces, police, fire services, journalists, doctors), groups at risk (refugees, asylum seekers).
Pre-trauma	• Previous trauma, history of mental illness, females, low socio-economic background, childhood abuse.
Peri-trauma	• Severity of trauma, perceived threat to life, adverse emotional reaction during or immediately after event.
Post-trauma	• Concurrent life stressors, absence of social support.

Clinical features

PTSD symptoms must occur **within 6 months** of the event and can be divided into **four** categories:

1. **Reliving** the situation (persistent, intrusive, involuntary): Flashbacks, vivid memories, nightmares, distress when exposed to similar circumstances as the stressor.

2. **Avoidance:** Avoiding reminders of trauma (e.g. associated people or locations), excessive rumination about the trauma, inability to recall aspects of the trauma.

3. **Hyperarousal:** Irritability or outbursts, difficulty with concentration, difficulty with sleep, hypervigilance, exaggerated startle response.

4. **Emotional numbing:** Negative thoughts about oneself, difficulty experiencing emotions, feeling of detachment from others, giving up previously enjoyed activities.

DSM-5 Criteria for post-traumatic stress disorder

Post-traumatic stress disorder

A. **NOTE:** The following criteria apply to adults, adolescents, and children older than 6 years. For children 6 years and younger, see corresponding criteria below.

Exposure to actual or threatened death, serious injury, or sexual violence in one (or more) of the following ways:

1. Directly experiencing the traumatic event(s).
2. Witnessing, in person, the event(s) as it occurred to others.
3. Learning that the traumatic event(s) occurred to a close family member or close friend. In cases of actual or threatened death of a family member or friend, the event(s) must have been violent or accidental.
4. Experiencing repeated or extreme exposure to aversive details of the traumatic event(s) (e.g. first responders collecting human remains; police officers repeatedly exposed to details of child abuse).

NOTE: Criterion A4 does not apply to exposure through electronic media, television, movies, or pictures, unless this exposure is work related.

B. Presence of one (or more) of the following intrusion symptoms associated with the traumatic event(s), beginning after the traumatic event(s) occurred:

1. Recurrent, involuntary, and intrusive distressing memories of the traumatic event(s).
NOTE: In children older than 6 years, repetitive play may occur in which themes or aspects of the traumatic event(s) are expressed.
2. Recurrent distressing dreams in which the content and/or affect of the dream are related to the traumatic event(s).
NOTE: In children, there may be frightening dreams without recognizable content.
3. Dissociative reactions (e.g. flashbacks) in which the individual feels or acts as if the traumatic event(s) were recurring. (Such reactions may occur on a continuum, with the most extreme expression being a complete loss of awareness of present surroundings.)
NOTE: In children, trauma-specific reenactment may occur in play.
4. Intense or prolonged psychological distress at exposure to internal or external cues that symbolize or resemble an aspect of the traumatic event(s).
5. Marked physiological reactions to internal or external cues that symbolize or resemble an aspect of the traumatic event(s).

DSM-5 Criteria for post-traumatic stress disorder *(continued)*

C. Persistent avoidance of stimuli associated with the traumatic event(s), beginning after the traumatic event(s) occurred, as evidenced by one or both of the following:
   1. Avoidance of or efforts to avoid distressing memories, thoughts, or feelings about or closely associated with the traumatic event(s).
   2. Avoidance of or efforts to avoid external reminders (people, places, conversations, activities, objects, situations) that arouse distressing memories, thoughts, or feelings about or closely associated with the traumatic event(s).
D. Negative alterations in cognitions and mood associated with the traumatic event(s), beginning or worsening after the traumatic event(s) occurred, as evidenced by two (or more) of the following:
   1. Inability to remember an important aspect of the traumatic event(s) (typically due to dissociative amnesia and not to other factors such as head injury, alcohol, or drugs).
   2. Persistent and exaggerated negative beliefs or expectations about oneself, others, or the world (e.g. "I am bad," "No one can be trusted," "The world is completely dangerous," "My whole nervous system is permanently ruined").
   3. Persistent, distorted cognitions about the cause or consequences of the traumatic event(s) that lead the individual to blame himself/herself or others.
   4. Persistent negative emotional state (e.g. fear, horror, anger, guilt, or shame).
   5. Markedly diminished interest or participation in significant activities.
   6. Feelings of detachment or estrangement from others.
   7. Persistent inability to experience positive emotions (e.g. inability to experience happiness, satisfaction, or loving feelings).
E. Marked alterations in arousal and reactivity associated with the traumatic event(s), beginning or worsening after the traumatic event(s) occurred, as evidenced by two (or more) of the following:
   1. Irritable behavior and angry outbursts (with little or no provocation) typically expressed as verbal or physical aggression toward people or objects.
   2. Reckless or self-destructive behavior.
   3. Hypervigilance.
   4. Exaggerated startle response.
   5. Problems with concentration.
   6. Sleep disturbance (e.g. difficulty falling or staying asleep or restless sleep).
F. Duration of the disturbance (Criteria B, C, D, and E) is more than 1 month.
G. The disturbance causes clinically significant distress or impairment in social, occupational, or other important areas of functioning.
H. The disturbance is not attributable to the physiological effects of a substance (e.g. medication, alcohol) or another medical condition.
Specify whether:
With dissociative symptoms: The individual's symptoms meet the criteria for post-traumatic stress disorder, and in addition, in response to the stressor, the individual experiences persistent or recurrent symptoms of either of the following:
1. **Depersonalization:** Persistent or recurrent experiences of feeling detached from, and as if one were an outside observer of, one's mental processes or body (e.g. feeling as though one were in a dream; feeling a sense of unreality of self or body or of time moving slowly).
2. **Derealization:** Persistent or recurrent experiences of unreality of surroundings (e.g. the world around the individual is experienced as unreal, dreamlike, distant, or distorted).
NOTE: To use this subtype, the dissociative symptoms must not be attributable to the physiological effects of a substance (e.g. blackouts, behavior during alcohol intoxication) or another medical condition (e.g. complex partial seizures).

DSM-5 Criteria for post-traumatic stress disorder *(continued)*

Specify if:

With delayed expression: If the full diagnostic criteria are not met until at least 6 months after the event (although the onset and expression of some symptoms may be immediate).

Post-traumatic stress disorder for children 6 years and younger

A. In children 6 years and younger, exposure to actual or threatened death, serious injury, or sexual violence in one (or more) of the following ways:

    1. Directly experiencing the traumatic event(s).

    2. Witnessing, in person, the event(s) as it occurred to others, especially primary caregivers.
       NOTE: Witnessing does not include events that are witnessed only in electronic media, television, movies or pictures.

    3. Learning that the traumatic event(s) occurred to a parent or caregiving figure.

B. Presence of one (or more) of the following intrusion symptoms associated with the traumatic event(s), beginning after the traumatic event(s) occurred:

    1. Recurrent, involuntary, and intrusive distressing memories of the traumatic event(s).
       NOTE: Spontaneous and intrusive memories may not necessarily appear distressing and may be expressed as play reenactment.

    2. Recurrent distressing dreams in which the content and/or affect of the dream are related to the traumatic event(s).
       NOTE: It may not be possible to ascertain that the frightening content is related to the traumatic event.

    3. Dissociative reactions (e.g. flashbacks) in which the child feels or acts as if the traumatic event(s) were recurring. (Such reactions may occur on a continuum, with the most extreme expression being a complete loss of awareness of present surroundings.) Such trauma-specific re-enactment may occur in play.

    4. Intense or prolonged psychological distress at exposure to internal or external cues that symbolize or resemble an aspect of the traumatic event(s).

    5. Marked physiological reactions to reminders of the traumatic event(s).

C. One (or more) of the following symptoms, representing either persistent avoidance of stimuli associated with the traumatic event(s) or negative alterations in cognitions and mood associated with the traumatic event(s), must be present, beginning after the event(s) or worsening after the event(s):

Persistent avoidance of stimuli

    1. Avoidance of or efforts to avoid activities, places, or physical reminders that arouse recollections of the traumatic event(s).

    2. Avoidance of or efforts to avoid people, conversations, or interpersonal situations that arouse recollections of the traumatic event(s).

Negative alterations in cognitions

    3. Substantially increased frequency of negative emotional states (e.g. fear, guilt, sadness, shame, confusion).

    4. Markedly diminished interest or participation in significant activities, including constriction of play.

    5. Socially withdrawn behavior.

    6. Persistent reduction in expression of positive emotions.

D. Alterations in arousal and reactivity associated with the traumatic event(s), beginning or worsening after the traumatic event(s) occurred, as evidenced by two (or more) of the following:

    1. Irritable behavior and angry outbursts (with little or no provocation) typically expressed as verbal or physical aggression toward people or objects (including extreme temper tantrums).

DSM-5 Criteria for post-traumatic stress disorder *(continued)*

   2. Hypervigilance.

   3. Exaggerated startle response.

   4. Problems with concentration.

   5. Sleep disturbance (e.g. difficulty falling or staying asleep or restless sleep).

E. The duration of the disturbance is more than 1 month.

F. The disturbance causes clinically significant distress or impairment in relationships with parents, siblings, peers, or other caregivers or with school behavior.

G. The disturbance is not attributable to the physiological effects of a substance (e.g. medication or alcohol) or another medical condition.

Specify whether:

With dissociative symptoms: The individual's symptoms meet the criteria for post-traumatic stress disorder, and the individual experiences persistent or recurrent symptoms of either of the following:

1. **Depersonalization:** Persistent or recurrent experiences of feeling detached from, and as if one were an outside observer of, one's mental processes or body (e.g. feeling as though one were in a dream; feeling a sense of unreality of self or body or of time moving slowly).

2. **Derealization:** Persistent or recurrent experiences of unreality of surroundings (e.g. the world around the individual is experienced as unreal, dreamlike, distant, or distorted).

NOTE: To use this subtype, the dissociative symptoms must not be attributable to the physiological effects of a substance (e.g. blackouts, behavior during alcohol intoxication) or another medical condition (e.g. complex partial seizures).

Specify if:

With delayed expression: If the full diagnostic criteria are not met until at least 6 months after the event (although the onset and expression of some symptoms may be immediate).

Reprinted with permission from the *Diagnostic and Statistical Manual of Mental Disorders*, 5th Edition, (© 2013). American Psychiatric Association.

Diagnosis and investigations

Hx
- 'Has there been any traumatic incident or event in your life recently which may account for how you are feeling?' **(exposure to stressful event)**
- 'Do you ever get any flashbacks, vivid memories or nightmares about the events that took place?' **(reliving the situation)**
- 'Do you find yourself constantly thinking about the same thing?' **(rumination)**
- 'Have you had any problems with sleep since the event?', 'Are you feeling more irritable or having trouble concentrating?', 'Do you get startled easily?' **(hyperarousal)**

OSCE tips: Normal bereavement reaction *(Fig. 6.1)*

In an OSCE, you may have a patient with severe symptoms after the loss of a loved one. Remember whilst it may be tempting to diagnose PTSD, **bereavement is a unique traumatic stress** which is a **normal human experience**. Bereavement reactions are natural and not coded for in *ICD-10*. Normal bereavement should not extend over **6 months**; if it does, **abnormal bereavement** or **adjustment disorder** should be considered.

MSE		
	Appearance & Behavior	Hypervigilance ('on edge'), exaggerated startle reaction, may have features of anxiety or depression, e.g. poor eye contact.
	Speech	Slow rate. Trembling. Non-spontaneous.
	Mood	Anxious.
	Thought	Pessimistic. Reliving or remembering of the event.
	Perception	No hallucinations. May have illusions.
	Cognition	Poor attention and concentration.
	Insight	Good.

Ix
- **Questionnaires:** Trauma Screening Questionnaire (TSQ), Post-traumatic diagnostic scale.
- **CT head:** if head injury suspected.

DDx
- **Psychiatric:** Adjustment disorder, acute stress reaction, bereavement, dissociative disorder, mood or anxiety disorders, personality disorder.
- **Organic:** Head injury (result of traumatic event), alcohol/substance misuse.

Stages of Grief
'DABDA'

DENIAL:
Temporary denial of reality as emotionally overwhelmed

↓

ANGER:
Intense emotions expressed as anger

↓

BARGAINING:
Negotiating a compromise in order to reduce grief

↓

DEPRESSION:
Depressed mood

↓

ACCEPTANCE:
Acceptance and reorganization of life

Fig. 6.1: Kübler–Ross stages of grief.

Management

Key facts 1: Acute stress disorder and adjustment disorder

Acute stress disorder
Exposure to **actual or threatened death, serious injury, or sexual violence**. At least 9 symptoms described in the five categories of PTSD I: intrusion, avoidance, negative mood, arousal, and dissociation. Symptoms last 3 days to 1 month.

Adjustment disorder
Identifiable (non-catastrophic) psychosocial stressor (e.g. job loss, divorce) **within three months** of onset of symptoms. The stressor results in marked distress and/or impairment in functioning.

PTSD where symptoms are present within 3 months of a trauma

- **Watchful waiting** may be used for mild symptoms lasting <4 weeks.
- Military personnel have access to treatment provided by the armed forces.
- **Trauma-focused CBT** can be given at least once a week for 8–12 sessions.
- **Short-term drug treatment** may be considered in the acute phase for management of **sleep disturbance** (e.g. trazodone, prazosin). Benzodiazepines should be avoided.
- **Risk assessment** is important to assess risk for neglect or suicide.

PTSD where symptoms have been present >3 months after a trauma

- All sufferers should be offered a course of **trauma-focused psychological intervention**.
- Among the options for psychological intervention are **CBT** and **exposure therapy** (see *Section 15.1*, Psychotherapies).
- **Drug treatment** should be considered when: (1) **little benefit** from **psychological therapy**; (2) **patient preference** not to engage in psychological therapy; (3) **co-morbid depression** or **severe hyperarousal** which would benefit from psychological interventions.
- Clonidine and guanfacine may help with hyperarousal symptoms.
- Sedating antidepressants such as mirtazapine and trazodone help with sleep.

Self-assessment

A 35-year-old lady presents to you with her husband. She does not speak much English and it transpires that she has recently arrived in the country (3 months ago) from Syria to be with her husband. The husband describes that she has been increasingly detached since she has been in the country and has given up activities that she previously enjoyed. She is easily startled, for instance when the cat makes a noise. On further questioning you discover that in her last few days in Syria, she saw her close friend being brutally assaulted to the point of hospitalization. You suspect PTSD.

1. Name six symptoms of PTSD. *(3 points)*
2. Within how many months of the traumatic event do symptoms have to occur? *(1 point)*
3. Name two distinguishing features between PTSD and adjustment disorder. *(2 points)*
4. Name two non-pharmacological management strategies for PTSD. *(2 points)*
5. Give two examples of antidepressants which are commonly used to treat PTSD. *(2 points)*

Answers to self-assessment questions are to be found in *Appendix B*.

Chapter 7

Obsessive-compulsive and related disorders

Definition

Obsessive–compulsive disorder (OCD) is characterized by **recurrent obsessional thoughts** or **compulsive acts**, or commonly both. It is ranked by the WHO as one of the top ten most disabling illnesses in terms of impact upon quality of life.

Obsessions: **Unwanted intrusive thoughts**, **images**, or **urges** that **repeatedly** enter the individual's mind. They are **distressing** for the individual who attempts to **resist** them and recognizes them as absurd (**egodystonic**) and a product of their **own mind**.

Compulsions: **Repetitive**, **stereotyped behaviors** or **mental acts** that a person feels **driven** into performing. They are **overt** (observable by others) or **covert** (mental acts not observable).

Pathophysiology/Etiology

There are a number of theories for the etiology of OCD:

- Biological: Related to ↓ **serotonin** and abnormalities of the frontal cortex and basal ganglia. Twin and family studies suggest a **genetic contribution** to OCD, particularly with pediatric onset. **Childhood group A beta-hemolytic streptococcal infection** may have a role in causing OCD symptoms by setting up an autoimmune reaction which damages the basal ganglia (this is called PANDAS).
- Psychoanalytic: Filling the mind with obsessional thoughts in order to prevent undesirable ideas from entering consciousness.
- Behavioral: Compulsive behavior is learned and maintained by **operant conditioning**. The anxiety created by the obsession is reduced by performing the compulsion, and subsequently the need to perform the compulsion is increased.

OCD has strong associations with other psychiatric disorders: **depression (30%)**, **schizophrenia (3%)**, **Sydenham's chorea**, **Tourette's syndrome**, and **anorexia nervosa**.

Epidemiology and risk factors

- The prevalence of OCD ranges from **0.8–3%**.
- It is **most common in early adulthood** and is **equally common in ♂ and ♀**.
- OCD is **more common** in the **relatives of OCD patients** than it is in the general population.
- **Carrying out the compulsive act** (e.g. washing) is likely to exacerbate the obsession and is thus a maintaining factor.
- **Developmental factors** such as neglect, abuse, bullying, and social isolation may have a role.

Clinical features

- Common obsessions and compulsions are illustrated in *Fig. 7.1*. The most common *obsession* is that of being **contaminated (38%)** and the most common *compulsion* is **checking (29%)** followed closely by **washing/cleaning (27%)**.

- Obsessions or compulsions must share **ALL** of the following features (**FORD Car**):
  1. **Failure to resist:** At least one obsession or compulsion is present which is unsuccessfully resisted.
  2. **Originate** from patient's mind: Acknowledged that the obsessions or compulsions originate from their own mind, and are not imposed by outside persons or influences.
  3. **Repetitive and Distressing:** At least one obsession or compulsion must be present which is acknowledged by the patient as excessive or unreasonable.
  4. **Carrying out the obsessive thought** (or compulsive act) is **not in itself pleasurable**, but reduces anxiety levels.
- Obsessions create **anxiety** which continues to build until a compulsion is carried out in order to provide **relief**. This vicious cycle is known as the **OCD cycle** (*Fig. 7.2*).

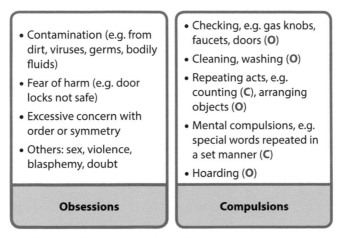

Obsessions	Compulsions
• Contamination (e.g. from dirt, viruses, germs, bodily fluids) • Fear of harm (e.g. door locks not safe) • Excessive concern with order or symmetry • Others: sex, violence, blasphemy, doubt	• Checking, e.g. gas knobs, faucets, doors (**O**) • Cleaning, washing (**O**) • Repeating acts, e.g. counting (**C**), arranging objects (**O**) • Mental compulsions, e.g. special words repeated in a set manner (**C**) • Hoarding (**O**)

Fig. 7.1: Obsessions and compulsions (**C** = covert; **O** = overt).

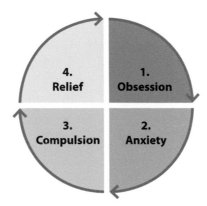

Fig. 7.2: The OCD cycle.

DSM-5 Criteria for OCD

A. Presence of obsessions, compulsions, or both:
   Obsessions are defined by (1) and (2):
   1. Recurrent and persistent thoughts, urges, or images that are experienced, at some time during the disturbance, as intrusive and unwanted, and that in most individuals cause marked anxiety or distress.
   2. The individual attempts to ignore or suppress such thoughts, urges, or images, or to neutralize them with some other thought or action (i.e. by performing a compulsion).
   Compulsions are defined by (1) and (2):
   1. Repetitive behaviors (e.g. hand washing, ordering, checking) or mental acts (e.g. praying, counting, repeating words silently) that the individual feels driven to perform in response to an obsession or according to rules that must be applied rigidly.
   2. The behaviors or mental acts are aimed at preventing or reducing anxiety or distress, or preventing some dreaded event or situation; however, these behaviors or mental acts are not connected in a realistic way with what they are designed to neutralize or prevent, or are clearly excessive.
   NOTE: Young children may not be able to articulate the aims of these behaviors or mental acts.
B. The obsessions or compulsions are time-consuming (e.g. take more than 1 hour per day) or cause clinically significant distress or impairment in social, occupational, or other important areas of functioning.
C. The obsessive-compulsive symptoms are not attributable to the physiological effects of a substance (e.g. a drug of abuse, a medication) or another medical condition.
D. The disturbance is not better explained by the symptoms of another mental disorder (e.g. excessive worries, as in generalized anxiety disorder; preoccupation with appearance, as in body dysmorphic disorder; difficulty discarding or parting with possessions, as in hoarding disorder; hair pulling, as in trichotillomania [hair-pulling disorder]; skin picking, as in excoriation [skin-picking] disorder; stereotypies, as in stereotypic movement disorder; ritualized eating behavior, as in eating disorders; preoccupation with substances or gambling, as in substance-related and addictive disorders; preoccupation with having an illness, as in illness anxiety disorder; sexual urges or fantasies, as in paraphilic disorders; impulses, as in disruptive, impulse-control, and conduct disorders; guilty ruminations, as in major depressive disorder; thought insertion or delusional preoccupations, as in schizophrenia spectrum and other psychotic disorders; or repetitive patterns of behavior, as in autism spectrum disorder).

Reprinted with permission from the *Diagnostic and Statistical Manual of Mental Disorders*, 5th Edition, (© 2013). American Psychiatric Association.

Diagnosis and investigations

Hx
- 'Do you have any distressing thoughts that enter your mind despite trying hard to resist them?', 'Is there any unwanted thought that keeps bothering you that you would like to get rid of but cannot?' **(obsessions)**
- 'Do you worry about contamination with germs even after washing?', 'Do you repeatedly check things you have already done?', 'Do you find yourself having to touch, count, and arrange things many times?', 'How often do you wash your hands each day?', 'Do you check things a lot?', 'Are you concerned about putting things in a specific order, or do you get upset by not completing tasks?' **(compulsions)**
- 'Do your daily activities take a long time to finish?' **(due to carrying out compulsions)**

MSE
- Patient may be on edge (easily startled). May look visibly worried or lost in thought. May be constantly checking doors or fidgety with hands (as they can't wash them).
- May demonstrate increasing levels of **anxiety** if unable to succumb to compulsion (*Fig. 7.2*).
- **Thoughts** are **unwanted**, **intrusive**, and **uncomfortable** for the patient.
- Obsessions can be distracting and lead to **poor concentration**.
- **Insight** is usually very **good** (as they recognize the thoughts are a product of their own mind).

OSCE tips 1: Exploring risk and co-existing psychiatric conditions

After exploring the patient's main obsessive–compulsive features, it is important to assess the impact of the obsessions and compulsions on the person's life and to assess risk, because these often are very distressing for the patient. Patients commonly have co-existing depression, anxiety disorders, substance misuse, eating disorders, and body dysmorphic disorder, and therefore these should also be assessed for.

Ix **Questionnaires:** Yale–Brown obsessive–compulsive scale (Y-BOCS) → 10-item questionnaire with each item graded from 0–4; e.g. Time occupied by obsessive thoughts (0 = none, 4 = extreme, >8 hours/day).

DDx	Obsessions *and* compulsions	Primarily obsessions	Primarily compulsions	Organic
	- **Eating disorders** (AN and BN) - **Obsessive–compulsive personality disorder** - **Body dysmorphic disorder:** Preoccupation with an imagined defect in physical appearance, resulting in time-consuming behaviors, e.g. mirror gazing	- **Anxiety disorders** (e.g. phobic anxiety) - **Depressive disorder** - **Illness anxiety** - **Schizophrenia**	- **Tourette's syndrome** - **Kleptomania** (inability to refrain from stealing items)	- **Dementia** - **Epilepsy** - **Head injury**

Management

There are two main strategies to the treatment of OCD:

1. CBT (including ERP – exposure and response prevention)

- **ERP** is a technique in which patients are repeatedly exposed to the situation which causes them anxiety (e.g. exposure to dirt) and are prevented from performing the repetitive actions which lessen that anxiety (e.g. washing their hands). After initial anxiety on exposure, the levels of anxiety gradually decrease.

2. Pharmacological therapy

- **SSRIs** are the drug of choice in OCD. **Fluoxetine, fluvoxamine, paroxetine, sertraline** or **esitalopram** are recommended.

- **Clomipramine** (a serotonergic TCA) is a second line drug therapy. This can be combined with citalopram in more severe cases. Alternatively, an **antipsychotic** can be added in with an SSRI or clomipramine.

- Deep brain stimulation (DBS) is used in refractory OCD.

General points

- **Psychoeducation, distracting techniques,** and **self-help books** can be used.

- Any potential **suicide risk** should be identified and managed.

- **Co-morbid depression** should be identified and treated.

- Method of treatment depends upon the **degree of functional impairment** (*Fig. 7.3*). This ranges from **mild** (limited impact on ADL) to **severe** (obsessional slowness that greatly impacts performance).

Low intensity psychological intervention (defined as <10 hours of therapist input per patient)

Mild

SSRI or high intensity psychological intervention

Moderate

Combined SSRI or clomipramine and CBT

Severe

Fig. 7.3: Management of OCD based on severity of functional impairment.

Self-assessment

A 22-year-old male student presents with his girlfriend who is worried about him as he spends at least 4 hours in the bathroom every day. He reluctantly describes a 6-month history of recurrent thoughts that he has specks of blood on his hands and feet. He has to shower exactly 12 times a day to be cleansed of this blood. He realizes that this is abnormal.

1. What is the most likely diagnosis? *(1 point)*
2. Provide two differential diagnoses. *(2 points)*
3. What further questions may you want to ask in order to confirm the diagnosis? *(2 points)*
4. What is the main difference in thought process here compared to in schizophrenia? *(1 point)*
5. What group of pharmacological agents would you give to this patient? Give an example of a drug belonging to this category that is commonly used. *(2 points)*
6. What psychotherapy would you suggest for this patient and what sub-type? *(2 points)*

Answers to self-assessment questions are to be found in *Appendix B*.

Chapter 8

Somatic symptom disorders

Definitions

Somatic symptom disorders are a group of disorders whose symptoms are suggestive of, or take the form of, a **physical disorder** but are not consistent with or explained by an underlying medical illness, leading to the presumption that they are caused by **psychological factors**. Sufferers **repeatedly seek medical attention** even when it has consistently failed to benefit them. The diagnosis of a somatic symptom disorder is made only after a medical etiology is ruled out.

Pathophysiology/Etiology

- The cause of **somatic symptom disorders** is **multifactorial** (see *Table 8.1*). Patients adopt the **sick role**, which provides relief from stressful or unachievable interpersonal expectations (**primary gain**). This offers attention, care from others and sometimes even financial rewards (**secondary gain**) in many societies.

Table 8.1: Pathophysiology of somatic symptom disorders	
Biological	• Possible implication of neuroendocrine genes. Studies indicate a genetic component.
Psychological	• A high proportion of those with PTSD suffer from somatic symptom disorders. • Association between somatization and physical or sexual abuse.
Social	• Adopting of the 'sick role' in order to gain relief from stress.

- As the name suggests, conversion disorder require **two** processes to occur:
  1. **Dissociation:** A process of 'separating off' certain memories from normal consciousness. This is a **psychological defense mechanism** that is used to cope with emotional conflict that is so distressing for the patient, that it is prevented from entering their conscious mind.
  2. **Conversion:** Distressing events are transformed into physical symptoms. This, like somatic symptom disorders, can lead to **primary** and **secondary gain** (*Fig. 8.1*).

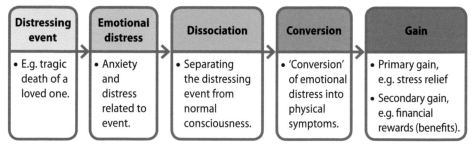

Fig. 8.1: Sequence of events in conversion disorders.

DSM-5 Criteria for conversion disorder

A. One or more symptoms of altered voluntary motor or sensory function.
B. Clinical findings provide evidence of incompatibility between the symptom and recognized neurological or medical conditions.
C. The symptom or deficit is not better explained by another medical or mental disorder.
D. The symptom or deficit causes clinically significant distress or impairment in social, occupational or other important areas of functioning or warrants medical evaluation.

Reprinted with permission from the *Diagnostic and Statistical Manual of Mental Disorders*, 5th Edition, (© 2013). American Psychiatric Association.

Epidemiology and risk factors (*Table 8.2*)

- The prevalence of somatic symptom disorders in the USA is **5–7%**.

- They are **more common in** ♀ than in ♂ and are likely to begin **before the age of 30**.

Table 8.2: Risk factors for somatic symptom disorders ('CRAMPS')
Childhood abuse
Reinforcement of illness behaviors
Anxiety disorders
Mood disorders
Personality disorders
Social stressors

Clinical features

- **Somatic symptom disorders** present as physical disorders but have a psychological basis.

- Somatic symptom disorders commonly present to primary care physicians.

- There is a significant danger of iatrogenic damage to patients with somatic symptom disorders from unneeded medical assessments and treatment including surgeries.

Somatic symptom disorder

- Also known as **Briquet's syndrome**.

- **Multiple**, **recurrent**, and **frequently changing** physical symptoms **not explained by a physical illness**.

- More common in ♀ (♀:♂ ratio is **10:1**).

- Common symptoms are listed in *Fig. 8.2*.

- **Long history of contact** with **medical services**.

- Often dependent on analgesics with a degree of functional impairment.

DSM-5 Criteria for somatic symptom disorder

A. One or more somatic symptoms that are distressing or result in significant disruption of daily life.

B. Excessive thoughts, feelings, or behaviors related to the somatic symptoms or associated health concerns as manifested by at least one of the following:
   1. Disproportionate and persistent thoughts about the seriousness of one's symptoms.
   2. Persistently high level of anxiety about health or symptoms.
   3. Excessive time and energy devoted to these symptoms or health concerns.

C. Although any one somatic symptom may not be continuously present, the state of being symptomatic is persistent (typically more than 6 months).

Specify if:

With predominant pain (previously pain disorder): This specifier is for individuals whose somatic symptoms predominantly involve pain.

Specify if:

Persistent: A persistent course is characterized by severe symptoms, marked impairment, and long duration (more than 6 months).

Specify current severity:

Mild: Only one of the symptoms specified in Criterion B is fulfilled.

Moderate: Two or more of the symptoms specified in Criterion B are fulfilled.

Severe: Two or more of the symptoms specified in Criterion B are fulfilled, plus there are multiple somatic complaints (or one very severe somatic symptom).

Reprinted with permission from the *Diagnostic and Statistical Manual of Mental Disorders*, 5th Edition, (© 2013). American Psychiatric Association.

Gastrointestinal	Cardiovascular	Genitourinary	Others
• Abdominal pain • Nausea and vomiting • Bloating • Regurgitation • Loose bowel motions • Swallowing difficulty	• Chest pain • Breathlessness at rest • Palpitations	• Dysuria • Frequency • Incontinence • Vaginal discharge • Menstrual problems	• Discoloration or itching of skin • Arthralgia • Paresthesia in limbs • Headaches • Visual disturbance

Fig. 8.2: Common symptoms in somatic symptom disorder.

Illness anxiety disorder (hyperchondriasis)

- Patient **misinterprets normal bodily sensations**, which leads them to the **non-delusional preoccupation** that they have a **serious physical disease**, e.g. cancer.
- They **refuse to accept reassurances** from doctors.
- **Dysmorphophobia** (body dysmorphic disorder) is a variant where there is an **excessive preoccupation** with **barely noticeable or imagined defects** in their **physical appearance** (e.g. the size and shape of their nose). The preoccupation causes significant distress (*Fig. 8.3*).

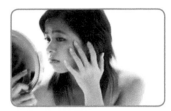

Fig. 8.3: An illustration of dysmorphophobia.

DSM-5 Criteria for illness anxiety disorder

A. Preoccupation with having or acquiring a serious illness.

B. Somatic symptoms are not present or, if present, are only mild in intensity. If another medical condition is present or there is a high risk for developing a medical condition (e.g. strong family history is present), the preoccupation is clearly excessive or disproportionate.

C. There is a high level of anxiety about health, and the individual is easily alarmed about personal health status.

D. The individual performs excessive health-related behaviors (e.g. repeatedly checks his or her body for signs of illness) or exhibits maladaptive avoidance (e.g. avoids doctor appointments and hospitals).

E. Illness preoccupation has been present for at least 6 months, but the specific illness that is feared may change over that period of time.

F. The illness-related preoccupation is not better explained by another mental disorder, such as somatic symptom disorder, panic disorder, generalized anxiety disorder, body dysmorphic disorder, obsessive-compulsive disorder, or delusional disorder, somatic type.

Specify whether:

Care-seeking type: Medical care, including physician visits or undergoing tests and procedures, is frequently used.

Care-avoidant type: Medical care is rarely used.

Reprinted with permission from the *Diagnostic and Statistical Manual of Mental Disorders*, 5th Edition, (© 2013). American Psychiatric Association.

Diagnosis and investigations

Hx
- 'How much do you worry about your health?'
- 'Are you worried about having a potentially serious medical condition?'
- 'Do you get frustrated when doctors tell you that you are fit and well?'
- 'Have there been any stressful events in your life that may have triggered your symptoms?'

MSE MSE findings in the areas of **appearance**, **behavior**, and **mood** may reflect underlying mood or anxiety disorders. **Thoughts** will show preoccupation with physical symptoms and overvalued ideas of having a serious medical condition. **Insight** into having a *psychiatric* illness will likely be clouded.

Ix **NOTE:** Somatic symptom disorders are often a **diagnosis of exclusion**. However, certain features point in the direction of a somatic symptom disorder. These include: (1) Multiple symptoms, often occurring in different organ systems; (2) Vague symptoms that exceed objective findings; (3) Chronic course; (4) Presence of a mental health disorder; (5) History of extensive diagnostic testing; and (6) Rejection of previous physicians.

- A **thorough physical examination** and **investigations** are performed to rule out an organic cause depending on the symptoms present.
- **Blood tests: CBC** (anemia, infection), **U&Es** (electrolyte disturbance), **LFTs** (liver or biliary pathology), **CRP** (infection, inflammation), **TFTs** (thyroid dysfunction).
- **Further investigations:**
  A. Gastrointestinal symptoms: AXR, stool culture, OGD, colonoscopy, diagnostic laparoscopy.
  B. Cardiovascular symptoms: ECG, 24 hr tape, ECHO, angiogram.
  C. Genitourinary symptoms: urine dipstick, MSU, cystoscopy.

DDx
- **Somatic symptom disorders:** Somatization disorder, illness anxiety disorder, somatic symptom disorder, conversion disorder.
- **Factitious disorder.**
- **Malingering.**
- **Other psychiatric disorders:** Mood disorder, psychotic disorder, anxiety disorder, PD.
- **Multi-systemic disease**, e.g. connective tissue disorders and inflammatory bowel disease.

Key facts 1: Malingering and factitious disorder

- In both malingering and factitious disorder (also known as Munchausen's syndrome) **physical or psychological symptoms are intentionally** produced, i.e. faked. The difference between the two is the patient's **motive** behind mimicking the symptoms (*Fig. 8.4*).
- **Malingering:** Patient **seeks advantageous consequences** of being diagnosed with a medical condition. For instance, evading criminal prosecution or receiving government benefits (i.e. **secondary gain**).
- **Factitious disorder (Munchausen's syndrome):** The individual wishes to **adopt the 'sick role'** in order to receive the care of a patient, for **internal emotional gain** (i.e. **primary gain**).

Factitious disorder	Malingering	Somatic symptom disorder	Conversion disorder
'I want to go to the hospital to be looked after.'	'If I go to the hospital, I can make a disability claim and won't have to work.'	'I think there is something seriously wrong and the doctors need to do more tests.'	'Ever since my father died, I have been paralyzed and can't walk.'

Fig. 8.4: Comparison between factitious disorder, malingering, somatic symptom disorders, and conversion disorder.

Management (Fig. 8.5)

Biological therapies

Unnecessary or aggressive medical interventions are to be avoided if there is a strong suspicion of a somatic symptom disorder. For somatic symptom disorders include **antidepressants** (primarily SSRIs) for any **underlying mood disorder or anxiety. Physical exercise** enhances self-esteem and can be helpful for many patients.

Psychological therapies

The **mainstay** of management is **cognitive behavioral therapy**, usually in short courses. Developing certain coping strategies can also be very useful.

Social therapies

From a **social** perspective, **stress-relieving activities** such as meditation and long walks can prove effective, as well as interventions reducing specific causes of stress (e.g. relationship counseling). It may be appropriate to interview/**involve family** members who serve to reinforce the sick role.

Biological
- **Antidepressants**
- **Physical exercise**

Psychological
- **CBT**
- **Coping strategies**

Social
- **Encourage pleasurable private time**
- **Involve family where appropriate**

Fig. 8.5: Bio-psychosocial management of medically unexplained symptoms.

OSCE tips: Explaining the diagnosis to a patient with a somatic symptom disorder

- A major obstacle in the management of patients with somatic symptom disorder or indeed any functional symptoms is that they often feel that doctors don't believe them and they feel that this brings into question their integrity. Therefore, good communication is of the utmost importance.
- **Discuss investigations** → 'The results of my examination and of the tests we conducted show that you do not have a life-threatening illness. However, what you are describing is something that I see often and may not have just one cause.'
- **Brief explanation** → 'We know that stress can cause physical illness. Have you been under stress recently?'
- **Placing a positive spin** → 'I would like to reassure you however, that there are still ways we can help you. We can help train your body to work normally again.'
- **Relate to a disorder they are more familiar with** → 'We know that most physical illnesses get worse if the patient feels tense or down, for example stress makes asthma worse, and therefore I feel that if we can reduce some of the stress in your life you are likely to feel better.'

NOTE: Allow the patient to query what you have said. Allow caregivers and relatives to be involved in the consultation.

Consultation for patient with medically unexplained symptoms

DO:	DO NOT:
• Focus on symptoms and their effect on the patient.	• Focus exclusively on a diagnosis or give a diagnosis when there is uncertainty.
• Match your explanation using their own words.	• Dismiss the symptoms as normal without matching your explanation to the patient's concerns.
• Share your uncertainty; discuss possible test results and their implications.	• Treat symptoms with medications anyway.
• Reach a shared understanding; listen to their ideas, concerns, and expectations.	• Assume what the patient wants.
• Acknowledge the importance of the patient's views and circumstances.	• Judge the patient or be critical of their behaviors.
• Agree to follow-up arrangements.	• Ignore or dismiss psychological cues.
	• Enforce psychosocial explanations, as this can lead to defensiveness.

Self-assessment

A 22-year-old female university student sought medical attention for recurrent physical symptoms which consisted of gastrointestinal difficulties, dysmenorrhea, nausea, weakness, malaise, fatigue, headaches, back pain, and insomnia. Her mother took her to numerous physicians in an attempt to find solutions to her complaints. As a result, she has had many investigations performed for which no biological cause has been identified. Both she and her mother refuse to accept reassurance that there is no physical cause for her symptoms.

1. List four differential diagnoses. *(2 points)*
2. What type of somatic symptom disorder is this lady likely to be suffering from and why? *(2 points)*
3. Name the three other types of somatic symptom disorders. *(3 points)*
4. What is the difference between a somatic symptom disorder and malingering or factitious disorder? *(3 points)*

Answers to self-assessment questions are to be found in *Appendix B*.

Chapter 9

Feeding and eating disorders

| 9.1 | Anorexia nervosa | 95 |
| 9.2 | Bulimia nervosa | 102 |

9.1 Anorexia nervosa

Eating disorders are a type of illness characterized by a disturbance in eating behaviors and associated thoughts and emotions. They are among the most life-threatening psychiatric disorders and include anorexia nervosa, bulimia nervosa, binge eating disorder (recurrent episodes of binge eating), rumination disorder (repeated regurgitation of food), and pica (persistent eating of non-nutritive substances such as dirt, paint chips, chalk, etc.). This chapter will focus on two of the more serious and common eating disorders, anorexia nervosa and bulimia nervosa.

Definition

Anorexia nervosa (AN) is an **eating disorder** characterized by **deliberate weight loss**, an **intense fear of weight gain**, **distorted body image**, and **endocrine disturbances**.

Pathophysiology/Etiology (Table 9.1.1)

The etiology of AN is generally considered to be **multifactorial**, and can be divided into predisposing, precipitating, and perpetuating factors (see *Table 9.1.1*).

Table 9.1.1: Etiological factors in AN

	Biological	Psychological	Social
Predisposing	• Genetics: Monozygotic twin studies have higher concordance rates than dizygotic twins. • Family history: First degree relatives have higher incidence of eating disorders. • Female. • Early menarche.	• Sexual abuse. • Preoccupation with slimness. • Dieting behaviors starting in adolescence. • Low self-esteem. • Premorbid anxiety or depressive disorder. • Perfectionism, obsessional/ anankastic personality.	• Western society: Pressure to diet in a society that emphasizes that being thin is beauty. • Bullying at school revolving around weight. • Stressful life events.
Precipitating	• Adolescence and puberty. • Dieting and exercise.	• Criticism regarding eating, body shape, or weight.	• Occupational or recreational pressure to be slim, e.g. ballet dancers, models.
Perpetuating (maintaining)	• Starvation leads to neuroendocrine changes that perpetuate anorexia.	• Perfectionism, obsessional personality.	• Occupation. • Western society.

Epidemiology and risk factors

- AN affects ♀ more than ♂ (**10:1**).
- Estimated incidence is **0.4 per 1000 yearly in** ♂ and approximately **9 in 1000** ♀ will experience it at some point in their lives.
- The typical **age of onset** is **mid-adolescence.**
- **Risk factors include dieting and exercise** in predisposed individuals.

DSM-5 Criteria for anorexia nervosa

A. Restriction of energy intake relative to requirements, leading to a significantly low body weight in the context of age, sex, developmental trajectory, and physical health. *Significantly low weight* is defined as a weight that is less than minimally normal or, for children and adolescents, less than that minimally expected.

B. Intense fear of gaining weight or of becoming fat, or persistent behavior that interferes with weight gain, even though at a significantly low weight.

C. Disturbance in the way in which one's body weight or shape is experienced, undue influence of body weight or shape on self-evaluation, or persistent lack of recognition of the seriousness of the current low body weight.

Specify whether:

Restricting type: During the last 3 months, the individual has not engaged in recurrent episodes of binge eating or purging behavior (i.e. self-induced vomiting or the misuse of laxatives, diuretics, or enemas). This subtype describes presentations in which weight loss is accomplished primarily through dieting, fasting, and/or excessive exercise.

Binge-eating/purging type: During the last 3 months, the individual has engaged in recurrent episodes of binge eating or purging behavior (i.e. self-induced vomiting or the misuse of laxatives, diuretics, or enemas).

Specify if:

In partial remission: After full criteria for anorexia nervosa were previously met, Criterion A (low body weight) has not been met for a sustained period, but either Criterion B (intense fear of gaining weight or becoming fat or behavior that interferes with weight gain) or Criterion C (disturbances in self-perception of weight and shape) is still met.

In full remission: After full criteria for anorexia nervosa were previously met, none of the criteria have been met for a sustained period of time.

Specify current severity:

The minimum level of severity is based, for adults, on current body mass index (BMI) (see below) or, for children and adolescents, on BMI percentile. The ranges below are derived from World Health Organization categories for thinness in adults; for children and adolescents, corresponding BMI percentiles should be used. The level of severity may be increased to reflect clinical symptoms, the degree of functional disability, and the need for supervision.

Mild: BMI ≥ 17 kg/m^2

Moderate: BMI 16–16.99 kg/m^2

Severe: BMI 15–15.99 kg/m^2

Extreme: BMI < 15 kg/m^2

Reprinted with permission from the *Diagnostic and Statistical Manual of Mental Disorders*, 5th Edition, (© 2013). American Psychiatric Association.

Clinical features

- The defining clinical features of AN are described in the *DSM-5* box.
- Other features include **PP**, **SS**:
  - **Physical:** Fatigue, hypothermia, bradycardia, arrhythmias, peripheral edema (due to hypoalbuminemia), headaches, lanugo hair (*Fig. 9.1.2*).
  - **Preoccupation with food:** Dieting, preparing elaborate meals for others.
  - **Socially isolated**, **Sexuality is feared.**
  - **Symptoms of depression and food obsessions.**

> **Key facts 1:** Working out BMI
>
> **Body mass index = weight (kg) ÷ [height (m)]²**
>
> BMI <18.5 kg/m² = **underweight**
> BMI 18.5–24.9 kg/m² = **normal**
> BMI 25–29.9 kg/m² = **overweight**
> BMI ≥30 kg/m² = **obese**
> BMI ≥35 kg/m² = **morbidly obese**

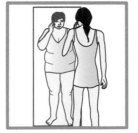

Fig. 9.1.1: Distorted body image.

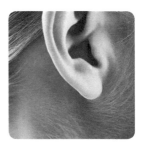

Fig. 9.1.2: Lanugo hair.

OSCE tips: Anorexia nervosa vs. bulimia nervosa

Anorexia nervosa	Bulimia nervosa
• Are significantly underweight. • Are more likely to have endocrine abnormalities such as amenorrhea. • Do not have strong cravings for food. • Do not binge eat. • May have compensatory weight loss behaviors (excluding purging).	• Are usually normal weight/overweight. • Are less likely to have endocrine abnormalities. • Have strong cravings for food. • Have recurrent episodes of binge eating. • Have compensatory weight loss behaviors.

Diagnosis and investigations

Hx
- 'Do you find yourself preoccupied with your weight?' **(fear of weight gain)**
- 'What would be your ideal target weight?' **(overvalued ideas about weight)**
- 'How much time do you spend exercising daily?' **(deliberate weight loss)**
- 'How much time do you spend counting calories or obsessing about the types of food you are eating?' (**food or eating obsessions**)
- 'When women lose significant weight, their periods have a tendency to stop. Has this happened in your case?' **(amenorrhea)**
- Also ask *specifically* about **physical symptoms** of anorexia nervosa, e.g. fatigue and headaches.

MSE	**Appearance & Behavior**	Thin, weak, slow, anxious. May try to disguise emaciation with makeup. Baggy clothes. Dry skin. Lanugo hair.
	Speech	May be slow, slurred, or normal.
	Mood	Can be low with co-morbid depression, or euthymic.
	Thought	Preoccupation with food, overvalued ideas about weight and appearance.
	Perception	No hallucinations.
	Cognition	Either normal or poor if physically unwell with complications.
	Insight	Often poor.

NOTE: A full systems examination should be carried out to find out the degree of emaciation, to exclude differential diagnoses and to look for possible complications (see *Key facts 2*).

Ix

- **Blood tests: CBC** (anemia, thrombocytopenia, leukopenia), **BUN/Cr** (↑ urea and creatinine if dehydrated, ↓ potassium, phosphate, magnesium and chloride), **TFTs** (↓ T_3 and T_4), **LFTs** (↓ albumin), **lipids** (↑ cholesterol), **cortisol** (↑), **sex hormones** (↓ LH, FSH, estrogens and progestogens), **glucose** (↓), **amylase** (pancreatitis is a complication).
- **Vitals:** hypotension, bradycardia.
- **Bone density scan:** To rule out osteoporosis (if suspected).
- **ECG:** Arrhythmias such as sinus bradycardia and prolonged QT are associated with AN patients.
- **Questionnaires:** e.g. eating attitudes test (EAT).

DDx

- **Bulimia nervosa.**
- **Other eating disorders** (see *Key facts 3*).
- **Depression.**
- **Obsessive–compulsive disorder.**
- **Schizophrenia:** Delusions about food.
- **Organic causes of low weight:** Diabetes, hyperthyroidism, malignancy.
- **Alcohol** or **substance misuse.**

Key facts 2: Complications of AN	
Metabolic	Hypokalemia, hypercholesterolemia, hypoglycemia, impaired glucose tolerance, deranged LFTs, ↑ urea and creatinine (if dehydrated), ↓ potassium, ↓ phosphate, ↓ magnesium, ↓ albumin and ↓ chloride.
Endocrine	↑ Cortisol, ↑ growth hormone, ↓ T_3 and T_4. ↓ LH, FSH, estrogens and progestogens leading to amenorrhea. ↓ Testosterone in men.
Gastrointestinal	Enlarged salivary glands, pancreatitis, constipation, peptic ulcers, hepatitis.
Cardiovascular	Cardiac failure, ECG abnormalities, arrhythmias, ↓ BP, bradycardia, peripheral edema.
Renal	Renal failure, renal stones.
Neurological	Seizures, peripheral neuropathy, autonomic dysfunction.
Hematological	Iron deficiency anemia, thrombocytopenia, leukopenia.
Musculoskeletal	Proximal myopathy, osteoporosis.
Others	Hypothermia, dry skin, brittle nails, lanugo hair, infections, suicide.

Key facts 3: Other eating disorders	
Bulimia nervosa	Recurrent episodes of binge eating and compensatory behavior (any one or a combination of vomiting, fasting, or excessive exercise) in order to prevent weight gain (see *Section 9.2*, Bulimia nervosa).
Binge eating disorder	Recurrent episodes of binge eating without compensatory behavior such as vomiting, fasting, or excessive exercise.
Other eating disorder	Approximately one-third of patients referred for eating disorders don't fit neatly in DSM categories. For example, some patients meet all the criteria for anorexia except have a normal weight, or patients with bulimia who have had the illness <3 months.

Management

- The management of AN is outlined using the **bio-psychosocial model** (*Fig. 9.1.3*).
- **Risk assessment** for suicide and medical complications is absolutely vital.
- **Psychological treatments** should normally be for at least **6 months' duration**.
- The aim of treatment as an **inpatient** is refeeding with a weight gain of **0.5–1 kg/week** and as an **outpatient** of **0.5 kg/week**.
- Patients are at risk of **refeeding syndrome** which causes metabolic disturbances (e.g. ↓ phosphate) and other complications (see *Key facts 4*).
- **Hospitalization** is necessary for **medical** (severe anorexia with BMI <14 or severe electrolyte abnormalities), bradycardia with HR <40, systolic BP <80, hypothermia <35.5°C, bowel obstruction, fainting spells, uncontrolled vomiting, severe hypoglycemia. Also for **psychiatric** (suicidal ideation) reasons.
- No medication has proven successful in the treatment of anorexia but antidepressants may help co-morbid depression/obessions. There may also be a limited role for antipsychotics to target ruminations.

> **Biological**
> - **Treatment of medical complications**, e.g. electrolyte disturbance
> - **SSRIs** for co-morbid depression or OCD

> **Psychological**
> - **Psycho-education** about nutrition
> - **Cognitive behavioral therapy**
> - **Family therapy** (Maudsley approach) in which the family monitors and facilitates refeeding at home. The family also monitors excessive exercise and other restrictive or obsessive behavior

> **Social**
> - **Voluntary organizations**
> - **Self-help groups**

Fig. 9.1.3: Bio-psychosocial approach to AN.

Key facts 4: Refeeding syndrome

- A potentially life-threatening syndrome that results from food intake (whether parenteral or enteral) after **prolonged starvation** or **malnourishment**, due to changes in **phosphate**, **magnesium**, and **potassium**.
- It occurs as a result of an **insulin surge** following increased food intake.
- Biochemical features include fluid balance abnormalities, **hypokalemia**, **hypomagnesemia**, **hypophosphatemia**, and **abnormal glucose metabolism**.
- The phosphate depletion causes reduction in cardiac muscle activity which can lead to **cardiac failure**.
- Prevention: Measure serum electrolytes prior to feeding and **monitor refeeding bloods daily**, start at 1200 kcal/day and gradually increase every 5 days, monitor for signs such as **tachycardia** and **edema**.
- If electrolyte levels are low, they will need to be replaced either orally or intravenously depending upon the severity of electrolyte depletion.

Self-assessment

A 16-year-old girl, accompanied by her mother, presents to her GP complaining of fatigue for 6 months. The doctor observes the patient is rather petite and is wearing an oversized, baggy dress. No signs are found on examination. During the examination the patient mentions how fat she has become. She weighs 42 kg and measures 160 cm. Her mother is concerned as her daughter has been eating only one small meal a day and exercising excessively, and seems uninterested in her friends. Her periods have also stopped.

1. Work out the girl's BMI. *(2 points)*
2. What is the most likely diagnosis? Name two differential diagnoses. *(2 points)*
3. What are the defining features of this condition? *(4 points)*
4. Give four complications of this condition. *(4 points)*
5. Outline the management strategy for this patient. *(4 points)*

Answers to self-assessment questions are to be found in *Appendix B*.

9.2 Bulimia nervosa

9.2

Definition

Bulimia nervosa (BN) is an **eating disorder** characterized by **repeated episodes** of **uncontrolled binge eating** followed by **compensatory weight loss behaviors** and **overvalued ideas** regarding 'ideal body shape/weight'.

Pathophysiology/Etiology

- The etiology of BN is very similar to AN, but whereas there is a clear genetic component in AN, the **role of genetics in BN is less clear**.
- When patients with BN binge due to **strong cravings**, they tend to feel guilty and as a result undergo **compensatory purging behaviors** such as **vomiting**, using **laxatives**, **exercising excessively**, and **alternating with periods of starvation**. This may result in large fluctuations in weight, which reinforce the compensatory weight loss behavior, setting up a vicious cycle (*Fig. 9.2.1*).

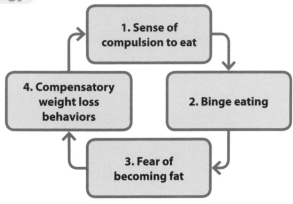

Fig. 9.2.1: The vicious cycle of BN.

Epidemiology and risk factors (Table 9.2.1)

- BN typically occurs in **young women**. The estimated prevalence in women aged **15–40** is **1–2%**.
- Whereas AN is thought to be more prevalent in higher socioeconomic classes, **BN has equal socioeconomic class distribution**.

Table 9.2.1: Risk factors for bulimia nervosa			
	Biological	**Psychological**	**Social**
Predisposing	• Female sex • Family history of eating disorder, mood disorder, substance misuse, or alcohol abuse • Early onset of puberty • Type 1 diabetes • Childhood obesity	• Physical or sexual abuse as a child • Childhood bullying • Parental obesity • Pre-morbid mental health disorder • Preoccupation with slimness • Parents with high expectations • Low self-esteem	• Living in a developed country • Profession (e.g. actors, dancers, models, athletes) • Difficulty resolving conflicts

Table 9.2.1: Risk factors for bulimia nervosa *(continued)*

	Biological	Psychological	Social
Precipitating	• Early onset of puberty/ menarche	• Perceived pressure to be thin may come from culture (e.g. Western society, media, and profession) • Criticism regarding body weight or shape	• Environmental stressors • Family dieting
Perpetuating	• Co-morbid mental health problems	• Low self-esteem, perfectionism • Obsessional personality	• Environmental stressors

OSCE tips 1: BN and other co-morbid psychiatric conditions

BN commonly co-exists with the following psychiatric disorders and it is hence important to screen for them:
1. Depression
2. Anxiety
3. Deliberate self-harm
4. Substance misuse
5. Borderline personality disorder.

Clinical features

Other features include:

- **Normal weight:** Usually the potential for weight gain from bingeing is counteracted by the weight loss/purging behaviors.
- **Depression and low self-esteem.**
- Loss of tooth enamel from excessive vomiting.
- Swollen (chipmunk) cheeks from salivary gland hypertrophy with excessive vomiting.
- **Signs of dehydration:** ↓ blood pressure, dry mucous membranes, ↑ capillary refill time, ↓ skin turgor, sunken eyes.
- **Consequences of repeated vomiting and hypokalemia** (see *Key facts 2* and *3*).

DSM-5 Criteria for bulimia nervosa

A. Recurrent episodes of binge eating. An episode of binge eating is characterized by both of the following:
1. Eating, in a discrete period of time (e.g. within any 2-hour period), an amount of food that is definitely larger than what most individuals would eat in a similar period of time under similar circumstances.
2. A sense of lack of control over eating during the episodes (e.g. a feeling that one cannot stop eating or control what or how much one is eating).
B. Recurrent inappropriate compensatory behaviors in order to prevent weight gain, such as self-induced vomiting; misuse of laxatives, diuretics, or other medications; fasting; or excessive exercise.
C. The binge eating and inappropriate compensatory behaviors both occur, on average, at least once a week for 3 months.
D. Self-evaluation is unduly influenced by body shape and weight.
E. The disturbance does not occur exclusively during episodes of anorexia nervosa.

Specify if:

In partial remission: After full criteria for bulimia nervosa were previously met, some, but not all, of the criteria have been met for a sustained period of time.

In full remission: After full criteria for bulimia nervosa were previously met, none of the criteria have been met for a sustained period of time.

Specify current severity:

The minimum level of severity is based on the frequency of inappropriate compensatory behaviors (see below). The level of severity may be increased to reflect other symptoms and the degree of functional disability.

Mild: An average of 1–3 episodes of inappropriate compensatory behaviors per week.

Moderate: An average of 4–7 episodes of inappropriate compensatory behaviors per week.

Severe: An average of 8–13 episodes of inappropriate compensatory behaviors per week.

Extreme: An average of 14 or more episodes of inappropriate compensatory behaviors per week.

Reprinted with permission from the *Diagnostic and Statistical Manual of Mental Disorders*, 5th Edition, (© 2013). American Psychiatric Association.

Key facts 1: Subtypes of bulimia nervosa

There are **two** subtypes of BN:
1. **Purging type:** The patient uses self-induced vomiting and other ways of purging food from the body, e.g. use of laxatives, diuretics, and enemas.
2. **Non-purging type:** Much less common. Patients use excessive exercise or fasting after a binge. Purging-type bulimics may also exercise and fast but this is not the main form of weight control for them.

OSCE tips 2: Anorexia vs. bulimia

Amenorrhea	Binge eating
No friends (socially isolated)	Use of drugs to prevent weight gain
Obvious weight loss	Low potassium
Restriction of food intake	Irregular periods
Emaciated	Mood disturbances
Xerostomia (dry mouth)	Irrational fear of fatness
Irrational fear of fatness	Alternating periods of starvation
Abnormal hair growth (lanugo hair)	

Key facts 2: Hypokalemia ($\downarrow$ K$^+$)

- A potentially life-threatening complication of excessive vomiting.
- Low potassium (<3.5 mmol/L) can result in muscle weakness, cardiac arrhythmias and renal damage.
- Mild hypokalemia requires oral replacement with potassium-rich foods (e.g. bananas) and/or oral supplements.
- Severe hypokalemia requires hospitalization and intravenous potassium replacement.

Diagnosis and investigations

Hx
- 'Do you ever feel that your eating is out of control?' **(binge eating)**
- 'After an episode of eating what you feel is too much, do you ever make yourself throw up so that you feel better?' **(compensatory self-induced vomiting)**
- 'Have you ever used diuretics or laxatives to help control your weight?' **(self-induced purging)**
- 'How do you feel about your weight?' **(body image)**
- 'Do you ever have the sensation that your heart is beating abnormally fast?' **(complications of hypokalemia)**
- Ask specifically about complications of repeated vomiting (see *Key facts 3*).
- Screen for other co-morbid psychiatric conditions (see *OSCE tips 1*).

MSE

Appearance & Behavior	May have appearance and behavior consistent with depression or anxiety. Likely normal weight. Parotid swelling. Russell's sign (*Fig. 9.2.2*). Sunken eyes (dehydration). Tooth erosion.
Speech	Slow or normal.
Mood	Low.
Thought	Preoccupation with body size and shape. Preoccupation with eating. Guilt.
Perception	Normal.
Cognition	Either normal or poor.
Insight	Usually has good insight.

Ix
- **Blood tests:** CBC, electrolytes, BUN/Cr amylase, lipids, glucose, TFTs, magnesium, calcium, phosphate.
- **Venous blood gas:** May show metabolic alkalosis.
- **ECG:** Arrhythmias as a consequence of hypokalemia (ventricular arrhythmias are life-threatening), classic ECG changes (prolongation of the PR interval, flattened or inverted T waves, prominent U waves after T wave).

DDx
- **Anorexia nervosa** – with bulimic symptoms.
- **Unspecified eating disorder.**
- **Kleine–Levin syndrome:** Sleep disorder in adolescent males characterized by recurrent episodes of binge eating and hypersomnia.
- **Depression.**
- **Obsessive–compulsive disorder.**
- **Organic causes of vomiting**, e.g. gastric outlet obstruction.

Key facts 3: Physical complications of repeated vomiting	
Cardiovascular	Arrhythmias, mitral valve prolapse, peripheral edema.
Gastrointestinal	Mallory–Weiss tears, ↑ size of salivary glands especially parotid (*Fig. 9.2.2*).
Metabolic/Renal	Dehydration, hypokalemia, renal stones, renal failure.
Dental	Permanent erosion of dental enamel secondary to vomiting of gastric acid (*Fig. 9.2.2*).
Endocrine	Amenorrhea, irregular menses, hypoglycemia, osteopenia.
Dermatological	Russell's sign (calluses on back of hand due to abrasion against teeth).
Pulmonary	Aspiration pneumonitis.
Neurological	Cognitive impairment, peripheral neuropathy, seizures.

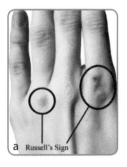 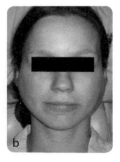 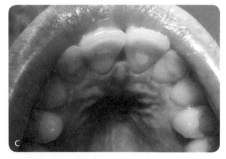

Fig. 9.2.2: Complications of repeated vomiting. (a) **Russell's sign**; (b) **Bilateral parotid swelling (chipmunk cheeks)**; and (c) **Dental erosion**.

Management

- The management of BN is based on the bio-psychosocial model:
  - **Biological:** A trial of antidepressant should be offered and can ↓ frequency of binge eating/purging. **Fluoxetine** is FDA-approved for the treatment of bulimia. Treat medical complications of repeated vomiting, e.g. potassium replacement. Treat co-morbid conditions (see *OSCE tips 1*).
  - **Psychological: Psychoeducation** about nutrition, CBT for bulimia nervosa (**CBT-BN** is a specifically adapted form of CBT). **Interpersonal psychotherapy** is an alternative.
  - **Social: Food diary** to monitor eating/purging patterns, **techniques to avoid bingeing** (eating in company, distractions), **small**, **regular meals**, **self-help programs**.
- From a biological perspective, **electrolytes should be monitored carefully** for any potential disturbances, and should be replaced accordingly where appropriate.
- **Risk assessment** for suicide. Co-morbid depression and substance misuse are common.
- **Inpatient treatment** is required for cases of **suicide risk** and **severe electrolyte imbalances**.
- Approximately **50%** of BN patients make a **complete recovery** in comparison with AN where roughly 20% make a full recovery.

Self-assessment

A 25-year-old female vegetarian presents to you very distressed. She describes a 3-year history of strong cravings for food, resulting in sessions of binge eating. To make herself feel better she states that she deliberately vomits five times a day and compulsively exercises for 2 hours a day.

1. Which eating disorder is the most likely diagnosis? Name two differentials. *(3 points)*
2. What are the four diagnostic features of this condition based on DSM-5? *(4 points)*
3. What is the most important complication of repeated vomiting? How would you test for this in a laboratory? *(2 points)*
4. Give two further complications for repeated episodes of vomiting. *(2 points)*
5. Outline the management of this condition in the community. *(3 points)*

Answers to self-assessment questions are to be found in *Appendix B*.

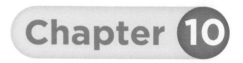

Chapter 10

Substance-related and addictive disorders

10.1   Substance misuse   109
10.2   Alcohol-use disorders   116

10.1 Substance misuse

Definitions

The **DSM-5** classifies substance misuse disorders according to the **type of substance** (see *Table 10.1.1*), the **state of the disorder** (intoxication vs. withdrawal), and the level of severity (mild, moderate, severe).

Common terms used in describing substance use disorders

1. **Acute intoxication:** The acute, usually transient, effect of the substance.
2. **Dependence syndrome** (see *Key facts 1*): Prolonged, compulsive substance use leading to addiction, tolerance and the potential for withdrawal syndromes.
3. **Withdrawal state:** Physical and/or psychological effects from complete (or partial) cessation of a substance after prolonged, repeated, or high level of use.
4. **Residual disorder:** Specific features (flashbacks, personality disorder, affective disorder, dementia, persisting cognitive impairment) *subsequent* to substance misuse.

Pathophysiology/Etiology (*Fig. 10.1.1*)

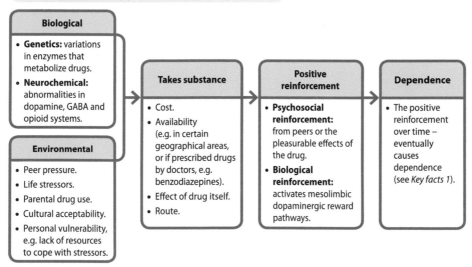

Fig. 10.1.1: Factors involved in, and chain of events leading to, substance dependence.

Table 10.1.1: Drug misuse

Group	Examples	Route PO: oral IV: intravenous IN: intranasal	Intoxication (psychological)	Intoxication (physical)	Withdrawal state (if applicable) At least 3 signs needed
Opiates	Morphine, heroin, codeine, methadone, oxycontin, fentanyl	Morphine (PO, IV), heroin (IN, IV, smoked), codeine/ methadone (PO)	Apathy, disinhibition, psychomotor retardation, impaired judgement and attention, drowsiness, slurred speech	Respiratory depression, hypoxia, ↓ BP, hypothermia, coma, pupillary constriction	Craving, rhinorrhea, lacrimation, myalgia, abdominal cramps, N+V, diarrhea, pupillary dilatation, piloerection, ↑ HR/↑ BP
Cannabinoids	Cannabis	PO, smoked	Euphoria, disinhibition, agitation, paranoid ideation, temporal slowing (time passes slowly), impaired judgement/ attention/reaction time, illusions, hallucinations	Increased appetite, dry mouth, conjunctival injection, ↑ HR	Anxiety, irritability, tremor of outstretched hands, sweating, myalgia
Sedative-hypnotics	Benzodiazepines, barbiturates	PO, IV	Euphoria, disinhibition, apathy, aggression, anterograde amnesia, labile mood	Unsteady gait, difficulty standing, slurred speech, nystagmus, erythematous skin lesions, ↓ BP, hypothermia, depression of gag reflex, coma	Tremor of hands, tongue or eyelids, N+V, ↑ HR, postural ↓ BP, headache, agitation, malaise, transient illusions/ hallucinations, paranoid ideation, grand mal convulsions

Table 10.1.1: Drug misuse (continued)

Group	Examples	Route PO: oral IV: intravenous IN: intranasal	Intoxication (psychological)	Intoxication (physical)	Withdrawal state (if applicable) At least 3 signs needed
Stimulants	Cocaine, crack cocaine, ecstasy methamphetamine	Cocaine, crack cocaine (IN, IV, smoked), ecstasy (PO), methamphetamine (PO, IV, IN, smoked)	Euphoria, increased energy, grandiose beliefs, aggression, argumentative, illusions, hallucinations (intact orientation), paranoid ideation, labile mood	↑HR, ↑BP, arrhythmias, sweating, N+V, pupillary dilatation, psychomotor agitation, muscular weakness, chest pain, convulsions	Dysphoric mood (must be present), lethargy, psychomotor agitation, craving, increased appetite, insomnia (or hypersomnia), bizarre/unpleasant dreams
Hallucinogens	LSD (lysergic acid diethylamide), psilocybin (mushrooms), MDMA	PO	Anxiety, illusions, hallucinations, depersonalization, derealization, paranoia, ideas of reference, hyperactivity, impulsivity, inattention	↑HR, palpitations, sweating, tremor, blurred vision, pupillary dilatation, incoordination	n/a
Volatile solvents	Aerosols, paint, glue, gasoline	Inhaled	Apathy, lethargy, aggression, impaired attention and judgement, psychomotor retardation	Unsteady gait, diplopia, nystagmus, decreased consciousness, muscle weakness	n/a
Anabolic steroids	Testosterone, androstenedione, danazol	PO, IM	Euphoria, depression, aggression, hyperactivity, mood swings, hallucinations, delusions	Increased muscle mass, reduced fat, acne, male pattern baldness, reduced sperm count/infertility, stunted growth	n/a

Epidemiology and risk factors (Fig. 10.1.1)

- Substance misuse is more common in ♂ at a ratio of **3:1** (♂:♀).
- **Cannabis** is the **most consumed** illegal drug used (although recently made legal in many states), with at least 1% of the US population using it daily and up to 10% of the population admitting to at least one use in the previous 12 months.

Clinical features

- Clinical features vary depending on the drug consumed. Commonly misused substances are **opioids**, **cannabinoids**, **stimulants**, **sedative-hypnotics**, **hallucinogens**, **volatile solvents**, and **anabolic steroids**.
- Complications of substance misuse can be divided into physical, psychological, and social (*Fig. 10.1.2*).

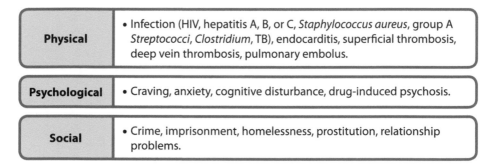

Physical	• Infection (HIV, hepatitis A, B, or C, *Staphylococcus aureus*, group A *Streptococci*, *Clostridium*, TB), endocarditis, superficial thrombosis, deep vein thrombosis, pulmonary embolus.
Psychological	• Craving, anxiety, cognitive disturbance, drug-induced psychosis.
Social	• Crime, imprisonment, homelessness, prostitution, relationship problems.

Fig. 10.1.2: Physical, psychological and social complications of drug misuse.

Key facts 1: Substance dependence [DRUG PROBLEMS WILL CONTINUE TO HARM]

- Substance dependence describes a syndrome including behavioral, physiological and psychological elements. Patients are physiologically dependent if they show tolerance or withdrawal.
- Manifestations of dependence may include the following: (1) Strong **Desire (compulsion)** to consume substance; (2) **Preoccupation** with substance use; (3) **Withdrawal state** when substance ingestion is **reduced** or **stopped**; (4) **Impaired ability** to **Control** substance-taking behavior (e.g. onset, termination, or level of use); (5) **Tolerance** to substance, requiring more consumption for desired effect; (6) Persisting with use, despite clear evidence to the **Harmful effects**.

Diagnosis and investigations

Hx The history may be difficult to elicit as people may not be honest about illegal activity (see *Key facts 2*). Obtain a collateral history to help determine the extent of substance misuse.

- 'Have you ever taken any recreational drugs? If so, how often do you take them, and for how long have you done this?', 'How much money do you spend, per week, on drugs?' **(quantity)**
- 'How does the drug affect you?' **(drug effects)**
- 'What impact has the drug had on your life?' **(occupation, relationships, forensic history)**
- 'Do you feel that taking the drug is always on your mind?' **(preoccupation)**
- 'Have you ever tried reducing the substance you're taking? Any problems with this?' **(withdrawal)**
- 'Are you able to control your consumption?' **(control)**
- 'Do you recently feel that you have to take more of the drug to get the same effect?' **(tolerance)**
- 'Are you aware of the harmful effects?' **(knowledge of harm)**

Key facts 2: United States Drug Enforcement Administration (DEA) drug schedules

Schedule	Examples
1	Crack cocaine, cocaine, ecstasy, heroin, LSD, psilocybin, peyote
2	Amphetamines, barbiturates, meperidine, oxycontin, methylphenidate, methadone, fentanyl
3	Ketamine, anabolic steroids, testosterone, low dose codeine (Tylenol 3)
4	Benzodiazepines, modafinil, armodafinil, zolpidem, eszopiclone

OSCE tips: History taking in substance misuse

- Substance misuse is often a sensitive issue to ask questions on. As such, in an OSCE you will be awarded points for **rapport and empathy**, **active listening**, and a **non-judgemental attitude**.
- It is useful to divide your history into **current use** (including **'TRAP'** [Type, Route, Amount, Pattern] and exploring the signs of dependency, see *Key facts 1*), **risk assessment** (suicide/self-harm as well as IV use/needle sharing), **possible triggers** or stressful life events, **past substance use**, **physical**, **psychological**, and **social complications** of drug abuse (e.g. future use), and **coping strategies**.

> **MSE** Dependent upon the drug consumed and whether patient is acutely intoxicated or withdrawing.

NOTE: Perform a **full systems examination** including respiratory, cardiovascular, gastrointestinal, and neurological, and a full set of **observations** is required including RR, HR, BP and neurological observations.

> **Ix**
> - **Bloods** including: (1) **HIV** screen, **Hep B**, **Hep C** and tuberculosis testing → risk of blood-borne infections is thought to be greater through needle sharing; (2) **Electrolytes**, **BUN/Cr** to check renal function; (3) **LFTs and clotting** to check hepatic function; (4) **Drug levels**.
> - **Urinalysis:** drug metabolites (e.g. cannabis, opioids) can be detected in urine.
> - **ECG** for arrhythmias, **ECHO** if endocarditis suspected (secondary to needle sharing).

> **DDx**
> - **Psychiatric disorders:** Psychosis, mood disorders, anxiety disorders, delirium.
> - **Organic disorders:** Hyperthyroidism, CVA, intracranial hemorrhage, neurological disorders (e.g. cerebellar pathology).

Management

- A **case worker** with a **therapeutic alliance** is best placed to offer psychosocial support.
- **Hep B immunization** must be considered for those at risk.
- **Motivational interviewing** to help with controlling the substance misuse and **CBT** (for co-morbid depression or anxiety) may be offered.
- **Contingency management** is a technique that focuses on changing specified behaviors by offering incentives (e.g. financial) for positive behaviors such as abstinence.

> **Key facts 3:** Detoxification vs. maintenance
>
> **Detoxification** refers to a process in which the effects of the drug are eliminated in a safe manner (a replacement drug is weaned) such that withdrawal symptoms are avoided, in an attempt to attain abstinence. In **maintenance** therapy abstinence is not the priority, rather the aim is to minimize harm (e.g. from IV drug use).

- **Supportive help** can be in **housing, finance**, and **employment**. Help with co-existing **alcohol misuse** and **smoking cessation** should be offered.
- **Self-help groups**, e.g. **Narcotics Anonymous** and **Cocaine Anonymous**.
- Consider the **issue of driving** and review local guidelines.

Opioid dependence

- **Biological therapies** include **methadone** (first-line) or **buprenorphine** for **detoxification** AND **maintenance** (see *Key facts 3*).
- **Naltrexone** is recommended for those who were formerly opioid-dependent but have now stopped and are motivated to continue abstinence.
- **Intravenous naloxone** (opioid antagonist) can be used as an **antidote** to opioid overdose.

Self-assessment

A 20-year-old man presents to the ER with a Glasgow Coma Score of 10 (obtunded), respiratory depression, and miosis (1 mm pupils). His friends state that the man was seen injecting something intravenously at a party, shortly after which he became unresponsive. He is deeply unresponsive to pain and is unable to give a history. The patient is a known drug user and has track marks on both upper extremities and syringes are found among his belongings.

1. What type of drug is the man most likely to have taken? *(1 point)*
2. Under what schedule of drugs would this drug be categorized? *(1 point)*
3. What antidote should be given to this patient and how is this administered? *(2 points)*
4. Name four features of drug dependence. *(4 points)*
5. Name three psychosocial interventions for his long-term management. *(3 points)*

Answers to self-assessment questions are to be found in *Appendix B.*

Alcohol-use disorders

Alcohol-use disorders involve a pattern of alcohol use that causes impairment or distress. Alcohol abuse is characterized by a number of features including cravings, tolerance, unsuccessful efforts to cut back, drinking more than intended, spending excessive time in activities to obtain alcohol or recover from its use, drinking despite physically hazardous circumstances, vocational and interpersonal activities negatively affected by the drinking, and/or continued use despite problems from drinking.

Pathophysiology/Etiology

- Alcohol affects several **neurotransmitter systems** in the brain (e.g. its effect on **GABA** causes **anxiolytic** and **sedative** effects).
- The pleasurable and stimulant effects of alcohol are mediated by a **dopaminergic pathway** in the brain. Repeated, excessive alcohol ingestion sensitizes this pathway and leads to the development of dependence.

> **Key facts 1:** Recommended maximum intake of alcohol
>
> | MALE ♂ | FEMALE ♀ |
> |---|---|
> | 14 drinks per week | 7 drinks per week |
>
> For information on the different types of alcohol content of drinks in the USA see: https://health.gov/dietaryguidelines/2015/guidelines/appendix-9/

- Long-term exposure to alcohol causes adaptive changes in several neurotransmitter systems, including **down-regulation** of **inhibitory neuronal GABA** receptors and **up-regulation** of **excitatory glutamate** receptors, so when alcohol is withdrawn, it results in central nervous system **hyper-excitability**.
- Patients with alcohol-use disorders often experience **craving** (a conscious desire or urge to drink alcohol). This has been linked to **dopaminergic**, **serotonergic**, and **opioid systems** that mediate **positive reinforcement**, and to the **GABA**, **glutamatergic**, and **noradrenergic systems** that mediate **withdrawal**.
- The **social learning theory** suggests that drinking behavior is modeled on **imitation** of relatives or friends. **Operant conditioning** states that **positive** or **negative reinforcement** from the effects of drinking will either perpetuate or deter drinking habits, respectively.

Epidemiology and risk factors (Table 10.2.1)

- The 12 month and lifetime prevalence of DSM-5 alcohol-use disorder in the US is 13% and 29%, respectively.
- Alcohol-use disorder is more common among white and Native American males than other ethnic groups.
- Previously and never-married individuals have higher rates of alcohol-use disorder than those currently married or cohabitating.

Table 10.2.1: Risk factors for alcohol abuse

Male	• Males are at **increased risk** of alcohol abuse and have **increased metabolism** of alcohol, thus allowing them to have higher quantities.
Younger adults	• 16.2% among 18–29 year olds; 9.7% among 30–44 year olds have alcohol-related disorders.
Genetics	• **Monozygotic twins** have **higher concordance** rates than dizygotic. Studies show increased risk of dependence in relatives of those affected.
Antisocial behavior	• Pre-morbid antisocial behavior has been found to predict alcoholism.
Lack of facial flushing	• The risk of alcoholism is ↓ in individuals who show alcohol-induced facial flushing due to a mutation of gene coding for aldehyde dehydrogenase so that it metabolizes acetaldehyde more slowly. More common in some East Asian populations.
Life stressors	• E.g. **Financial problems**, **relationship issues**, and **certain occupations** can increase the risk.

Clinical features

- Clinical features vary depending on the alcohol-related disorder.

Alcohol intoxication

- Characterized by **slurred speech**, **labile affect**, **impaired judgement**, and **poor co-ordination**.
- In severe cases, there may be **hypoglycemia**, **stupor** and **coma**.

Alcohol dependence (Edward and Gross Criteria – 'SAW DRINk')

- **Subjective awareness** of compulsion to drink.
- **Avoidance or relief of withdrawal symptoms** by further drinking (also known as relief drinking).
- **Withdrawal symptoms**.
- **Drink-seeking behavior** predominates.
- **Reinstatement** of drinking after attempted abstinence.
- **Increased tolerance** to alcohol.
- **Narrowing of drinking repertoire** (i.e. a stereotyped pattern of drinking – individuals have fixed as opposed to variable times for drinking, with reduced influence from environmental cues).

Alcohol withdrawal

- Symptoms such as malaise, tremor, nausea, insomnia, transient hallucinations, and autonomic hyperactivity occur at 6–12 hours after abstinence. Peak incidence of seizures at 36 hours.
- The severe end of the spectrum of withdrawal is also termed **delirium tremens** and the peak incidence is at **72 hours** (see *Key facts 2*).
- Alcohol abuse has many **long-term effects** (*Fig. 10.2.1*).

Medical
• **Hepatic:** fatty liver, hepatitis, cirrhosis, hepatocellular carcinoma (*Fig. 10.2.2*). • **Gastrointestinal:** peptic ulcer disease, esophageal varices, pancreatitis, esophageal carcinoma. • **Cardiovascular:** hypertension, cardiomyopathy, arrhythmias. • **Hematological:** anemia, thrombocytopenia. • **Neurological:** seizures, peripheral neuropathy, cerebellar degeneration, Wernicke's encephalopathy, Korsakoff's psychosis, head injury (secondary to falls). • **Obstetrics:** fetal alcohol syndrome.

Psychiatric	
• Morbid jealousy.	• Alcohol-related dementia.
• Self-harm and suicide.	• Alcoholic hallucinosis.
• Mood disorders.	• Delirium tremens.
• Anxiety disorders.	

Social	
• Domestic violence.	• Homelessness.
• Drink driving (see *Key facts 4*).	• Accidents.
• Employment difficulties.	• Relationship problems.
• Financial problems.	

Fig. 10.2.1: Negative effects of alcohol consumption.

DSM-5 Criteria for alcohol-use disorder

A. A problematic pattern of alcohol use leading to clinically significant impairment or distress, as manifested by at least two of the following, occurring within a 12-month period:
1. Alcohol is often taken in larger amounts or over a longer period than was intended.
2. There is a persistent desire or unsuccessful efforts to cut down or control alcohol use.
3. A great deal of time is spent in activities necessary to obtain alcohol, use alcohol, or recover from its effects.
4. Craving, or a strong desire or urge to use alcohol.
5. Recurrent alcohol use resulting in a failure to fulfill major role obligations at work, school, or home.
6. Continued alcohol use despite having persistent or recurrent social or interpersonal problems caused or exacerbated by the effects of alcohol.
7. Important social, occupational, or recreational activities are given up or reduced because of alcohol use.
8. Recurrent alcohol use in situations in which it is physically hazardous.
9. Alcohol use is continued despite knowledge of having a persistent or recurrent physical or psychological problem that is likely to have been caused or exacerbated by alcohol.
10. Tolerance, as defined by either of the following:
    a. A need for markedly increased amounts of alcohol to achieve intoxication or desired effect.
    b. A markedly diminished effect with continued use of the same amount of alcohol.

DSM-5 Criteria for alcohol-use disorder *(continued)*

11. Withdrawal, as manifested by either of the following:
    a. The characteristic withdrawal syndrome for alcohol (refer to Criteria A and B of the criteria set for alcohol withdrawal).
    b. Alcohol (or a closely related substance, such as a benzodiazepine) is taken to relieve or avoid withdrawal symptoms.

Specify if:

In early remission: After full criteria for alcohol use disorder were previously met, none of the criteria for alcohol use disorder have been met for at least 3 months but for less than 12 months (with the exception that Criterion A4, "Craving, or a strong desire or urge to use alcohol," may be met).

In sustained remission: After full criteria for alcohol use disorder were previously met, none of the criteria for alcohol use disorder have been met at any time during a period of 12 months or longer (with the exception that Criterion A4, "Craving, or a strong desire or urge to use alcohol," may be met).

Specify if:

In a controlled environment: This additional specifier is used if the individual is in an environment where access to alcohol is restricted.

Code based on current severity: Note for ICD-10-CM codes: If an alcohol intoxication, alcohol withdrawal, or another alcohol-induced mental disorder is also present, do not use the codes below for alcohol use disorder. Instead, the comorbid alcohol use disorder is indicated in the 4th character of the alcohol-induced disorder code (see the coding note for alcohol intoxication, alcohol withdrawal, or a specific alcohol-induced mental disorder). For example, if there is comorbid alcohol intoxication and alcohol use disorder, only the alcohol intoxication code is given, with the 4th character indicating whether the comorbid alcohol use disorder is mild, moderate, or severe: F10.129 for mild alcohol use disorder with alcohol intoxication or F10.229 for a moderate or severe alcohol use disorder with alcohol intoxication.

Specify current severity:

305.00 (F10.10) Mild: Presence of 2–3 symptoms.

303.90 (F10.20) Moderate: Presence of 4–5 symptoms.

303.90 (F10.20) Severe: Presence of 6 or more symptoms.

Reprinted with permission from the *Diagnostic and Statistical Manual of Mental Disorders*, 5th Edition, (© 2013). American Psychiatric Association.

Key facts 2: Delirium tremens

- This **withdrawal delirium** develops between **24 hours and one week** after alcohol cessation. Peak incidence of delirium tremens is at **72 hours**.
- Physical illness is a predisposing factor.
- **Dehydration** and **electrolytic disturbances** are a feature.
- It is characterized by:
  - **Cognitive impairment**
  - **Vivid perceptual abnormalities** (hallucinations and/or illusions)
  - **Paranoid delusions**
  - **Marked tremor**
  - **Autonomic arousal** (e.g. tachycardia, fever, pupillary dilatation, and increased sweating).
- Medical treatment can be with large doses of **benzodiazepines** (e.g. chlordiazepoxide), **haloperidol** for any psychotic features, and **intravenous Pabrinex**.

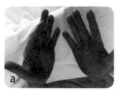 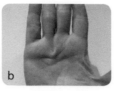 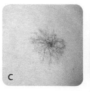 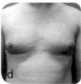

Fig. 10.2.2: Peripheral stigmata of chronic liver disease in alcoholics. (a) palmar erythema; (b) Dupuytren's contracture; (c) spider nevi; (d) gynecomastia. Other features include clubbing, caput medusa, and esophageal varices.

Diagnosis and investigations

Hx
- See *OSCE tips 2*.

NOTE: A collateral history is important.

OSCE tips 1: CAGE questionnaire

A useful screening tool for alcohol dependence in an OSCE setting are the **'CAGE' questions**. The patient has a problem if they answer yes to any of the following questions:
- **C** – Have you ever felt you should **Cut** down on your drinking?
- **A** – Have people **Annoyed** you by criticizing your drinking?
- **G** – Have you ever felt **Guilty** about your drinking?
- **E** – Do you ever have a drink early in the morning to steady your nerves or wake you up? (**Eye opener**)

MSE		Intoxication	Withdrawal
	Appearance & Behavior	Poor coordination, secondary injuries (e.g. lacerations), smell of alcohol.	Agitated, sweaty, tremor. May have seizures.
	Speech	Slurred.	Confused.
	Mood	May be elevated or depressed. Labile affect.	Anxious.
	Thought	Variable. Disinhibited.	Paranoid delusions.
	Perception	No abnormalities.	Visual hallucinations, illusions.
	Cognition	Impaired judgement, reduced concentration.	Delirium, inattention.
	Insight	Poor.	Poor.

NOTE: It is important to carry out neurological, cardiovascular, and GI examinations (*Fig. 10.2.1*).

OSCE tips 2: Specific alcohol history

1. **Screen for alcohol dependence**
   - See *CAGE questionnaire* above.
2. **Establish drinking pattern and quantity consumed**
   - 'Can you describe what drinks you have in a typical day?'
   - 'How much alcohol do you consume in an average week?' (quantify number of drinks)
   - 'How much money do you spend on drinking?'
   - 'How often have you drunk 6 or more drinks at one time in the past year?'
   - 'Do you drink steadily or have periods of binge drinking?'
   - 'Is there anything in particular which causes you to drink more?'
3. **Explore features of alcohol dependence**
   - 'When and where do you normally drink?' **(narrowing of drinking repertoire)**
   - 'Do you often feel the urge to drink?' **(compulsive need to drink)**
   - 'Have you noticed that alcohol has less effect on you than it had in the past?' **(↑ tolerance)**
   - 'Is alcohol the first thing that comes into your mind when planning a social gathering?' **(drink-seeking behavior predominates)**
   - 'Do you ever feel shaky and anxious when you haven't had a drink?', 'Have you ever tried to give up drinking, if so what happened?' **(withdrawal effects)**
   - 'Do you ever drink to get rid of this feeling?' **(prevention of withdrawal effects)**
4. **Explore possible risk factors**
   - 'Is there any family history of alcohol-related problems?'
   - Explore other risk factors, e.g. financial difficulties, relationship difficulties, etc.
5. **Establish impact**
   - 'Has alcohol affected your mental health?' **(psychiatric impact)**
   - 'Has alcohol affected your medical health?' Ask about alcohol-related disorders, e.g. liver disease, cardiovascular disease, neurological disorders **(physical impact)**
   - 'Has alcohol caused any problems with work, relationships, or the law?' **(social impact)**

Ix

- **Bloods** including: blood alcohol level, **CBC** (anemia), electrolytes and BUN/Cr (dehydration, ↓ urea), **LFTs** including gamma GT (may be ↑), **blood alcohol concentration**, **MCV** (macrocytosis), **vitamin B$_{12}$/folate/TFTs** (alternative causes of ↑MCV), **amylase** (pancreatitis), **hepatitis serology**, **glucose** (hypoglycemia).
- **Alcohol questionnaires:** CAGE questionnaire, Severity of Alcohol Dependence Questionnaire (SADQ), FAST screening tool (4 items, designed for busy settings).
- **CT head** (if head injury is suspected).
- **ECG** (for arrhythmias).

DDx

Psychiatric disorders:	Medical disorders:
• Psychosis.	• Head injury.
• Mood disorders (including bipolar).	• Cerebral tumor.
• Anxiety disorders.	• Cerebrovascular accident (e.g. stroke).
• Delirium.	

Key facts 3: Neuropsychiatric complications (Wernicke's encephalopathy and Korsakoff's psychosis)

- *Wernicke's encephalopathy:* An **acute encephalopathy** due to **thiamine deficiency**, presenting with **delirium**, **nystagmus**, **ophthalmoplegia**, **hypothermia**, and **ataxia**. Requires urgent treatment and may progress to **Korsakoff's psychosis** (AKA amnesic syndrome). Treated with **parenteral thiamine**.
- *Korsakoff's psychosis:* Profound, irreversible **short-term memory loss** with **confabulation** (the unconscious filling of gaps in memory with imaginary events) and **disorientation to time**.

OSCE tips 3: Quantifying the amount of alcohol consumed

- **One drink** of alcohol is defined as a drink containing **10 ml (8g)** of **ethanol**.

  Alcohol drinks = [strength (alcohol by volume) × volume (ml)] ÷ 1000

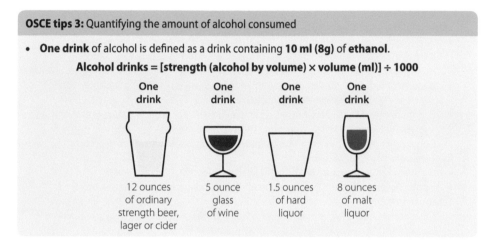

One drink	One drink	One drink	One drink
12 ounces of ordinary strength beer, lager or cider	5 ounce glass of wine	1.5 ounces of hard liquor	8 ounces of malt liquor

Management

See *Fig. 10.2.3* for an overview of the **bio-psychosocial management** of alcohol abuse.

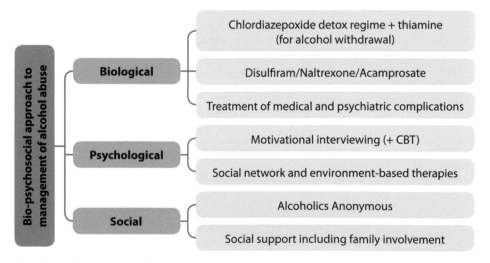

Fig. 10.2.3: Bio-psychosocial management for alcohol abuse.

For alcohol withdrawal

- It is important to recognize signs of alcohol dependence as the withdrawal syndrome is associated with significant morbidity and mortality.
- An alcohol detoxification regime offers controlled withdrawal, and can be carried out in the community or as an inpatient in more severe cases, in order to achieve **abstinence**. **Inpatient** detoxification is recommended in patients at **risk of suicide**, those with **poor social support** or those with a **history of severe withdrawal reactions**.
- **High dose benzodiazepines** (commonly **chlordiazepoxide**) are given initially, and the dose is **tapered down** over 5–9 days or titrated to BP and HR (see *Table 10.2.2*).
- Thiamine (Vitamin B$_1$) is also given in order to prevent **Wernicke's encephalopathy and Korsakoff's psychosis**. This can be given **orally** (200–300 mg daily in divided doses) or **intravenously**.

Table 10.2.2: An example of a chlordiazepoxide regime

DRUG chlordiazepoxide		Time	Day 1 Dose	Day 2 Dose	Day 3 Dose	Day 4 Dose	Day 5 Dose	Day 6 Dose	Day 7 Dose	Day 8 Dose	Day 9 Dose
Dose variable	**Route** oral	8	20 mg	20 mg	15 mg	15 mg	10 mg	10 mg	5 mg	5 mg	–
		12	20 mg	15 mg	15 mg	10 mg	10 mg	5 mg	5 mg	–	–
Signature		18	20 mg	15 mg	15 mg	10 mg	10 mg	5 mg	5 mg	–	–
		22	20 mg	20 mg	15 mg	15 mg	10 mg	10 mg	5 mg	5 mg	5 mg

For alcohol dependence (long term)

- Pharmacological therapies include:
  1. **Disulfiram:** Works by causing a build-up of acetaldehyde on consumption of alcohol, causing unpleasant symptoms e.g. anxiety, flushing and headache.
  2. **Acamprosate:** Reduces craving by enhancing GABA transmission.
  3. **Naltrexone:** Blocks opioid receptors (antagonist) in the body, thus reducing the pleasurable effects of alcohol.
- Motivational interviewing guides the person into wanting to change (*Fig. 10.2.4*). Motivational interviewing is most effective during the pre-contemplation and contemplation phases.
- CBT can be effective in managing alcohol problems and focuses specifically on alcohol-related beliefs and behaviors.

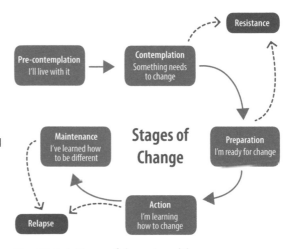

Fig. 10.2.4: 'Stages of change' model.

- **Alcoholics Anonymous (AA)** is a popular supportive program for patients who accept that they have a drinking problem. It is a **12-step approach** that utilizes **psychosocial techniques** in order to change behavior (e.g. social support networks, rewards). Each new member is assigned a 'sponsor' (a supervisor recovering from alcoholism).

General points

- Preventive measures include **raising taxation** on alcohol, **restricted advertising** or **sales**, and more **education** on alcohol issues in schools.
- **Prophylactic oral thiamine** (50 mg once daily) should be offered to harmful drinkers if they are **malnourished** (or at risk of malnourishment) or have **decompensated liver disease**.

Self-assessment

A 32-year-old man presents for a routine check-up for his blood pressure. He is found to have a BP of 172/88. You notice that he appears unkempt with an obvious odour of alcohol and that his speech is slurred. His concerned partner states she is worried about his drinking which is out of control and that he has been requiring more and more alcohol recently.

1. Aside from ↑ tolerance to alcohol, name four other features of alcohol dependence. *(4 points)*
2. Name two medical, two psychiatric, and two social complications of excess alcohol intake. *(3 points)*
3. Define delirium tremens and state its five features. *(6 points)*
4. What is the pharmacological management for alcohol withdrawal? *(2 points)*

Answers to self-assessment questions are to be found in *Appendix B*.

Chapter 11

Personality disorders

Definition

A personality disorder can be thought of as a **deeply ingrained** and **enduring pattern of inner experience and behavior** that deviates markedly from expectations in the individual's culture, is **pervasive** and **inflexible**, has an **onset** in **adolescence** or **early adulthood**, is **stable** over time, and leads to **distress** or **impairment**.

Pathophysiology/Etiology

- The cause of personality disorders (PD) involves both **biological** and **environmental** factors (*Table 11.1*).
- **Biological** factors can be **genetic** and **neurodevelopmental** (abnormal cerebral maturation).
- **Environmental** factors encompass both **adverse social circumstances** and **difficult childhood experiences** such as abuse.
- PDs can be classified into **three clusters** assigned **A**, **B** and **C** based on symptoms (*Fig. 11.1*).

Table 11.1: Risk factors for personality disorders	
Society	• Both **low socioeconomic status** and social reinforcement of abnormal behavior are linked to PDs.
Genetics	• **Monozygotic twin studies** show a **higher concordance rate** for PD than dizygotic studies. Incidence is higher in those with a **positive family history** of PD.
Dysfunctional family	• **Poor parenting** and **parental deprivation** are risks for the development of PD.
Abuse during childhood	• This includes physical, sexual (particularly linked to emotionally unstable PD), and emotional **abuse**, as well as neglect.

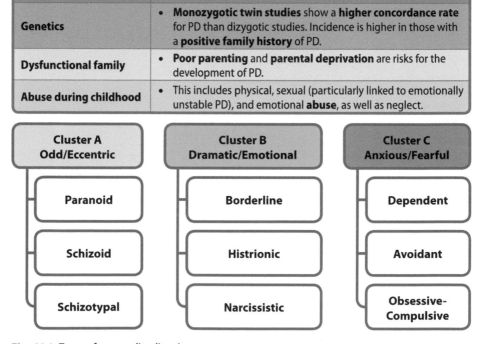

Cluster A Odd/Eccentric	Cluster B Dramatic/Emotional	Cluster C Anxious/Fearful
Paranoid	Borderline	Dependent
Schizoid	Histrionic	Avoidant
Schizotypal	Narcissistic	Obsessive-Compulsive

Fig. 11.1: Types of personality disorder.

Epidemiology and risk factors

- **4–13%** of the **adult population** has a PD of at least mild severity.
- **20%** of **PCP patients** who are adults suffer from a PD.
- The most prevalent PD is **antisocial (3%)** followed by **histrionic (2–3%)** and **paranoid (0.5–2.5%)**.

Clinical features

- The clinical features of the **specific PDs** are shown in *Table 11.2*.
- A useful mnemonic for remembering clusters is **WWW**: Cluster A = 'Weird'; Cluster B = 'Wild'; Cluster C = 'Worriers'.

Table 11.2: The features of personality disorders[1]

Cluster A (Weird)

Paranoid 'SUSPECTS'	• Suspicious of others • Unforgiving (bears grudges) • Spouse fidelity questioned • Perceives attack	• Envious (jealous) • Criticism not liked/Cold affect • Trust in others reduced • Self-reference
Schizoid 'DISTANT'	• Detached (flattened) affect • Indifferent to praise or criticism • Sexual drive reduced • Tasks done alone	• Absence of close friends • No emotion (cold) • Takes pleasure in few activities
Schizotypal	• Reduced capacity for close relationship • Cognitive or perceptual distortion • Eccentricity of behavior	

Cluster B (Wild)

Emotionally unstable (borderline) 'AM SUICIDE'	• Abandonment feared • Mood instability • Suicidal behavior • Unstable relationships • Intense relationships	• Control of anger poor • Impulsivity • Disturbed sense of self (identity) • Emptiness (chronic)
Antisocial 'CORRUPT'	• Callous • Others blamed • Reckless disregard for safety • Remorseless (lack of guilt)	• Underhanded (deceitful) • Poor planning (impulsive) • Temper/Tendency to violence
Histrionic 'PRAISE'	• Provocative behavior • Real concern for physical attractiveness • Attention seeking	• Influenced easily • Shallow/Seductive inappropriately • Egocentric (vain)/Exaggerated emotions

Cluster C (Worriers)

Dependent 'RELIANCE'	• Reassurance required • Expressing disagreement is difficult • Lack of self-confidence • Initiating projects is difficult	• Abandonment feared • Needs others to assume responsibility • Companionship sought • Exaggerated fears

Table 11.2: The features of personality disorders *(continued)*		
Avoidant **'CRIES'**	• Certainty of being liked needed before becoming involved with people • Restriction to lifestyle in order to maintain security • Inadequacy felt	• Embarrassment potential prevents involvement in new activities • Social inhibition
Obsessive-Compulsive **'LAW FIRMS'**	• Loses point of activity (due to preoccupation with detail) • Ability to complete tasks compromised (due to perfectionism) • Workaholic at the expense of leisure	• Fussy (excessively concerned with minor details) • Inflexible • Rigidity • Meticulous attention to detail • Stubborn

OSCE tips 1: Differentiating between 'Cluster A' PDs and psychotic disorders

'Cluster A' PDs (paranoid and schizoid) may present with similar features to psychotic disorders, e.g. schizophrenia, for instance with suspiciousness, odd beliefs, and social withdrawal. The differentiating factor is that hallucinations and true delusions are ABSENT in 'Cluster A' PDs.

Diagnosis and investigations

Hx
- 'How do you think your friends and family would describe your personality?' **(open question)**
- 'Do you worry that most people can't be trusted or have ill intent towards you?', 'Can you rely on friends and family?', 'How do you view your relationship with family?' **(paranoid)**
- 'Do you work well with others?', 'What activities do you enjoy?', 'Would you say you have many close friends?' **(schizoid)**
- 'How would you describe your relationships with the people in your life?', 'Do other people ever say you have a temper?', 'Do you ever feel life is not worth living?', 'Do you have any worries about being alone?' **(borderline)**
- 'Have you ever got into serious trouble, for instance with the police? If so, was it your fault?', 'Do people ever tell you that you have a temper?', 'Do you like to think things through properly before carrying out an act?' **(antisocial)**
- 'Do you feel that you are easily influenced by your friends?', 'Do you like to be the life and soul of a party?' **(histrionic)**
- 'Is there anything you worry about or fear?', 'Do you struggle to make an important decision?', 'Place yourself on a scale ranging from very shy to confident.' **(dependent)**
- 'Tell me about your social circle', 'Do you ever take risks or partake in brand new activities?', 'Do you feel contented with yourself?' **(anxious)**
- 'Do you feel that you are a perfectionist?', 'Do you need to make lists and have things in order?', 'Are other people bothered by your perfectionism?' **(Obsessive–compulsive)**
- **A reliable collateral history is imperative:** to determine the course of the symptoms, as well as identifying characteristic features which the patient may not have disclosed.

> **MSE** | MSE findings will vary depending on the type of PD and the features associated.

OSCE tips 2: Insight

Patients with PDs often have **no insight** into their psychiatric disorder. It is almost impossible to make a diagnosis of personality disorder without taking a **reliable collateral history** to elicit the pervasiveness and stability of the presentation. You need to complete a detailed personal and social history to understand the impact of the disorder on relationships, friendships, and occupation.

Ix
- **Questionnaires:** e.g. Personality Diagnostic Questionnaire, Eysenck Personality Questionnaire.
- **Psychological testing:** Minnesota Multiphasic Personality Inventory (MMPI).
- **CT head/MRI:** to rule out organic causes of personality change such as frontal lobe tumors and intracranial bleeds.

DDx
- **Mood disorders:** Mania, depression.
- **Psychotic disorders:** Schizophrenia, schizoaffective disorder.
- **Substance misuse.**

Management

- See *Fig. 11.2* for the principles of managing PD.
- Co-morbid **psychiatric illness** and **substance misuse** are common in patients with PD. Their recognition and treatment are essential.
- **Risk assessment** is crucial, particularly in cases of **borderline PD**, where patients may be suicidal. Potential **stressors** that induce crises should be identified and reduced.
- Several **psychosocial interventions** exist in the treatment of PD.
- **Pharmacological management** will not resolve the PD, but may be used to **control symptoms**. **Low-dose antipsychotics** for ideas of reference, impulsivity, and intense anger. **Antidepressants** may be useful in emotionally unstable personality disorder. **Mood stabilizers** can also be given. All of these are off-label indications for prescribing.
- Give the patient a **written crisis plan**. At times of crisis, if dangerous and violent or if there is a suicide risk consider an **involuntary commitment**.
- The management of people with PDs **can be outlined using** the **bio-psychosocial approach** (*Table 11.3*).

Identify and treat co-morbid **mental health disorders**

Treat any co-existing **substance misuse**

Help patient to deal with situations that **provoke problem behaviors or traits**

Provide **general support** to **reduce tension** and **anxieties**

Give **support and reassurance** to **family** and friends

Fig. 11.2: Main principles in managing PD.

Table 11.3: Bio-psychosocial management of personality disorders		
Biological	**Psychological**	**Social**
1. **2nd generation antipsychotics** may be used in the short term for transient psychotic periods in certain PDs (e.g. paranoid PD). 2. **Mood stabilizers** can be used in emotionally unstable PD for symptoms such as mood instability and aggression. 3. For mood symptoms consider **antidepressants**.	1. **Cognitive behavioral therapy.** 2. **Psychodynamic psychotherapy –** which may be individual or group. 3. **Dialectical behavioral therapy** – emphasis placed on developing coping strategies to improve impulse control and reduce self-harm in emotionally unstable PD.	1. **Support groups.** 2. **Substance misuse services.** 3. Assistance with social problems (e.g. housing, finance, and employment). 4. Help to access education, voluntary work, meaningful occupation, and work.

Self-assessment

A 34-year-old man presents feeling suicidal with a background of numerous acts of deliberate self-harm. He has a turbulent relationship with his girlfriend but tells you he plans to propose to her later that same day. He has been arrested on several occasions for attacking rival supporters at football games. He reports a difficult childhood, having been sexually abused by his step-father.

1. What is the most likely personality disorder? *(1 point)*
2. Name six other personality disorders based on the DSM-5 criteria. *(3 points)*
3. What are the features of antisocial personality disorder? *(3 points)*
4. Highlight three psychological interventions for personality disorders. *(3 points)*

Answers to self-assessment questions are to be found in *Appendix B*.

[1] Adapted from 'Mnemonics for DSM-IV Personality Disorders', Pinkofsky, H.B., *Psychiatric Services* (1997), **48**: 9.

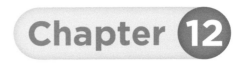

Chapter 12

Suicide and self-harm

12.1 Deliberate non-suicidal self-harm   132

12.2 Suicide and risk assessment   135

Deliberate non-suicidal self-harm

Definition

Deliberate self-harm (DSH) refers to an **intentional act** of **self-injury** (*Fig. 12.1.1*), without the clear or expressed intention of completing a suicide. It is usually an expression of **emotional distress** and may provide relief from a negative emotional state or even induce positive feelings.

- Cutting
- Burning
- Head banging
- Stabbing
- Swallowing objects
- Genital mutilation

Fig. 12.1.1: Methods of self-harm.

Pathophysiology/Etiology

- The etiology of DSH includes psychosocial and environmental factors (see *Table 12.1.1* and *OSCE tips*).

Epidemiology and risk factors (*Table 12.1.1*)

- DSH affects 15% of teens and up to 4% of adults.
- It is more common in ♀ at a ratio of 1.5:1, but this varies greatly with age.
- DSH is more common in **adolescents and young adults**. Incidence peaks in ♀ aged **15–19 years**, and in ♂ aged **20–24 years**.
- It is **20–30 times** more common than **suicide**.
- The **rate of suicide** in people who have self-harmed **increases** to between **50–100** times greater than that of the suicide rate in the general population.

Table 12.1.1: Risk factors for deliberate self-harm
Borderline personality
Severe life stressors
Harmful drug/alcohol use
Less than 35 (age)
Depression, OCD, psychosis
Violence (domestic) or childhood maltreatment
Socioeconomic disadvantage
Brain injury, intellectual disability

Clinical features

The most common forms of non-suicidal self-harm in the USA are skin cutting or scratching (70–90%), head banging or hitting (25–44%), and burning (25–35%).

- About half the men and a quarter of women who self-harm have taken alcohol in the 6 hours prior to the act, indicating that alcohol is a key risk factor.
- The most common complication of DSH is **permanent scarring of skin** and **damage to tendons** and **nerves** as a result of self-cutting.

Diagnosis and investigations

Hx
- What were their **intentions** before and during the act? **(intention)**
- Does the patient now wish to die? **(suicidal ideation)**
- What are the **current problems** in their life? **(severe life stressors)**
- How do they feel immediately after self-cutting, burning, etc. (relief, feel alive)? **(personality issues, other psychological factors)**
- **Collateral history** from relatives, friends or the PCP is important.
- For further details see *Section 12.2*, Suicide and risk assessment, *OSCE tips 1–3*.

OSCE tips: Motives behind deliberate self-harm (ask about these) – 'DRIPS'

- **Death wish:** genuine **wish to die**.
- **Relief:** seeking unconsciousness or pain as a means of **temporary relief** and escape from problems. Relief from feelings of emptiness.
- **Influencing others:** trying to **influence another person** to change their views or behavior (e.g. making a spouse feel guilty for not caring enough).
- **Punishment:** to **punish oneself**.
- **Seeking attention:** trying to get **help** or **seek attention** (expression of emotional distress).

MSE **General points** on assessment of the patient who has self-harmed:
- Obvious **self-inflicted injuries** may be seen (most commonly on the arms). The patient may be **tearful** or **indifferent**. **Behavior** may reflect an underlying mental disorder (depression, schizophrenia).
- Thoughts may include feelings of **emptiness**, **guilt**, **worthlessness**, or **helplessness**.
- **Hallucinations** may be present in cases of **schizophrenia** and **depression with psychosis** where DSH is triggered by **command hallucinations**.
- **Concentration** is often **impaired** and **insight can vary**.

Ix
- Electrolytes, BUN/Cr (renal function), **LFTs and clotting** (synthetic hepatic function).
- **Urinalysis** for possible toxicological analysis.
- **CT/MRI head** if an intracranial cause for altered consciousness is suspected.
- **Lumbar puncture** if intracranial infection (e.g. meningitis) suspected.

DDx **Psychiatric:** Borderline personality, schizophrenia or other psychotic disorder, major depression, OCD (skin picking), major depression.
Non-psychiatric: Clotting disorders (causing significant bruising or bleeding), delirium, brain injury, seizure disorder.

Management

The **bio-psychosocial management** of self-harm is outlined below:

- **Biological:** Medications to treat underlying disorders such as SSRIs for depression or OCD/skin picking, antipsychotics for psychotic disorders, etc.
- **Psychological:** Includes **counseling** and **CBT** for underlying **depressive illness. Dialectical behavior therapy** (DBT) to learn how to deal with destructive thoughts and impulses.
- **Social:** Evaluation of social circumstances and environmental stressor.

General points (Fig. 12.1.2)

- **Risk assessment is <u>mandatory</u>** as there is an immediate risk of suicide and risk of repeat acts of self-harm. Need for hospitalization should be assessed ± use of a **psychiatric hold**.
- There is often involvement of the Crisis team in the community as an alternative to hospital admission.
- If the patient refuses medical treatment for the consequences of self-harm (e.g. acute liver failure, deep lacerations) a **mental capacity assessment** may be required.
- Treat any **underlying psychiatric illness** with medication and/or psychological therapies.
- **Consider safety in overdose of antidepressants** for co-morbid depression. TCAs and MAOIs are most dangerous in overdose. Venlafaxine and citalopram carry a moderate risk of arrhythmia in overdose.
- **Psychosocial assessment** is required. Many patients have personal, relationship, or social problems for which they can be offered help (e.g. counseling and social service input).
- Ensure that the patient is **followed up** within 48 hours of discharge.
- **NOTE:** that approximately **1 in 6 people** who attend the ER following an act of self-harm will self-harm again **within a year**.

Acute management	Manage high suicide risk	Treat any psychiatric disorder	Enable patient to resolve any difficulties that led to the DSH	Enable patient to manage future crises
Medical assessment. Need for a hold or hospitalization.	Full risk assessment. Consider inpatient psychiatric assessment.	For instance antidepressants or CBT for depression.	Manage psychosocial needs. Refer to drug/alcohol services if appropriate. Offer financial and occupational rehabilitation advice.	Arrange for follow-up. Offer written and verbal information. Remove access to means of DSH.

Fig. 12.1.2: Principles behind managing deliberate self-harm.

12.2 Suicide and risk assessment

Definitions

- **Suicide:** A fatal act of self-harm initiated with the intention of ending one's own life.
- **Attempted suicide:** The act of intentionally trying to take one's own life with the primary aim of dying, but not completing this endeavor.
- **Parasuicide event:** An apparent attempt at suicide, commonly called a suicidal gesture, in which the aim is not death (e.g. a sublethal drug overdose).

Pathophysiology/Etiology

- The risk of someone taking their own life is increased by certain risk factors and reduced by certain protective factors (*Fig. 12.2.1*).

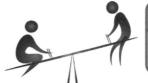

Protective factors	**Risk factors**
Dependent children at home, pregnancy, strong religious beliefs or spiritual belief that suicide is immoral, strong social support, positive coping skills, positive therapeutic relationship, supportive living arrangements, life satisfaction, fear of the physical act of suicide, responsibility for others, hope for the future.	• See *Tables 12.2.1* and *12.2.2*, and *OSCE tips 1*.

OSCE tips 1: Mnemonic for suicide risk factors ('**I'M A SAD PERSON**')

Institutionalized, **M**ental health disorders, **A**lone (lack of social support), **S**ex (male), **A**ge (middle aged or older), **D**epression, **P**revious attempts, **E**thanol use, **R**ational thinking lost, **S**ickness, **O**ccupation (see *Table 12.2.2*), **N**o job (unemployed)

Fig. 12.2.1: An imbalance between risk factors and protective factors predisposes to suicide.

Epidemiology and risk factors (*Tables 12.2.1* and *12.2.2*)

- Suicide is the **10th** leading cause of death overall in the USA and the second leading cause of death in those aged 10–34.
- In 2017, there were **14** suicides **per 100 000 population**:
  - Men completed suicide at 3.5x the rate in women (due to lethal methods: firearms).
  - 77% of completed suicides in the USA in 2017 were in white males.
- The most common methods of suicide in the USA are firearms (**50%**), followed by suffocation/hanging (28%), and poisoning/overdose (18%).

Key facts: Antidotes to overdose

Drug	Antidote
Paracetamol	**N-acetylcysteine**
Opiates	**Naloxone**
Benzodiazepines	**Flumazenil**
Warfarin	**Vitamin K**
Beta-blockers	**Glucagon**
TCAs (e.g. amitriptyline)	**Sodium bicarbonate**
Organophosphates	**Atropine**

- **Activated charcoal:** for the majority of drugs taken in overdose, early use of activated charcoal (within one hour of ingestion) can prevent or reduce absorption of the drug.
- There are 55 Poison Control Centers in the US. The American Association of Poison Control Centers can be reached 24 hours/day at 1-800-222-1222 for help in managing a specific overdose or ingestion. In addition, up-to-date information can also be found at www. poisonhelp.org.

Table 12.2.1: Clinical risk factors of suicide

History of DSH or attempted suicide	• The rate of suicide in people who have self-harmed increases and is **50–100** times greater than in the general population.
Psychiatric illness	• Including **depression, schizophrenia, substance misuse, alcohol abuse**, and **personality disorder**.
Childhood abuse	• History of childhood **sexual** or **physical** abuse.
Family history	• **Family history of suicide or suicide attempt** in first-degree relatives increases the risk.
Medical illness	• Physically **disabling, painful**, or **terminal** illness.

Table 12.2.2: Socio-demographic risk factors of suicide

Male gender	• Males are **3x** more likely than females. Male suicide attempts are more likely to be by lethal means from which survival is unlikely (firearms vs. overdose).
Age	• Highest in the age group **44** to **54** and over 75 in **men**.
Employment and financial status	• Those **unemployed** and who have **low socioeconomic** status are at higher risk.
Occupation	• **Doctors, dentists**, and **police officers** are at higher risk of suicide.
Access to lethal means	• The most lethal means of suicide are **firearms**, followed by **hanging, suffocation**, and **overdose**.
Social support	• **Low social support, living alone, institutionalized**, e.g. prisons, soldiers.
Marital status	• Those that are **single, widowed, separated**, or **divorced**.
Recent life crisis	• e.g. Bereavement, family breakdown.

Clinical features

Individuals who are suicidal usually have a number of characteristics, including the following:

- **Preoccupation with death:** Thoughts, fantasies, ruminations, and preoccupations with death, particularly self-inflicted death.
- **Sense of isolation and withdrawal from society.**
- **Emotional distance** from others.
- **Distraction and lack of pleasure:** Often are 'in their own world' and suffer from anhedonia.
- **Focus on the past:** They dwell on past losses and defeats and anticipate no future; they voice the notion of Beck's cognitive triad (see *Section 3.2*, Depressive disorder) that the world would be better off without them.
- **Feelings of hopelessness and helplessness.**

Diagnosis and investigations

Hx
- See *OSCE tips 2 and 3*.
- A **collateral history** may provide valuable information.

MSE See *OSCE tips 3*.

Ix
- Medical investigations according to the method, e.g. drug levels (see *Section 12.1*, Deliberate non-suicidal self-harm).
- Questionnaires - **Tool for Assessment of Suicide Risk (TASR)**, Beck Suicide Intent Scale.
- Suicide can be confirmed by **post-mortem**.

OSCE tips 2: Determining the risk of suicide following DSH '**Note: Planned Attempts Are Very Frightening!**' (The following ↑ risk).

1. Note left behind: usually written.
2. Planned attempt of suicide.
3. Attempts to avoid discovery.
4. Afterwards help was not sought.
5. Violent method.
6. Final acts: sorting out finances, writing a will.

DDx
- Self-harm (for attempted suicide).

Key facts: Self-harm vs. suicide

Suicide	Self-harm
More common in **males**	More common in **females**
Risk **increases with age**	More common in **young people**
Act may be **planned meticulously**	Act is **impulsive**
Act is more often **violent**	Usually in form of **overdose or cutting**
Physical and **psychiatric illness** is common	**Physical** and **psychiatric illness** is less common

OSCE tips 3: Risk assessment

1. **Exploring suicidal ideation:**
   - 'How do you feel about your future?'
   - 'Do you feel that life is worth living?'
   - 'Have you ever thought about taking your own life?'
2. **Exploring suicide intent:** (see *OSCE tips 2*)
   - What precipitated the attempt? Was it planned?
   - What method did they use?
   - Was a suicide note left? Did they make any other preparations before acting? e.g. writing a will.
   - Was the patient intoxicated with drugs or alcohol?
   - Was the patient alone?
   - Were there precautions taken to avoid discovery (e.g. they waited until the house was empty, locked doors, timed so that intervention would be highly unlikely)?
   - Did the patient think that they were certain to die even if they received medical attention?
   - What was the degree of premeditation? How long had they been contemplating suicide for? What plans had they made before acting?
   - Did the patient seek help after the attempt or were they found and brought in by someone else?
   - How does the patient feel about it now? Do they regret it or do they wish that they had succeeded?
   - How do they feel about being found? Are they relieved or are they angry?
3. **Exploring risk factors:**
   - 'Is there anything in particular that is making you feel this way?', 'Can you tell me about it?' (stress)
   - 'Have you ever tried anything like this before?', 'Can you tell me about it?' (previous suicide attempts)
   - 'Have you suffered from depression, substance use disorder, or had other psychiatric issues?' (psychiatric illness)
   - 'Do you have a gun or weapon in the house?' (access to lethal means)
   - 'Do you have any health problems that are bothering you at the moment?' (medical illness)
   - 'Is there any family history of suicide, depression, or substance abuse?' (family history)
4. **Perform mental status examination:**
   May indicate signs of underlying psychiatric disorder (usually depression):
   - **Appearance & behavior:** e.g. disheveled, unkempt and unclean clothing, evidence of suicidal behavior, such as wrist lacerations and neck rope burns.
   - **Mood:** Usually low mood and a flat affect.
   - **Thoughts:** May have delusions about the benefits of suicide (e.g. family will be better off), obsession with taking his or her own life.
   - **Perception** - Possibly second person auditory command hallucinations telling the patient to kill themself in psychotic depression or schizophrenia.
5. **Explore protective factors:** (see *Fig. 12.2.1*)
   - 'What would stop you from acting on suicidal thoughts?' What are the good things in your life? Do you have pets? (general protective factors)
   - 'Do you have someone to confide in, close family or friends?', 'Who do you live with?', 'Do you have company at home?' (establishing social support or lack of)

OSCE tips 3: Risk assessment *(continued)*

6. **Explore risk *to* others (including children) and risk *from* others:**
   - 'Do you ever have thoughts of harming others?'
   - Patients may have children/relatives that are in danger: 'Do you have close contact with any children?' Document the child's name, DOB, place of residence and enquire as to the nature of the relationship.
   - 'Do you ever feel threatened or at risk from others?'
7. **Formulate management plan:**
   - Determine whether the patient is low, medium or high risk and formulate a management plan accordingly, depending on the degree of planning, severity of the attempt and ongoing concerns about risk (see *Management section*).

Key facts 2: Psychiatric holds

Involuntary civil commitment of psychiatric patients may be necessary to protect both the patient and society from the consequences of a serious mental illness. A hold may allow for the involuntary hospitalization for purposes of psychiatric observation for a limited time period (up to 72 hours). Psychiatric holds do not typically allow for the administration of treatment other than emergency psychiatric medications against the will of the patient. A psychiatric hold may be initiated by a mental health professional, a police officer, an ER physician, or other professional designated by a particular county or municipality. Judicial oversight (a hearing) is typically necessary to extend the hold for up to 14 days. The hold may be released at any time a designated mental health professional (usually a licensed psychiatrist or psychologist) deems the patient no longer holdable.

Grounds for an involuntary hold on the basis of a psychiatric disorder:
1. Imminent danger to self (may include deliberate self-harm, misuse of medications, suicide risk, etc.).
2. Imminent danger to others (may include viable threats, assault, stalking, etc.).
3. Grave disability defined as the inability to provide for food, clothing and/or shelter on the basis of a psychiatric disorder.

Management

- **Ensure safety:** Immediate action should include removing means for suicide (guns) and ensuring the safety of the patient and others.
- Patients who have attempted suicide should be **medically stabilized,** e.g. management of drug overdose or treatment of physical injury.

OSCE tips 4: When to refer to secondary care for patient at risk of suicide: '**SUSP**icious'

Is usually considered if: (1) **S**uicidal ideation clearly stated; (2) **U**nderlying psychiatric illness is severe; (3) **S**ocial support (lack of); (4) **P**resentation change for an individual who has repeatedly self-harmed.

- **Risk assessment:** The risk of further suicide should then be assessed. People with a high degree of suicidal intent, specific plans, or chosen methods (particularly if lethal) should be assigned a higher level of risk (see *OSCE tips 3*).
- **Admission to hospital** (or observation in a safe place) is generally indicated if individuals pose a high and immediate risk of suicide. A **psychiatric hold** (see *Key facts 2* above) might be required if the patient refuses help and there is evidence of a mental illness.

- **Referral to secondary care** (see *OSCE tips 4*).
- **Psychiatric treatment:** Depression or psychosis should be detected and treated accordingly.
- **Outpatient and community treatment** may be more suitable for patients with chronic suicidal ideation but no history of previous significant suicide attempts. For this to succeed, a strong support network and easy access to outpatient and community facilities are required.
- **Prevention strategies** (*Fig. 12.2.2*).

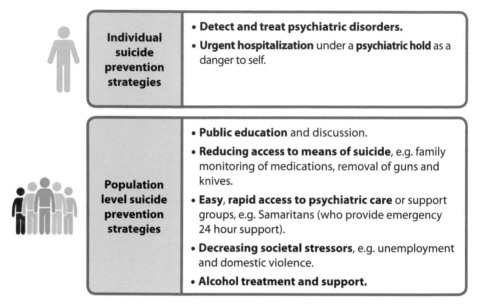

Individual suicide prevention strategies	• **Detect and treat psychiatric disorders.** • **Urgent hospitalization** under a **psychiatric hold** as a danger to self.
Population level suicide prevention strategies	• **Public education** and discussion. • **Reducing access to means of suicide**, e.g. family monitoring of medications, removal of guns and knives. • **Easy, rapid access to psychiatric care** or support groups, e.g. Samaritans (who provide emergency 24 hour support). • **Decreasing societal stressors**, e.g. unemployment and domestic violence. • **Alcohol treatment and support.**

Fig. 12.2.2: Individual vs. population suicide prevention strategies.

Self-assessment

A 75-year-old man in a rural community presents to his PCP with a 2-week history of constipation, headache, and fatigue. He has a past medical history of ischemic heart disease and insulin-dependent diabetes. He is the primary carer for his wife, who has recently been diagnosed with Alzheimer's disease. Upon further questioning, he admits to feelings of low mood, hopelessness, and persistent suicidal ideation. He feels overwhelmed by the burden of being his wife's care provider. He has made vague suicide plans but is worried about how his death would affect his wife's care.

1. What risk factors of suicide does he possess? *(3 points)*
2. Give four other risk factors of suicide. *(2 points)*
3. What protective factor of suicide does he possess? *(1 point)*
4. How should he be managed? *(3 points)*
5. Give two ways suicide can be prevented on a population level. *(2 points)*

Answers to self-assessment questions are to be found in *Appendix B*.

Chapter 13

Neurocognitive disorders

| 13.1 | Delirium | 142 |
| 13.2 | Dementia | 149 |

13.1 Delirium

Definition

Delirium is an **acute**, **transient**, **global brain disorder** resulting in **impaired consciousness** and **attention**. There are different types of delirium: **hypoactive**, **hyperactive**, and **mixed**, depending on the clinical presentation (*Fig. 13.1.1*).

Hypoactive (40%)
- Lethargy, ↓ motor activity, apathy and sleepiness.
- It is the **most common** type of delirium but often goes unrecognized.
- Can be confused with depression.

Hyperactive (25%)
- Agitation, irritability, restlessness, and aggression.
- Hallucinations and delusions prominent.
- May be confused with functional psychoses.

Mixed (35%)
- Both hypo- and hyperactive subtypes co-exist and therefore there are signs of both.

Fig. 13.1.1: Subtypes of delirium.

Pathophysiology/Etiology

- Delirium has a number of causes (see *Table 13.1.1*); however, most causes of delirium are **multifactorial**, each of which may be important at different time points of the illness. The causes can be remembered using the mnemonic 'HE IS NOT MAAD'.

Table 13.1.1: Causes of delirium ('HE IS NOT MAAD')	
Hypoxia	Respiratory failure, myocardial infarction, cardiac failure, pulmonary embolism.
Endocrine	Hyperthyroidism, hypothyroidism, hyperglycemia, hypoglycemia, Cushing's.
Infection	Pneumonia, UTI, encephalitis, meningitis.
Stroke and other intracranial events	Stroke, raised ICP, intracranial hemorrhage, space-occupying lesions, head trauma, epilepsy (post-ictal), intracranial infection.
Nutritional	↓ Thiamine, ↓ nicotinic acid, ↓ vitamin B_{12}.
Others	Severe pain, sensory deprivation (for example leaving the person without spectacles or hearing aids), relocation (such as moving people with impaired cognition to unfamiliar environments), sleep deprivation.
Theater (post-operative period)	Anesthetic, opiate analgesics, and other post-operative complications.

Table 13.1.1: Causes of delirium ('HE IS NOT MAAD') *(continued)*

Metabolic	Hypoxia, electrolyte disturbance (e.g. hyponatremia), hypoglycemia, hepatic impairment, renal impairment.
Abdominal	Fecal impaction, malnutrition, urinary retention, bladder catheterization.
Alcohol	Intoxication, withdrawal (delirium tremens).
Drugs	Benzodiazepines, opioids, anticholinergics, anti-parkinsonian medications, steroids.

OSCE tips 1: Medical sieves!

Since there are numerous causes for delirium work through the list systematically by always thinking of the **most common** causes first, e.g. infection (UTI is a very common cause of delirium in the elderly).

Epidemiology and risk factors (*Table 13.1.2*)

- Delirium occurs in about **15–20%** of all general admissions to hospital.
- Delirium is the **most common** complication of hospitalization in the **elderly population**.
- Up to **two-thirds** of delirium cases occur in inpatients with **pre-existing dementia**.
- **15%** of >65s are delirious **on admission** to hospital.
- Cardiovascular surgery and hip replacement in the elderly are commonly associated with delirium.

Table 13.1.2: Risk factors for delirium

Older age ≥65	Multiple co-morbidities
Dementia	Physical frailty
Renal impairment	Male sex
Sensory impairment	Previous episodes
Recent surgery	Severe illness (e.g. CCF)

Clinical features ('DELIRIUM')

Delirium has an **acute onset** and takes a **fluctuating course** (often worse at night). Other features include:

- **Disordered thinking:** Slowed, irrational, incoherent thoughts.
- **Euphoric**, **fearful**, **depressed**, or **angry**.
- **Language impaired:** Rambling speech, repetitive and disruptive.
- **Illusions**, **delusions** (transient persecutory or delusions of misidentification) and **hallucinations** (usually tactile or visual).
- **Reversal of sleep-wake pattern:** i.e. may be tired during day and hyper-vigilant at night.
- **Inattention:** Inability to focus, clouding of consciousness.
- **Unaware/disoriented:** Disoriented to time, place, or person.
- **Memory deficits.**

DSM-5 Criteria for delirium

A. A disturbance in attention (i.e. reduced ability to direct, focus, sustain, and shift attention) and awareness (reduced orientation to the environment).

B. The disturbance develops over a short period of time (usually hours to a few days), represents a change from baseline attention and awareness, and tends to fluctuate in severity during the course of a day.

C. An additional disturbance in cognition (e.g. memory deficit, disorientation, language, visuospatial ability, or perception).

D. The disturbances in Criteria A and C are not explained by another preexisting, established, or evolving neurocognitive disorder and do not occur in the context of a severely reduced level of arousal, such as coma.

E. There is evidence from the history, physical examination, or laboratory findings that the disturbance is a direct physiological consequence of another medical condition, substance intoxication or withdrawal (i.e. due to a drug of abuse or to a medication), or exposure to a toxin, or is due to multiple etiologies.

Specify whether:

Substance intoxication delirium: This diagnosis should be made instead of substance intoxication when the symptoms in Criteria A and C predominate in the clinical picture and when they are sufficiently severe to warrant clinical attention.

Reprinted with permission from the *Diagnostic and Statistical Manual of Mental Disorders*, 5th Edition, (© 2013). American Psychiatric Association.

Key facts: Delirium vs. dementia

	Delirium	Dementia
Sleep-wake cycle	Disrupted	Usually normal
Attention	Markedly reduced	Normal/reduced
Arousal	Increased/decreased	Usually normal
Autonomic features	Abnormal	Normal
Duration	Hours to weeks	Months to years
Delusions	Fleeting	Complex
Course	Fluctuating	Stable/slowly progressive
Consciousness level	Impaired	No impairment
Hallucinations	Common (especially visual)	Less common
Onset	Acute/subacute	Chronic
Psychomotor activity	Usually abnormal	Usually normal

OSCE tips 2: Beware of missing hypoactive delirium!

Delirium may be unrecognized by doctors and nurses in two-thirds of people. Healthcare professionals often do not recognize delirium and may misdiagnose hypoactive delirium as depression. Remember to always consider delirium in a person, particularly an elderly person who is apathetic, quiet, or withdrawn.

Diagnosis and investigations

NOTE: Before or during a history, a thorough physical examination should be performed: **ABC** (**A**irway/**B**reathing/**C**irculation), **conscious level**, and **vital signs**, e.g. oxygen saturations, pulse, blood pressure, temperature, capillary blood glucose. **Nutritional** and **hydration status**, **cardiovascular examination**, **respiratory examination**, **abdominal examination** (check for urinary retention and rectal exam for fecal impaction), **neurological examination** (including speech).

Hx	
	• **Much of the history may be collateral** as obtaining the history from the patient may prove very difficult.
	• Identify rate of onset and course of the confusion.
	• Any symptoms of underlying cause, e.g. symptoms of infection or of intracranial pathology?
	• Having an understanding of their premorbid mental state is important.
	• Are they hypo-alert or hyper-alert?
	• Do they have hypersensitivity to sound and light?
	• Is there any perceptual disturbance (misidentification, illusions, and hallucinations)?
	• Take a thorough drug history and a full alcohol history.

MSE		
	Appearance & Behavior	Hypo- or hyper-alert. Agitated, aggressive, purposeless behavior.
	Speech	Incoherent, rambling.
	Mood	Low mood, irritable, or anxious. Mood is often labile.
	Thought	Confused, ideas of reference, delusions.
	Perception	Illusions, hallucinations (mainly visual), misinterpretations.
	Cognition	Disoriented, impaired memory, reduced concentration/attention.
	Insight	Poor.

Ix

1. **Routine investigations: Urinalysis** (UTI); **Bloods: CBC** (infection); **BUN/Cr** (electrolyte disturbance); **LFTs** (alcoholism, liver disease); **calcium** (hypercalcemia); **glucose** (hypo-/hyperglycemia); **CRP** (infection/inflammation); **TFTs** (hyperthyroidism); **B$_{12}$, folate, ferritin** (nutritional deficiencies); **ECG** (cardiac abnormalities, acute coronary syndrome); **CXR** (chest infection); **infection screen: blood culture** (sepsis) and **urine culture** (UTI).

2. **Investigations based on history/examination: ABG** (hypoxia), **CT head** (head injury, intracranial bleed, CVA), and you may consider **lumbar puncture** (meningitis), **EEG** (epilepsy).

3. **Diagnostic questionnaire** (helps with diagnosis but also monitoring):
   - **Abbreviated Mental Test (AMT):** A quick easy tool (see *OSCE tips 3*).
   - **Confusion Assessment Method (CAM):** Usually performed after AMT (see *OSCE tips 3*).
   - **Mini-Mental State Examination (MMSE).**

DDx

- **Dementia.**
- **Mood disorders:** depression or mania (bipolar).
- **Late onset schizophrenia.**
- **Dissociative disorders.**
- **Hypothyroidism** and **hyperthyroidism** (may mimic hypo- and hyperactive delirium, respectively).

OSCE tips 3: Abbreviated Mental Test (AMT) and Confusion Assessment Method (CAM)

Abbreviated Mental Test	Confusion Assessment Method
1. Age? (1) 2. Time to the nearest hour? (1) 3. Recall address at end: '42 West Street' (1) 4. 'What year is it?' (1) 5. 'Where are you right now?' (1) 6. Identify two people. (1) 7. 'What is your date of birth?' (1) 8. 'Date of First World War?' (1) 9. 'Who is the current president of the USA?' (1) 10. 'Count backwards from 20 to 1.' (1) **≥8 → cognitive impairment unlikely.**	The Confusion Assessment tool (CAM) involves assessing a patient for four features. The diagnosis involves the presence of **1 and 2 + *either* 3 or 4:** 1. **Acute onset and fluctuating course.** 2. **Inattention** (e.g. using the serial 7s test where 7 is subtracted from 100 and then 7 is taken from each remainder, i.e. 100, 93, 86, 79, 72…). 3. **Disorganized thinking** (e.g. incoherent speech). 4. **Alteration in consciousness.**

Management (Fig. 13.1.2)

Treat the underlying cause

- Treat any infections. Correct any electrolyte disturbances.
- Stop any potential offending drugs.
- Laxatives for fecal impaction or temporary catheterization for urinary retention. Give analgesia if required.

Reassurance and re-orientation

- Reassure patients to reduce anxiety and disorientation.
- Patients should be reminded of the time, place, day and date regularly.

Provide appropriate environment

- Quiet, well-lit side room.
- Consistency in care and staff.
- Reassuring nursing staff.
- Encourage presence of friend or family member.
- Optimize sensory acuity, e.g. glasses, well-lit room, orientation aids (clock, calendar).

Managing disturbed, violent, or distressed behavior

- Encourage oral intake and pay attention to continence.
- Verbal and non-verbal de-escalation techniques (e.g. redirection).
- Oral low-dose haloperidol (0.5–4 mg), or olanzapine (2.5–10 mg).
- Avoid benzodiazepines (unless delirium due to alcohol withdrawal).
- Referral to a Care of the Elderly Consultant may be appropriate.

Fig. 13.1.2: Overview of the management of delirium.

OSCE tips 4: Medications are not the answer

Antipsychotics and benzodiazepines are never first-line for managing delirium and unfortunately this is a misconception amongst many clinicians. Treating the underlying cause, providing reassurance and re-orientation and an appropriate environment are the main means for treating delirium. Low-dose antipsychotics should only be used as a last resort in cases of violent or severely distressed behavior and when other ways of calming the patient have failed.

Self-assessment

You are paged in the middle of the night by a nurse who reports that an 83-year-old man has become disturbed and distressed two days after his abdominal surgery. The patient has been pulling out his cannulas, shouting, repeatedly getting out of bed despite being unsteady, and has been aggressive towards staff. You suspect the patient is suffering from delirium post-operatively.

1. State four differences between delirium and dementia. *(4 points)*
2. Name six common causes of delirium. *(3 points)*
3. What routine investigations would you perform on this patient? *(5 points)*
4. Name two tools you can use to test his cognition. *(2 points)*
5. How should this patient be managed? *(5 points)*

Answers to self-assessment questions are to be found in *Appendix B.*

13.2 Dementia

Definition

Dementia is a syndrome of generalized decline of **memory**, **intellect**, and **personality**, without impairment of **consciousness**, leading to **functional impairment**.

Pathophysiology/Etiology

- Dementia affects different areas of the brain (*Fig. 13.2.1*) depending on its cause (**reversible** or **irreversible**, see *Table 13.2.1*). **Alzheimer's disease (AD)** is the most common type (*Fig. 13.2.2*).
- In **Alzheimer's** disease there is degeneration of cholinergic neurons in the nucleus basalis of Meynert leading to a **deficiency of acetylcholine**. Other pathophysiological changes can be divided into microscopic (*Fig. 13.2.3*) and macroscopic:

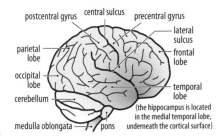

Fig. 13.2.1: Regions of the brain.

- Microscopic → **Neurofibrillary tangles** (intracellularly) and **β-amyloid plaque formation** (extracellularly).
- Macroscopic → **Cortical atrophy** (commonly hippocampal). **Widened sulci** and **enlarged ventricles**.

Table 13.2.1: Causes of dementia	
IRREVERSIBLE causes of dementia	**REVERSIBLE causes of dementia**
• **Neurodegenerative:** Alzheimer's disease, fronto-temporal dementia, Pick's disease, dementia with Lewy bodies (DLB), Parkinson's disease with dementia, Huntington's disease. • **Infections:** HIV, encephalitis, syphilis, CJD. • **Toxins:** Alcohol, barbiturates, benzodiazepines. • **Vascular:** Vascular dementia, multi-infarct dementia, CVD. • **Traumatic head injury.**	• **Neurological:** Normal pressure hydrocephalus, intracranial tumors, chronic subdural hematoma. • **Vitamin deficiencies:** B_{12}, folic acid, thiamine, nicotinic acid (pellagra). • **Endocrine:** Cushing's syndrome, hypothyroidism.

NOTE: A useful mnemonic for **reversible/preventable** causes of dementia 'DEMENTIA': **D**rugs (e.g. barbiturates), **E**yes and **E**ars (visual/hearing impairment may be confused with dementia), **M**etabolic (Cushing's, hypothyroidism), **E**motional (depression can present as a pseudodementia), **N**utritional deficiencies/**N**ormal pressure hydrocephalus, **T**umors/**T**rauma, **I**nfections (e.g. encephalitis), **A**lcoholism/**A**therosclerosis (vascular).

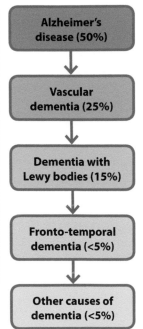

Fig. 13.2.2: The dementias in order of prevalence.

- **Vascular** dementia (VaD) occurs as a result of **cerebrovascular disease**, either due to stroke, multi-infarcts (multiple smaller unrecognized strokes), or chronic changes (arteriosclerosis) in the small vessels. Vascular dementia and Alzheimer's disease often co-exist.

- In **Lewy body** dementia (DLB), there is **abnormal deposition of a protein** (Lewy body) within the neurons of the brainstem, substantia nigra, and neocortex. Outside the brainstem LBs are associated with more profound cholinergic loss than in AD. Within the brainstem, they are associated with dopaminergic loss and parkinsonian-like symptoms.

- In **fronto-temporal** dementia there is specific degeneration **(atrophy)** of the **frontal** and **temporal** lobes of the brain. One type of fronto-temporal dementia is **Pick's disease**, where protein tangles (Pick's bodies) are seen histologically.

- Dementias can be divided on the basis of predominance of **cortical**, **subcortical**, or **mixed** dysfunction (see *Table 13.2.2*). Cortical dementias include AD and fronto-temporal dementia. Subcortical dementias include DLB. Vascular dementia is mixed.

Table 13.2.2: Cortical vs. subcortical dementias

	Cortical	Subcortical
Memory loss	Severe	Moderate
Mood	Normal	Low
Speech and language	Early aphasia	Can be dysarthria
Personality	Indifferent	Apathetic
Coordination	Normal	Impaired
Praxis	Apraxia	Normal
Motor speed	Normal	Slow

Plaques   Neurofibrillary Tangles

Fig. 13.2.3: Microscopic changes in brain of a patient with AD.

Epidemiology and risk factors

- There are currently 5.7 million people with dementia in the USA and it is estimated that there will be **over 8 million** by **2021**.

- Dementia increases with age (rare if <55 years; **5–10%** if **>65 years**; and **20%** if **>80 years**).

- Overall prevalence is similar in ♂ and ♀, but AD is more common in ♀, whereas vascular and mixed dementias are more common in ♂.

- See *Table 13.2.3* and *Key facts 2* for risk factors and genes associated with AD.

Key facts 1: Potentially reversible causes of a major cognitive deficits or dementia

- Hypo- and hyper-thyroidism
- Normal pressure hydrocephalus
- Cushing's/Addison's
- Infections (neurosyphilis, Lyme disease, meningitis, etc.
- Chronic renal, respiratory, or liver failure
- Encephalitis (HIV, limbic, equine, etc.)
- Vitamin deficiency (B_1, B_6, B_{12}, folate)
- Depression (pseudodementia)
- Severe obstructive sleep apnea
- Drug intoxication or withdrawal (CNS depressants, opiates, etc.).

Table 13.2.3: Risk factors for Alzheimer's disease	
Advancing age	• The incidence of AD increases with **advancing age**.
Psychiatric illness	• Depression, bipolar disorder, alcohol dependence.
Family history	• The lifetime risk of AD in first degree relatives of those affected is **25–50%**.
Genetics	• See *Key facts 2*.
Down's syndrome	• The mutations in **trisomy 21** are associated with the development of **early onset AD**.
Low IQ	• Lower educational attainment and **lower IQ** scores are associated with higher risks of developing dementia.
Cerebrovascular disease	• Strong risk factor for **vascular dementia** which can co-exist with AD.
Vascular risk factors	• e.g. Past stroke/MI, smoking, hypertension, diabetes, and high cholesterol are risk factors for both AD and vascular dementia.

Key facts 2: Genetics and Alzheimer's disease

There are several genes which play a role in Alzheimer's disease:
- **Presenilin 1** (chromosome 14), **Presenilin 2** (chromosome 2) and **amyloid precursor protein** (chromosome 21) are genes associated with early onset AD.
- **ApoE-4** (chromosome 19) is a susceptibility gene that contributes to late onset AD. The **ApoE-2** variant is thought to be protective.

Clinical features

DSM-5 Criteria for major neurocognitive disorder

A. Evidence of significant cognitive decline from a previous level of performance in one or more cognitive domains (complex attention, executive function, learning and memory, language, perceptual-motor, or social cognition) based on:
  1. Concern of the individual, a knowledgeable informant, or the clinician that there has been a significant decline in cognitive function; and
  2. A substantial impairment in cognitive performance, preferably documented by standardized neuropsychological testing or, in its absence, another quantified clinical assessment.
B. The cognitive deficits interfere with independence in everyday activities (i.e. at a minimum, requiring assistance with complex instrumental activities of daily living such as paying bills or managing medications).
C. The cognitive deficits do not occur exclusively in the context of a delirium.
D. The cognitive deficits are not better explained by another mental disorder (e.g. major depressive disorder, schizophrenia).

DSM-5 Criteria for major neurocognitive disorder *(continued)*

Specify whether due to:

Alzheimer's disease	**HIV infection**
Frontotemporal lobar degeneration	**Prion disease**
Lewy body disease	**Parkinson's disease**
Vascular disease	**Huntington's disease**
Traumatic brain injury	**Another medical condition**
Substance/medication use	**Multiple etiologies**
Unspecified	

Reprinted with permission from the *Diagnostic and Statistical Manual of Mental Disorders*, 5th Edition, (© 2013). American Psychiatric Association.

Mild neurocognitive disorder occurs when the cognitive deficits are more modest and do not interfere with activities of daily living.

Alzheimer's disease

See *Figs. 13.2.4* and *13.2.5*.

Early stages	Disease progression	Later stages
Memory lapses, difficulty finding words, forgetting names of people/places.	Apraxia, confusion, language problems, difficulty with executive thinking.	Disorientation to time and place, wandering, apathy, incontinence, eating problems, depression, agitation.

Fig. 13.2.4: Symptomatic progression of Alzheimer's disease.

- AD can be classified into **early onset** (<65 yrs, familial) and **late onset** (>65 yrs, sporadic), but it usually occurs after the age of 65. It has an **insidious onset** over years.
- **Loss of memory** is the commonest presenting symptom. Initially there is inability to recall new information, and remote memory (long-term memory) declines with disease progress.
- **Disorientation to time and place** is closely related to memory impairment.

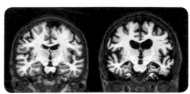

Fig. 13.2.5: MRI scan showing clear evidence of hippocampal atrophy and enlarged ventricles in Alzheimer's disease (right side) compared to control subject (left side).

- **Impairment** of **cognitive** and **executive functions**:
  - **Executive functions:** Problem solving, abstract thinking, reasoning, decision making, judgement, planning, organization and processing.
  - **Visuospatial abilities:** Getting lost, impaired driving, copying figures.
  - **Language disturbances (dysphasia):** Word finding difficulties, decreased vocabulary, perseveration (uncontrollable repetition of a particular response, such as a word, phrase, or gesture), global aphasia (impairment of language, affecting the production or comprehension of speech and the ability to read or write).
  - **Apraxia:** Inability to carry out previously learned purposeful movements despite normal coordination and strength, e.g. dressing, unbuttoning shirt.

> ### Criteria for Alzheimer's disease
>
> A. The general criteria for dementia A–D must be met.
> B. No evidence for any other possible cause of dementia or systemic disorder.
>
> **Early onset Alzheimer's disease**
> A. General criteria for Alzheimer's met and age of onset is <65.
> B. At least one of the following must be met:
> (1) relatively **rapid onset** and **progression;**
> (2) in addition to memory impairment there is **aphasia, agraphia** (↓ ability to communicate through writing), **alexia** (↓ ability to read), **acalculia** (↓ ability to perform mathematical tasks) or **apraxia.**
>
> **Late onset Alzheimer's disease**
> A. General criteria for Alzheimer's met and age of onset is >65.
> B. At least one of the following must be met:
> (1) slow, gradual onset and progression;
> (2) predominance of memory impairment over intellectual impairment.

- **Agnosia:** Impaired recognition of sensory stimuli not attributed to sensory loss or language disturbance, e.g. object agnosia, auditory agnosia.
- **Non-cognitive symptoms: Perception** (hallucinations), **thought content** (delusions), **emotion** (depression, apathy), **behavior** (wandering, aggression, restlessness).

Other common types of dementia (Table 13.2.4)

Table 13.2.4: Clinical features of different types of dementia	
Vascular dementia	• Usually presents in the **late sixties** or **early seventies**. • **Stepwise** rather than continuous deterioration, i.e. stepwise increases in severity of symptoms. • **Memory loss.** • **Emotional** (depression, apathy) and **personality changes** (earlier than memory loss). • **Confusion** is common. • **Neurological symptoms or signs** (e.g. unilateral spastic weakness of the limbs or increased tendon reflexes, an extensor plantar response, or pseudobulbar palsy). • On examination there may be **focal neurology** (often upper motor neuron signs) and **signs of cardiovascular disease** elsewhere.

Table 13.2.4: Clinical features of different types of dementia *(continued)*

Mixed dementia	• Features of both Alzheimer's disease and vascular dementia.
Dementia with Lewy bodies (DLB)	• **Day to day fluctuations** in **cognitive performance.** • Recurrent **visual hallucinations.** • Motor signs of **parkinsonism** (tremor, rigidity, bradykinesia). • **Recurrent falls, syncope, depression.** • Severe sensitivity to neuroleptic drugs. • People with Parkinson's disease who develop dementia **after 12 months** are diagnosed as having **Parkinson's disease with dementia** as opposed to **DLB** where dementia and parkinsonian features occur **within 12 months** of one another.
Fronto-temporal dementia (including Pick's disease)	• Usually occurs between the ages of **50** and **60** and develops insidiously. • **Family history** is positive in 50% of cases. • Early personality changes: e.g. **disinhibition** (reduced control over one's behavior), **apathy/restlessness** (see *Key facts 4* for frontal lobe tests). • **Worsening of social behavior.** • **Repetitive behavior.** • **Language problems:** e.g. difficulty finding word, problems naming/ understanding words. • **Memory is preserved** in early stages whereas insight is lost early.
Huntington's disease	• **Autosomal dominant**, therefore strong family history. • **Abnormal choreiform movements** of face, hands, and shoulders and **gait abnormalities**. • Dementia presents later.
Creutzfeldt– Jakob disease (CJD; prion disease)	• Onset usually **before 65**. • **Rapid progression** with death within 2 years. • **Disintegration** of virtually all **higher cerebral functions**. • Dementia associated with **neurological signs** (pyramidal, extrapyramidal, cerebellar).

OSCE tips 1: A mnemonic for the areas of impairment in dementia (My Cat Loves Eating Pigeons)

Memory, Cognition, Language, Executive functioning, Personality.

Diagnosis and investigations

Hx | **Questions to ask the patient**
- 'Do you find yourself forgetting things? Can you give some examples? When did it begin?'
- 'Do you find yourself forgetting familiar people's names?'
- 'Do you get lost more easily than you used to?', 'Are you able to handle money confidently?'
- 'Do you think being forgetful is stopping you from doing anything?'

Collateral history from informant (Also ask about functional status. See *Key facts 2*)
- 'Are they repetitive in conversation?'
- 'Has their personality changed, for example, are they more irritable or anxious?'
- 'Have you noticed any change in their behavior, for instance being more isolated?'
- 'Are their memory problems getting in the way of their daily life?'
- 'Do you have any concerns about their safety?'

MSE

Appearance & Behavior	May appear unkempt with poor self-care. Behavior may be inappropriate, e.g. in fronto-temporal dementia due to disinhibition. Uncoordinated or restless.	
Speech	Slow, confused. Difficulty finding right word. Repetitive.	
Mood	Low or normal. Disturbance of affect more common in VaD.	
Thought	May have delusions.	
Perception	Hallucinations are a core feature in DLB. May have illusions.	
Cognition	Affected in all dementias but to varying degrees depending on the type and severity of dementia. Memory impairment is most severe in cortical dementias. There is usually impaired attention and disorientation.	
Insight	May be preserved initially but is invariably lost in the latter stages of the disease.	

NOTE: MSE findings will vary depending on the type of dementia and its severity.

Ix

(**NOTE:** Patients presenting with memory impairment are often referred to the **memory clinic**.)

Routine investigations

- **Blood tests: CBC** (infection, anemia); **CRP** (infection, inflammation); **BUN/Cr** (renal disease); **calcium** (hypercalcemia); **LFTs** (alcoholic liver disease); **glucose** (hypoglycemia); **vitamin B$_{12}$** and **folate** (nutritional deficiencies); **TFTs** (hypothyroidism).

Non-routine investigation (guided by clinical assessment)

1. **Urine dipstick:** Rule out UTI.
2. **Chest X-ray:** Pneumonia, lung tumor.
3. **Syphilis serology and HIV testing:** Only if there are atypical features or special risks.
4. **Brain imaging:** Imaging is only indicated for dementia if there is early onset (<60 years), sudden decline, high risk of structural pathology, focal CNS signs or symptoms (to rule out space-occupying lesions, e.g. subdural hematoma, abscess and tumor), or to monitor disease progression.
   - **CT scan:** usual imaging modality. Can identify hippocampal atrophy.
   - **MRI:** identifies posterior circulation vascular pathology with much greater sensitivity.
   - **SPECT:** rarely used in specialist centers to reliably differentiate between Alzheimer's disease, vascular dementia, and fronto-temporal dementia.
5. **ECG:** If cardiovascular disease suspected.
6. **EEG:** If fronto-temporal lobe dementia or CJD is suspected, or where seizure activity is a possibility.
7. **Lumbar puncture:** If meningitis or CJD is suspected.
8. **Genetic tests:** For Huntington's disease and familial dementia.
9. **Cognitive assessment:** Folstein Mini-Mental State Examination (MMSE, see *Key facts 4*), the Abbreviated Mental Test (AMT), General Practitioner Assessment of Cognition (GPCOG), or the Montreal Cognitive Assessment (MOCA).

DDx

- **Normal aging** and **mild cognitive impairment.**
- **Delirium.**
- **Trauma:** Stroke, hypoxic, or traumatic brain injury.
- **Depression ('pseudodementia'):** Poor concentration and impaired memory are common in depression in the elderly. Identify whether the low mood or poor memory came first.

- **Late onset schizophrenia.**
- **Amnesic syndrome:** Severe disruption in memory with minimal deterioration in cognitive functioning.
- **Learning/intellectual disability.**
- **Substance misuse.**
- **Drug side effects:** Opiate, benzodiazepine.

OSCE tips 2: Mini-Mental State Examination and AD

- Normal: MMSE 25–30
- **Mild:** MMSE 21–24
- **Moderate:** MMSE 10–20
- **Moderate–severe:** MMSE 10–14
- **Severe:** MMSE <10.

Key facts 3: Assessment of functional status in dementia patients

Enquire about **functional capacity** in dementia patients. The following areas of functional capacity should be explored: **dressing, continence, self-care, shopping/housework**, ability to manage **financial affairs, social contacts, safety** in the home, **ability to cook, nutrition, orientation**.

Key facts 4: The Folstein Mini-Mental State Examination (MMSE)

Generally speaking, a quick and informal cognitive assessment can be carried out by recording the following:
- Orientation in time, place, and person
- Attention and concentration, e.g. serial sevens test. Record the time taken and the number of errors
- Memory:
  - short-term memory
  - recent memory
  - remote memory
- Grasp, e.g. name the current president

If cognitive impairment is suspected, you can carry out the Folstein Mini-Mental State Examination (MMSE). The MMSE is scored out of 30. Scores of less than 22 are indicative of significant cognitive impairment, while scores of 22 to 25 are indicative of moderate cognitive impairment. The result is invalid if the patient is delirious or has an affective disorder. Due to recent copyright restrictions only some of the items on the MMSE can be reproduced here.

Sample items from the Folstein Mini-Mental State Examination
Orientation to time
"What is the date?"

Registration
"Listen carefully. I am going to say three words. You say them back after I stop. Ready? Here they are . . .
APPLE (pause), PENNY (pause), TABLE (pause). Now repeat those words back to me." [Repeat up to five times, but score only the first trial.]

Naming
"What is this?" [Point to a pencil or pen.]

Reading
"Please read this and do what it says." [Show examinee the words on the stimulus form.]
CLOSE YOUR EYES

Key facts 5: Frontal lobe tests

- There are a number of frontal lobe tests that are useful adjuncts when considering a diagnosis of fronto-temporal dementia.
- *Verbal fluency and initiation:* Ask the patient to recall as many words as possible in one minute starting with the letter 'S'. Fewer than 10 words is abnormal. Should aim for >15.
- *Cognitive estimates:* Ask the patient to make educated guesses to questions which they are unlikely to know the specific answer to, e.g. 'what is the age of the oldest person in the country?'
- *Clock drawing test:* Tests executive function. Ask the patient to draw a large clock face, put the numbers in and then make the clock show ten after five.
- *Similarities (conceptualization):* Ask in what way two objects are alike e.g. banana and orange (both fruits), table and chair (both items of furniture), tulip and rose (both types of flower).
- *Motor sequencing (Luria's 3 step test):* Tell the patient you are going to show them a series of hand movements. Demonstrate fist, edge, palm 5 times without verbal prompts and ask them to repeat.

NOTE: When talking to the patient you may register an expressive dysphasia due to involvement of Broca's area in the frontal lobe.

Management

General points

- After a diagnosis of dementia is made, patients may need, depending on the state they live in, to notify the Department of Motor Vehicles (DMV). They may then be required to report to the DMV for a driver re-examination.
- Early discussions should take place to allow **advance planning** prior to cognition deteriorating. Topics include **advance statements or decisions**, **lasting power of attorney**, and preferred place of care plans.
- In the later stages of the disease, if patients are not competent to make a decision, a capacity evaluation is required.
- **Vascular dementia** is **modifiable** and somewhat **preventable** by targeting cardiovascular risk factors.
- A summary of management strategies in AD is illustrated in *Fig. 13.2.6*.

Non-pharmacological management

- The aims of treatment are to **promote independence**, **maintain function**, and **treat symptoms** including cognitive, non-cognitive (hallucinations, delusions, anxiety, marked agitation, and associated aggressive behavior), behavioral, and psychological (*Fig. 13.2.7*):

First-line

- Supportive treatment (e.g. OT input for home safety evaluation)
- Environmental control measures (e.g. motion sensors for patients at risk of wandering)
- Acetylcholinesterase inhibitors

Adjuncts

- Antidepressants
- Antipsychotics
- Management of insomnia (e.g. trazodone)
- Management of behavioral and psychological symptoms
- Adding in or switching to memantine (initially 5 mg OD)

Fig. 13.2.6: Management strategies in AD.

- **Social support** including support groups such as Alzheimer's Association.
- **Increasing assistance with day-to-day activities**
- **Information and education**
- **Community dementia teams**
- **Home nursing and personal care**
- **Community services** such as Meals on Wheels, befriending services, day centers, respite care, and care homes.
- For non-cognitive symptoms or behavior that challenges, **aromatherapy, massage, therapeutic use of music**, or **animal-assisted therapy** may be considered.

Pharmacological management

- The three **acetylcholinesterase (AChE) inhibitors (donepezil, galantamine, and rivastigmine)** are recommended as options for managing **mild to moderate** Alzheimer's disease (see *Key facts 6*). They can also be used in dementia with Lewy bodies, in cases where non-cognitive symptoms cause significant distress.
- **Memantine** is an **NMDA (*N*-methyl-ᴅ-aspartate) receptor antagonist** and is an option for Alzheimer's disease in the following circumstances:
  - **Moderate** Alzheimer's disease in those who are **intolerant** of or have a **contraindication to AChE inhibitors**.
  - **Severe** Alzheimer's disease.
- For **behavior that challenges**, if non-pharmacological strategies have proved ineffective, a short course of an **antipsychotic** (e.g. risperidone) can be used. However, antipsychotics are associated with increased morbidity and mortality in elderly patients with dementia and are not approved for this purpose. Pimavanserin is approved for hallucinations associated with Parkinson's disease. For **low mood**, **antidepressants** (e.g. sertraline) can be initiated.

NOTE: Use of antipsychotics in dementia with Lewy bodies can cause severe adverse effects including neuroleptic sensitivity reactions or worsening of extrapyramidal features.

Fig. 13.2.7: Principles of dementia management.

Key facts 6: Acetylcholinesterase inhibitors (*BNF*)

- Acetylcholinesterase inhibitors are **centrally acting agents** that work by **compensating for the depletion of acetylcholine** in the **cerebral cortex** and **hippocampus** in AD.
- They are cautioned in arrhythmias (sick sinus syndrome and other supraventricular conduction abnormalities), peptic ulcer disease, and asthma/COPD. Galantamine is contraindicated in severe renal or hepatic impairment.
- Side effects include gastrointestinal disturbances, bradycardia, and muscle spasms. Rivastigmine may cause extrapyramidal side effects.
- Doses: donepezil (5–10 mg OD), rivastigmine (1.5–6 mg BD), galantamine (4–12 mg BD).

Self-assessment

A 75-year-old woman is brought to the memory clinic by her children because she is becoming more forgetful. She used to pay her bills independently and enjoyed cooking but has recently received overdue notices from utility companies and found it difficult to prepare a balanced meal. She left the water running in her bathtub and flooded the bathroom. She denies anything is wrong with her when her children express their concerns. Her Mini-Mental State Examination (MMSE) score is 19/30. You suspect dementia.

1. What is the most likely type of dementia? *(1 point)*
2. What are the microscopic and macroscopic changes in the brain with this disorder? *(4 points)*
3. What routine blood tests should be performed on this patient? *(5 points)*
4. What is the severity of her dementia? *(1 point)*
5. Give six preventable causes of dementia. *(3 points)*
6. Name four non-pharmacological management options for this patient. *(4 points)*
7. Name two pharmacological agents for this patient. *(2 points)*

Answers to self-assessment questions are to be found in *Appendix B*.

Chapter 14

Child psychiatry

14.1	Autism spectrum disorders	162
14.2	Attention deficit hyperactivity disorder	169
14.3	Learning disability	175

Autism spectrum disorders

Child psychiatry encompasses many disorders. This chapter focuses on three of the more common and serious pediatric disorders including disorders in the autism spectrum, ADHD, and intellectual disability.

Definition

Autism spectrum disorders (ASDs) are a type of **pervasive developmental disorder** characterized by deficits in **social interactions** and **communication**, as well as **restricted, stereotyped interests** and **behaviors. Autism spectrum disorders range from mild with minimal deficits (formerly called Asperger's) to severe with profound intellectual, language, and behavioral deficits.**

Pathophysiology/Etiology

The etiology of autism spectrum disorders can be divided into **prenatal**, **perinatal**, and **postpartum**.

Prenatal

- **Genetics:** There is a complex polygenic relationship, with a number of chromosomes implicated, such as **chromosome 7**. There is a significantly increased risk of autism associated with genetic syndromes such as **fragile X syndrome** and **tuberous sclerosis**.
- **Parental age:** A study found that women who are **40 years old** have a **50%** greater chance of having a child with autism as compared with women aged **20–29 years**.
- **Drugs:** Babies who have been exposed to certain medications in the womb have a greater risk of developing autism. These include **sodium valproate** in particular.
- **Infection:** Prenatal viral infections (e.g. **rubella**) increase the risk of autism.

Antenatal

- **Obstetric complications** such as **hypoxia** during childbirth, ↓ **gestational age** at birth, as well as very **low birthweight** offer increased risk of autism.

Postpartum

- **Toxins** such as **lead** and **mercury** may increase the risk of autism.
- **Pesticide exposure** may affect those genetically predisposed to autism.

NOTE: There is no proven link between the MMR vaccine or other vaccines and the development of autism (*Medical Research Council*).

Epidemiology and risk factors (*Table 14.1.1*)

- Autism spectrum disorders affect approximately **1.1%** of the population. The ♂ to ♀ ratio is 4:1.

Table 14.1.1: Risk factors for autism spectrum disorders	
Male	• **Males** are **4 ×** more likely to be affected than females.
Genetics/Family history	• There is an **88% concordance rate** in **monozygotic** twins, indicating a strong genetic component.
Advancing parental age	• Recent studies have suggested that **advancing parental age** is a significant risk factor for ASD.
Parental psychiatric disorders	• Evidence suggests a link between **parental psychiatric disorders** such as schizophrenia and the child having autism.
Prematurity	• Born before **35 weeks'** gestation.
Maternal medication use	• ↑ with mothers receiving sodium valproate during pregnancy.

Clinical features

- The triad of clinical features associated with autism as mentioned in DSM-5 fit the mnemonic '**ABC**' (see *Table 14.1.2*).

Table 14.1.2: Autism triad	
Asocial	• Few social gestures, e.g. waving, nodding, and pointing at objects. • Lack of: Eye contact (gaze avoidance), social smile, response to name, interest in others, emotional expression, sustained relationships, and awareness of social rules.
Behavior restricted	• Restricted, repetitive, and stereotyped behavior, e.g. rocking and twisting. • Upset at any change in daily routine. • Insists on eating the same foods, wearing the same clothes and playing the same games. • Obsessively pursued interests. • Fascination with sensory aspects of environment.
Communication impaired	• Distorted and delayed speech (often the first sign which is noticed). • Echolalia (repetition of words).

- **50%** of parents have cause for concern by **12–18 months** of age. The diagnosis is usually made before the age of 3.

- Other features include: **Intellectual disability (NOTE:** if one includes all on the autistic spectrum, the majority will not have an intellectual disability), **temper tantrums**, **impulsivity**, **cognitive impairment** may be present as associated conditions (see *Key facts 1*).

Key facts 1: Other conditions associated with autism

- **Epileptic seizures:** ~20% develop these.
- **Visual impairment.**
- **Hearing impairment.**
- **Infections.**
- **Pica:** Eating inedible objects.
- **Constipation.**
- **Sleep disorders.**
- **Underlying medical conditions:** PKU, fragile X, tuberous sclerosis, congenital rubella, CMV, or toxoplasmosis.
- **Psychiatric:** ADHD, depression, bipolar affective disorder, anxiety, psychosis, OCD, DSH.

Diagnosis and investigations

Hx
- 'Does your child ever engage in pretend play alone or with others?', 'Does your child struggle to interact with others and make friends?' **(social interaction poor)**
- 'Have you noticed any patterns in their behavior?', 'Does your child insist on the same toys, activities, or foods?', 'Have you noticed them making any abnormal movements such as flapping their hands or walking on tiptoes?' **(repetitive, stereotypical behavior)**
- 'Do they struggle to communicate with you?', 'Have you noticed that their speech is monotonous or repetitive?' **(impaired communication)**
- 'What sort of games does your child play and with what toys?' **(unimaginative play)**
- 'Do you have any concerns about your child's development?' **(developmental history)**

DSM-5 Criteria for autism spectrum disorder

A. Persistent deficits in social communication and social interaction across multiple contexts, as manifested by the following, currently or by history (examples are illustrative, not exhaustive; see text):
  1. Deficits in social-emotional reciprocity, ranging, for example, from abnormal social approach and failure of normal back-and-forth conversation; to reduced sharing of interests, emotions, or affect; to failure to initiate or respond to social interactions.
  2. Deficits in nonverbal communicative behaviors used for social interaction, ranging, for example, from poorly integrated verbal and nonverbal communication; to abnormalities in eye contact and body language or deficits in understanding and use of gestures; to a total lack of facial expressions and nonverbal communication.
  3. Deficits in developing, maintaining, and understanding relationships, ranging, for example, from difficulties adjusting behavior to suit various social contexts; to difficulties in sharing imaginative play or in making friends; to absence of interest in peers.
Specify current severity:
Severity is based on social communication impairments and restricted, repetitive patterns of behavior.
B. Restricted, repetitive patterns of behavior, interests, or activities, as manifested by at least two of the following, currently or by history (examples are illustrative, not exhaustive; see text):
  1. Stereotyped or repetitive motor movements, use of objects, or speech (e.g. simple motor stereotypies, lining up toys or flipping objects, echolalia, idiosyncratic phrases).
  2. Insistence on sameness, inflexible adherence to routines, or ritualized patterns of verbal or nonverbal behavior (e.g. extreme distress at small changes, difficulties with transitions, rigid thinking patterns, greeting rituals, need to take same route or eat same food every day).
  3. Highly restricted, fixated interests that are abnormal in intensity or focus (e.g. strong attachment to or preoccupation with unusual objects, excessively circumscribed or perseverative interests).
  4. Hyper- or hyporeactivity to sensory input or unusual interest in sensory aspects of the environment (e.g. apparent indifference to pain/temperature, adverse response to specific sounds or textures, excessive smelling or touching of objects, visual fascination with lights or movement).

DSM-5 Criteria for autism spectrum disorder *(continued)*

Specify current severity:
Severity is based on social communication impairments and restricted, repetitive patterns of behavior.

C. Symptoms must be present in the early developmental period (but may not become fully manifest until social demands exceed limited capacities, or may be masked by learned strategies in later life).

D. Symptoms cause clinically significant impairment in social, occupational, or other important areas of current functioning.

E. These disturbances are not better explained by intellectual disability (intellectual developmental disorder) or global developmental delay. Intellectual disability and autism spectrum disorder frequently co-occur; to make comorbid diagnoses of autism spectrum disorder and intellectual disability, social communication should be below that expected for general developmental level.

NOTE: Individuals with a well-established DSM-IV diagnosis of autistic disorder, Asperger's disorder, or pervasive developmental disorder not otherwise specified should be given the diagnosis of autism spectrum disorder. Individuals who have marked deficits in social communication, but whose symptoms do not otherwise meet criteria for autism spectrum disorder, should be evaluated for social (pragmatic) communication disorder.

Specify if:
With or without accompanying intellectual impairment
With or without accompanying language impairment
Associated with a known medical or genetic condition or environmental factor
(Coding note: Use additional code to identify the associated medical or genetic condition.)
Associated with another neurodevelopmental, mental, or behavioral disorder
(Coding note: Use additional code[s] to identify the associated neurodevelopmental, mental, or behavioral disorder[s].)
With catatonia (refer to the criteria for catatonia associated with another mental disorder for definition)

Reprinted with permission from the *Diagnostic and Statistical Manual of Mental Disorders*, 5th Edition, (© 2013). American Psychiatric Association.

MSE		
Appearance & Behavior	Ritualized, stereotyped behavior, e.g. clapping, rocking. Poor eye contact, detached. Lack of facial expression and gestures. May attach to unusual items.	
Speech	Delayed speech. Difficulty initiating and maintaining conversation. Repetitive language. May have unusual rate, rhythm, and volume.	
Mood	Normal or have erratic mood changes (can appear to have a labile mood).	
Thought	Obsessions and compulsions. Intense preoccupation with special interests.	
Perception	May be very sensitive to noise, touch, or smell.	
Cognition	Impaired attention but may also be able to concentrate on special interests.	
Insight	May be poor but they may be distressed if aware they are different/don't fit in.	

Ix
- **Full developmental assessment** including family history, pregnancy, birth, medical history, developmental milestones, daily living skills, and assessment of communication, social interaction, and stereotyped behaviors (see *OSCE tips*).
- **Hearing tests** if required.
- **Screening tools** including **CHAT** (**CH**ecklist for **A**utism in **T**oddlers).

DDx
- **Intellectual disability disorder***
- **Rett's syndrome***
- **Childhood disintegrative disorder***

- **Learning disorder**
- **Deafness**
- **Childhood schizophrenia**

*See *Key facts 2*

Key facts 2: Eponymous syndromes: the pervasive developmental disorders

- **Mild autism spectrum disorder** (Asperger's syndrome): Milder abnormalities in social interaction and restricted, stereotyped, repetitive interests and behaviors. Typically there is **no significant impairment in language, cognition, or intelligence (IQ normal)**. It is more prevalent in boys.
- **Rett's syndrome:** Severe, progressive disorder starting in early life. Results in language impairment, repetitive stereotyped hand movements, loss of fine motor skills, irregular breathing, and seizures. Almost exclusively seen in girls. The *MECP2* gene's role in Rett's syndrome has been identified.
- **Childhood disintegrative disorder (Heller's syndrome):** Characterized by two years of normal development followed by loss of previously learned skills (language, social, and motor). Also associated with repetitive, stereotyped interests and behaviors as well as cognitive deterioration.

OSCE tips: The developmental assessment

A full developmental assessment is essential in any child with suspected autism, paying particular attention to **communication** and **social interaction**.
SPEECH and HEARING developmental milestones:
- **3 months** → turns towards sound, quietens to parent's voice.
- **6 months** → double syllables e.g. 'adah'.
- **9 months** → says 'mama' and 'dada'.
- **12 months** → knows and responds to own name.
- **12–15 months** → knows about 2–6 words, understands simple commands.
- **2 years** → combines two words.
- **3 years** → talks in short sentences (e.g. 3–5 words), asks 'what?' and 'who?' questions.
- **4 years** → asks 'when?', 'how?' and 'why?' questions.

SOCIAL BEHAVIOR developmental milestones:
- **6 weeks** → smiles (refer at 10 weeks if not smiling).
- **6 months** → enjoys interaction.
- **1 year** → waves bye-bye.
- **2 years** → interested in other children.
- **3 years** → make-believe play.
- **4 years** → plays with other children.

NOTE: Delays in language and social interaction alone indicate likely autism. Global developmental delay indicates a likely alternative pathology.

Management

General points (*Fig. 14.1.1*)

- Diagnosis should be by a **specialist** (e.g. child psychiatrist) and can be reliably made by **age 3**.
- **Community-based multidisciplinary teams** including pediatricians, psychiatrists, educational psychologists, speech and language therapists, and occupational therapists. A **case manager** to manage and coordinate treatment can be extremely helpful if available.
- **CBT** can be used if the child has the verbal and cognitive ability to engage and is motivated.
- Interventions for life skills include support developing their **daily living skills**, their **coping strategies**, and **enabling access to education and community facilities** such as those related to leisure and sports.
- Ensure all **physical health**, **mental health**, and **behavioral issues** are addressed (*Key facts 1*).
- **Families** and **care-givers** should also be offered personal, social, and emotional **support**. Groups such as the **Autism Association** can point to support groups and other resources for families.
- **Special education programs** may be considered.
- **Melatonin** may be considered for sleep disorders that persist despite behavioral interventions.
- Antipsychotics (risperidone, paliperidone) are FDA approved for treating irritability in autism spectrum disorders.

Interventions for the core features of autism

- **Social-communication intervention** (e.g. play-based strategies).

BIOLOGICAL

- Treat co-existing disorders (e.g. methylphenidate for ADHD).
- Antipsychotics for irritability or disruptive behavior.
- Melatonin.

PSYCHOLOGICAL

- Psychoeducation for families or care-givers.
- Full assessment of the functions of behavior, to understand the child fully.
- CBT.

SOCIAL

- Modification of environmental factors.
- Social-communication intervention.
- Self-help groups such as the National Autism Association.
- Special schooling.

Fig. 14.1.1: Bio-psychosocial approach to management of autism.

Interventions for behavior that challenges

- **Treat co-existing physical disorders** (e.g. epilepsy and constipation) and **mental health** (e.g. anxiety, depression) and **behavioral problems** (e.g. ADHD).
- **Modification of environmental factors** which initiate or maintain challenging behavior, is the **first line** in management (e.g. lighting, noise, social circumstances, and inadvertent reinforcement of challenging behavior).
- **Antipsychotics** may be considered for disruptive behavior or irritability when psychosocial interventions are insufficient or if the features are severe. Risperidone and aripiprazole are FDA-approved for the treatment of irritability associated with autism.

Self-assessment

A mother presents with her 3-year-old boy following concerns about language development. He spoke his first words at 17 months but still does not combine two words. He also seems uninterested in engaging with other children. He occasionally engages with his parents but less than they think he should do, and he has difficulty maintaining eye contact. When he wants something he pulls them to where the object is and screams; he doesn't point like other children. His parents have also noticed that he does not play in the same way as other children of his age; he tends to line toys up, or plays with certain aspects of them, such as the toy car doors.

1. What is the most likely diagnosis? *(1 point)*
2. What other questions would you like to ask in your history? *(3 points)*
3. What is the clinical triad of this condition? *(3 points)*
4. Name three medical conditions associated with this syndrome. *(3 points)*
5. Name four non-pharmacological management approaches to this syndrome. *(2 points)*

Answers to self-assessment questions are to be found in *Appendix B.*

14.2 Attention deficit hyperactivity disorder

Definition

Attention deficit hyperactivity disorder (commonly referred to as ADHD) is characterized by an early onset, persistent pattern of **inattention**, **hyperactivity**, and **impulsivity** that are more frequent and severe than in individuals at a comparable stage of development, and are present in more than one situation. Children may present with difficulties at **school** and at **home**.

NOTE: Adults are now also presenting, wondering whether they have ADHD which was not identified at school.

Pathophysiology/Etiology

- The etiology of ADHD is **multifactorial** (see *Table 14.2.1*).
- It can be divided into **genetic, neurochemical, neurodevelopmental**, and **social**.

Table 14.2.1: Etiology of ADHD	
Genetic	Twin and adoption studies indicate a **genetic predisposition** (concordance rate of **82%** for monozygotic twins). The *DRD4* and *DRD5* genes are thought to play a role.
Neurochemical	There are reports of a link between ADHD and the genes coding for the dopamine system, suggesting an abnormality in the **dopaminergic pathways**.
Neurodevelopmental	Neurodevelopmental abnormalities of the **pre-frontal cortex** are hypothesized based on symptoms of recklessness, inattention, and learning difficulties.
Social	There is an association with **social deprivation** and **family conflict**.

Epidemiology and risk factors (see *Table 14.2.2*)

- The prevalence of ADHD in children is estimated to be around **5–11%** according to the CDC.
- It is **three times** more common in ♂ than ♀.
- The **age of diagnosis** is commonly between **3** and **7** years.

Table 14.2.2: Risk factors for ADHD	
Male	• Males are **three times** more likely to be affected than females.
Family history	• Family history is a strong determinant of ADHD with twin studies reporting about 70% heritability.
Environmental risk factors	• Social deprivation and family conflict as well as parental cannabis and alcohol exposure.

Clinical features (Fig. 14.2.1)

- The **three core features** of ADHD are **inattention**, **hyperactivity**, and **impulsivity**.

Inattention
• Not listening when spoken to.
• Highly distractible (moving from one activity to the next).
• Reluctant to engage in activities that require persistent mental effort, e.g. school work which contains careless mistakes.
• Forgetting or regularly losing belongings.

Hyperactivity
• Restlessness and fidgeting or tapping with hands or feet.
• Recklessness.
• Running and jumping around in inappropriate places.
• Difficulty engaging in quiet activities.
• Excessive talking or noisiness.

Impulsivity
• Difficulty waiting their turn.
• Interrupting others.
• Prematurely blurting out answers.
• Temper tantrums and aggression.
• Disobedient.
• Running into the street without looking.

Fig. 14.2.1: Core features of ADHD: '**I H**appily **I**nterrupt'.

DSM-5 Criteria for attention-deficit/hyperactivity disorder

A. A persistent pattern of inattention and/or hyperactivity-impulsivity that interferes with functioning or development, as characterized by (1) and/or (2):

   1. **Inattention:** Six (or more) of the following symptoms have persisted for at least 6 months to a degree that is inconsistent with developmental level and that negatively impacts directly on social and academic/occupational activities:

   NOTE: The symptoms are not solely a manifestation of oppositional behavior, defiance, hostility, or failure to understand tasks or instructions. For older adolescents and adults (age 17 and older), at least five symptoms are required.

      a. Often fails to give close attention to details or makes careless mistakes in schoolwork, at work, or during other activities (e.g. overlooks or misses details, work is inaccurate).
      b. Often has difficulty sustaining attention in tasks or play activities (e.g. has difficulty remaining focused during lectures, conversations, or lengthy reading).

DSM-5 Criteria for attention-deficit/hyperactivity disorder *(continued)*

    c. Often does not seem to listen when spoken to directly (e.g. mind seems elsewhere, even in the absence of any obvious distraction).

    d. Often does not follow through on instructions and fails to finish schoolwork, chores, or duties in the workplace (e.g. starts tasks but quickly loses focus and is easily sidetracked).

    e. Often has difficulty organizing tasks and activities (e.g. difficulty managing sequential tasks; difficulty keeping materials and belongings in order; messy, disorganized work; has poor time management; fails to meet deadlines).

    f. Often avoids, dislikes, or is reluctant to engage in tasks that require sustained mental effort (e.g. schoolwork or homework; for older adolescents and adults, preparing reports, completing forms, reviewing lengthy papers).

    g. Often loses things necessary for tasks or activities (e.g. school materials, pencils, books, tools, wallets, keys, paperwork, eyeglasses, mobile telephones).

    h. Is often easily distracted by extraneous stimuli (for older adolescents and adults, may include unrelated thoughts).

    i. Is often forgetful in daily activities (e.g. doing chores, running errands; for older adolescents and adults, returning calls, paying bills, keeping appointments).

2. Hyperactivity and impulsivity: Six (or more) of the following symptoms have persisted for at least 6 months to a degree that is inconsistent with developmental level and that negatively impacts directly on social and academic/occupational activities:

    NOTE: The symptoms are not solely a manifestation of oppositional behavior, defiance, hostility, or a failure to understand tasks or instructions. For older adolescents and adults (age 17 and older), at least five symptoms are required.

    a. Often fidgets with or taps hands or feet or squirms in seat.

    b. Often leaves seat in situations when remaining seated is expected (e.g. leaves his or her place in the classroom, in the office or other workplace, or in other situations that require remaining in place).

    c. Often runs about or climbs in situations where it is inappropriate.

    (**NOTE:** In adolescents or adults, may be limited to feeling restless.)

    d. Often unable to play or engage in leisure activities quietly.

    e. Is often "on the go," acting as if "driven by a motor" (e.g. is unable to be or uncomfortable being still for extended time, as in restaurants, meetings; may be experienced by others as being restless or difficult to keep up with).

    f. Often talks excessively.

    g. Often blurts out an answer before a question has been completed (e.g. completes people's sentences; cannot wait for turn in conversation).

    h. Often has difficulty waiting his or her turn (e.g. while waiting in line).

    i. Often interrupts or intrudes on others (e.g. butts into conversations, games, or activities; may start using other people's things without asking or receiving permission; for adolescents and adults, may intrude into or take over what others are doing).

B. Several inattentive or hyperactive-impulsive symptoms were present prior to age 12 years.

C. Several inattentive or hyperactive-impulsive symptoms are present in two or more settings (e.g. at home, school, or work; with friends or relatives; in other activities).

D. There is clear evidence that the symptoms interfere with, or reduce the quality of, social, academic, or occupational functioning.

E. The symptoms do not occur exclusively during the course of schizophrenia or another psychotic disorder and are not better explained by another mental disorder (e.g. mood disorder, anxiety disorder, dissociative disorder, personality disorder, substance intoxication or withdrawal).

DSM-5 Criteria for attention-deficit/hyperactivity disorder *(continued)*

Specify whether:

Combined presentation: If both Criterion A1 (inattention) and Criterion A2 (hyperactivity-impulsivity) are met for the past 6 months.

Predominantly inattentive presentation: If Criterion A1 (inattention) is met but Criterion A2 (hyperactivity-impulsivity) is not met for the past 6 months.

Predominantly hyperactive/impulsive presentation: If Criterion A2 (hyperactivity-impulsivity) is met but Criterion A1 (inattention) is not met over the past 6 months.

Specify if:

In partial remission: When full criteria were previously met, fewer than the full criteria have been met for the past 6 months, and the symptoms still result in impairment in social, academic, or occupational functioning.

Specify current severity:

Mild: Few, if any, symptoms in excess of those required to make the diagnosis are present, and symptoms result in only minor functional impairments.

Moderate: Symptoms or functional impairment between "mild" and "severe" are present.

Severe: Many symptoms in excess of those required to make the diagnosis, or several symptoms that are particularly severe, are present, or the symptoms result in marked impairment in social or occupational functioning.

Reprinted with permission from the *Diagnostic and Statistical Manual of Mental Disorders*, 5th Edition, (© 2013). American Psychiatric Association.

Diagnosis and investigations

Hx   'Do you find that your child...'

1. **Inattention:** '...is reluctant to engage in activities which need sustained mental effort, such as school work?', '...often leaves play activities unfinished?', '...regularly loses their possessions?', '...does not listen when spoken to?'

2. **Hyperactivity:** '...is constantly fidgeting, jumping, or running around?', '...is unable to remain still?', '...is difficult to engage in quiet activities?'

3. **Impulsivity:** '...cannot wait their turn when playing in groups?', '...blurts out answers to questions before the question has been completed?'

OSCE tips: Assessment of ADHD

In a clinical setting, three approaches can be used to assess for ADHD:

1. **Observe the child:** Hyperactivity is relatively easy to elicit but be aware that a child may be overawed by the clinical context, and so any evidence of hyperactivity will be missed if the session is very brief. The child may demonstrate impulsivity by interrupting the parents or blurting out answers.

2. **Speak to the child:** Is the child able to engage in a conversation with you and do they make eye contact? Offer them a toy and see whether they get bored or are easily distracted.

3. **Speak to the parents:** Speaking to the parents will allow you to explore all three core features in more detail and to elicit whether symptoms are present in more than one environment.

MSE		
Appearance & Behavior	Fidgety. Unable to sit still. Running around, jumping, or climbing inappropriately. If toys offered, will flit from one to another. If parents are asked a question, the child replies with the answer before the parents can.
Speech	Talks loudly, even at inappropriate times and makes excessive noise.
Mood	Normal but may be low if co-morbid depressive disorder.
Thought	No disorders of thought.
Perception	No hallucinations.
Cognition	Poor attention levels. Lack of concentration.
Insight	Poor.

Ix

NOTE: As problem behaviors vary in different settings, it is important to obtain information from teachers, as well as the parents and the child. For *adults* seeking a diagnosis, school reports are usually reviewed and a collateral history from parents is helpful.

- **Blood tests** including **TFTs** (to rule out thyroid disease).
- **Hearing tests:** Examine middle/inner ear with an otoscope and consider a pure tone audiogram.
- **Rating scales:** e.g. Conners' rating scale and the Strengths and Difficulties questionnaire.

DDx

- **Learning disorders**
- **Oppositional defiant disorder** (see *Key facts 1*)
- **Conduct disorder** (see *Key facts 1*)
- **Autism**
- **Sleep disorders**
- **Mood disorders** (particularly bipolar)
- **Anxiety disorder**
- **Hearing impairment**

Key facts 1: Co-morbidities including conduct disorder and oppositional defiant disorder

- **70%** of ADHD patients have co-morbidities including **learning difficulties** (e.g. ASD, dyslexia), **dyspraxia**, **Tourette's syndrome**, and **mood/anxiety disorders**.
- **Conduct disorder** (co-exists in **50%** of ADHD children) is a repetitive and severe pattern of antisocial behavior including aggression, destruction of property, deceitfulness (or stealing), and major violations of age-appropriate social expectations. Risk factors include being male, abuse as a child, poor socioeconomic status and parental psychiatric disorders. It is the most common psychiatric disorder of childhood.
- **Oppositional defiant disorder** is defiant and disruptive behavior against authoritative figures but is less severe than conduct disorder, in that violations of law and physical abuse of others are far less common.

Management

General points

- ADHD is diagnosed by specialists and treatment depends on whether the patient is **pre-school**, **school-age**, or **adult**, as well as the **severity** of symptoms.
- **Support** for **parents** and **teachers** is crucial.
- If there is a *clear link* between food or drink consumed and behavior, parents should be advised to keep a food diary and a referral to a dietitian can be made if appropriate.

Pre-school

- **Parent-training** and **education programs** (psychoeducation) are first-line.
- **Parent-training** is **behavioral** with parents being helped to reinforce positive behavior and to find alternative ways of managing disruptive behavior.
- Drug treatments are not recommended.

School-age

- **Psychoeducation** and **CBT** (and/or **social skills training**) should be provided.
- In **severe** ADHD in *school-age* children, **drug treatment is first-line** with the CNS stimulant **methylphenidate** (Ritalin) being a common choice.
- Side effects of CNS stimulants include headache, insomnia, loss of appetite, and weight loss.
- Recent studies show no clear link between *extended* stimulant use and growth retardation.
- Non-stimulant drugs approved for ADHD include atomoxetine, clonidine, and guanfacine.

Self-assessment

An 8-year-old boy presents to the PCP with his father. The father reports that his son has recently been trying to avoid school. His teachers are starting to get frustrated as he stands up unexpectedly in class, disrupts others, seldom finishes work, and shouts out answers without raising his hand. His parents report that he is uncontrollable at home and does not listen.

1. What is the most likely diagnosis? *(1 point)*
2. What are the three core clinical features of this condition? *(3 points)*
3. What questions would you ask the parents? *(3 points)*
4. What is the pharmacological management in school-aged children? *(3 points)*

Answers to self-assessment questions are to be found in *Appendix B.*

14.3 **Learning disability**

14.3 **Learning disability**

Definition (*World Health Organization*)

- An intellectual disability (ID) is a developmental disorder in which an individual has both intellectual and adaptive functioning deficits.
- Deficits occur in three domains: Practical, social, and conceptual.
- DSM-5 divides ID into four levels of severity: Mild, moderate, severe, and profound (see *DSM-5 box*).
- A **triad** must exist to constitute an intellectual disability. This includes (1) **Deficits in intellect** (previously defined as IQ below 70). (2) **Onset at birth** or **during early childhood**. (3) **Wide range of functional impairment** including social handicap due to reduced ability to acquire adaptive skills (activities of daily living).

Pathophysiology/Etiology

- ID can be due to a number of different causes which are highlighted below (*Table 14.3.1*).

Table 14.3.1: Etiology of intellectual disability	
Genetic	Down's syndrome, fragile X syndrome, Cri du chat, Prader–Willi, neurofibromatosis, tuberous sclerosis, Angelman syndrome, homocystinuria, galactosemia (carbohydrate), phenylketonuria (protein), Tay–Sachs disease (lipid), hydrocephaly.
Prenatal	Congenital infection (rubella, CMV, toxoplasmosis), nutritional deficiency, intoxication (alcohol, cocaine, lead), endocrine disorders (hypothyroidism, hypoparathyroidism), physical damage (injury, radiation, hypoxia), antepartum hemorrhage, pre-eclampsia.
Perinatal	Birth asphyxia, intraventricular hemorrhage.
Neonatal	Hypoglycemia, meningitis, neonatal infections, kernicterus, neonatal sepsis.
Postpartum	Infection (e.g. meningitis, encephalitis), anoxia, metabolic (e.g. hypothyroidism, hypernatremia), cerebral palsy.
Environmental	Neglect/non-accidental injury, malnutrition, socioeconomically deprived.
Psychiatric	Autism, Rett's syndrome.

Epidemiology and risk factors

- The prevalence of ID in the US population is 0.5-1%.
- The most common risk factor is a **positive family history** of ID.

Clinical features

- The clinical features of ID vary depending on its degree (see *Table 14.3.2*) as well as if there is any underlying cause, e.g. a congenital syndrome (see *Key facts 1*).
- Common physical disorders include **motor disabilities** (e.g. ataxia, spasticity), **epilepsy**, **impaired hearing and/or vision**, and **incontinence** (fecal and urinary).
- Specific causes are uncommon in mild LD whereas they are usually identifiable in severe or profound LD.

Table 14.3.2: Clinical features of intellectual disability according to severity

Mild ID	Usually identified at a later age when the child starts school. They have **adequate language abilities**, **social skills**, and **self-care**. There may be **difficulties in academic work**. Most **live independently** but may need some support in housing and employment.
Moderate ID	Able to communicate but **language is limited**. May need supervision for self-care but able to do simple work.
Severe ID	There is a **marked degree of motor impairment**. **Little or no speech** in early childhood but may eventually use simple communication. May be able to perform simple tasks under supervision. They may have associated **physical disorders**.
Profound ID	**Severe motor impairment** and **severe difficulties in communication**. Have **little or no self-care**. Frequently have **physical disorders** and require residential care.

Key facts 1: Specific congenital syndromes associated with intellectual disability

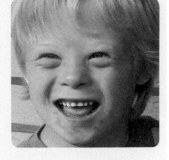

Fig. 14.3.1: Typical facial features of a child with Down's syndrome.

- **Down's syndrome:** A genetic disorder (trisomy 21) characterized by ID, dysmorphic facial features, and multiple structural abnormalities. It is the commonest cause of ID.
  - **Physical features** ('**PROBLEMS**'): **P**alpebral fissure (up slanting), **R**ound face, **O**ccipital + nasal flattening, **B**rushfield spots (pigmented spots on iris)/**B**rachycephaly, **L**ow-set small ears, **E**picanthic folds, **M**outh open + protruding tongue, **S**trabismus (squint)/**S**andal gap deformity/**S**ingle palmar (Simian) crease (*Fig. 14.3.1*).
  - **Medical problems:** heart defects (ventricular and atrial septal defects, ToF), hearing loss, visual disturbance (cataracts, strabismus, keratoconus), GI problems (esophageal/duodenal atresia, Hirschsprung's, celiac), hypothyroidism and hematological malignancies (AML, ALL), increased incidence of Alzheimer's.
- **Fragile X syndrome:** The second most common cause of ID. A sex-linked disorder with developmental, physical, and behavioral problems.
  - **Physical features:** Large, protruding ears, long face, high arched palate, flat feet, soft skin, lax joints.
  - **Medical problems:** Mitral valve prolapse.
- **Prader–Willi:** Due to a deletion of part of chromosome 15. Characterized by hypotonia and developmental delay as an infant, and obesity, hypogonadism, and behavioral problems (compulsive eating, disruptive behavior) in later years.
- **Cri du chat:** Caused by a partial deletion of chromosome 5. Those affected have a high-pitched cry like a cat. Low birth weight and feeding difficulties are also characteristic.

Diagnosis and investigations

DSM-5 Criteria for diagnosis of intellectual disability

Intellectual disability (intellectual developmental disorder) is a disorder with onset during the developmental period that includes both intellectual and adaptive functioning deficits in conceptual, social, and practical domains. The following three criteria must be met:

A. Deficits in intellectual functions, such as reasoning, problem solving, planning, abstract thinking, judgement, academic learning, and learning from experience, confirmed by both clinical assessment and individualized, standardized intelligence testing.

B. Deficits in adaptive functioning that result in failure to meet developmental and sociocultural standards for personal independence and social responsibility. Without ongoing support, the adaptive deficits limit functioning in one or more activities of daily life, such as communication, social participation, and independent living, across multiple environments, such as home, school, work, and community.

C. Onset of intellectual and adaptive deficits during the developmental period.

Specify current severity:

- **Mild**
- **Moderate**
- **Severe**
- **Profound**

The various levels of severity are defined on the basis of adaptive functioning, and not IQ scores, because it is adaptive functioning that determines the level of supports required. Moreover, IQ measures are less valid in the lower end of the IQ range.

Reprinted with permission from the *Diagnostic and Statistical Manual of Mental Disorders*, 5th Edition, (© 2013). American Psychiatric Association.

Hx
- 'Did you have any issues during your pregnancy?', 'Were all of the prenatal scans normal?', 'Was the baby premature?', 'Were there any complications during the delivery?', 'What was the condition of the baby when he/she was born?' (**pregnancy-related factors**)
- 'Is there any history of conditions, specifically learning disability, which run in the family?', 'Do you and your partner have any mutual relatives?' (**family-related factors**)
- Depending on age: 'How does your child cope with daily activities?', 'Did they reach their milestones at the proper time, for instance at what age did they start walking?', 'Do they have any known medical problems?' (**clinical features**)
- Ask about associated medical problems and screen for co-morbid psychiatric problems.

MSE
- **Appearance** will vary depending on the cause of intellectual disability, for example the type of genetic disorder (see *Key facts 1*).
- The extent of **behavior** problems is determined by the level of ID. In more severe cases there may be motor impairment. There is often **speech** disturbance and **mood** can be low or normal.

- **Examinations to be performed:** Cardiovascular, respiratory, neurological (cranial nerves and peripheral), weight/height/head circumference, developmental assessment.

OSCE tips: Tips for communicating with ID patients

- Always greet the patient before greeting the accompanying individual and ensure communication is clear with simple language used.
- Give appropriate time for the patient to respond.
- Use gestures or pictures to explain your point if they struggle to understand.
- **NOTE:** Focus on their abilities not their disabilities.

Key facts 2: Common psychiatric co-morbidities in ID

The following psychiatric disorders are more common in patients with intellectual disability: Early-onset **Alzheimer's disease**, **schizophrenia**, **anxiety** and **depressive** disorders, **autism**, **ADHD**, **eating disorders**, **personality disorders**.

Ix
- **Before birth:** Amniocentesis, chorionic villus sampling, genetic testing, and karyotyping.
  - **For Down's syndrome:** Two methods, (1) Serum screening (β-hCG and pregnancy-associated plasma protein A) + nuchal translucency; (2) Quad test (β-hCG, α-fetoprotein, inhibin A, estriol).
- **After birth:**
  - **Bloods:** CBC (infection), TFTs (hypothyroidism), glucose (hypoglycemia), serology (ToRCH infections).
  - **Brain imaging:** CT head and/or MRI.
  - **IQ** (intelligence quotient) **test**.

DDx See *Table 14.3.1*.

Management

- A **multidisciplinary approach** is vital. Care is provided by a variety of health care professionals including a **psychiatrist, speech and language therapist, specialist nurses, psychologist, occupational therapist, social worker**, and even **teachers** (for educational support).
- The **PCP** must be involved in the care of the individual as **physical health problems are common**. Treatment of co-morbid medical conditions and psychiatric problems is vital.
- **Antipsychotics** are **somewhat effective** in reducing aggressive behavior in children with ID, but carry significant side effects (EPSE, metabolic syndrome, elevations in prolactin, etc.)
- **Behavioral techniques** such as **applied behavioral analysis**, social skills training, and **positive behavior support**, as well as **CBT** can be used. Psychiatrists, mental health nurses, and psychologists can support care providers with these strategies.
- **Family education** is essential and support should be offered through **educational programs** and **voluntary organizations**.
- **Prevention** can be attempted through **genetic counseling** and **prenatal diagnosis**.

Self-assessment

A couple are offered Down's screening for their unborn child. They decide against this. Eight months later after a smooth delivery, you are the doctor who performs the baby check. You note the baby is hypotonic, he has low-set ears and oblique palpebral fissures. You also observe a single palmar crease and auscultate a heart murmur. You suspect trisomy 21.

1. Give three other physical features of Down's syndrome. *(3 points)*
2. Give five other causes of intellectual disability. *(5 points)*
3. Define mild, moderate, and severe ID in terms of intellectual performance. *(3 points)*
4. Name four healthcare professionals that may be involved in patients with LD. *(4 points)*

Answers to self-assessment questions are to be found in *Appendix B.*

Chapter 15

Management

15.1	Psychotherapies	181
15.2	Antidepressants	187
15.3	Antipsychotics	194
15.4	Mood stabilizers	202
15.5	Anxiolytics and hypnotics	207
15.6	Electroconvulsive therapy (ECT)	210
15.7	Transcranial magnetic stimulation (TMS)	213
15.8	Vagus nerve stimulation (VNS)	215

15.1 Psychotherapies

Introduction to psychotherapies

- The basis of **psychological therapy** (or **psychotherapy**) is to help people better understand the way that they feel (*Fig. 15.1.1*).
- The aim of the therapy is to support patients in changing the way they interact with and perceive the world, to come to terms with past stressors and to cope more effectively with current and future stressors.
- Psychotherapies can be used for a variety of psychiatric illnesses, including mild to moderate **depressive illness**, **bipolar affective disorder, schizophrenia**, **eating disorders**, and **personality disorders**.
- Specific therapies also have a place in the management of patients with **learning disabilities, psychosexual problems, substance misuse disorders**, and **chronic psychotic symptoms**.
- The most commonly used forms of psychotherapy are **cognitive behavioral therapy (CBT)** and **psychodynamic psychotherapy**. There are many other psychotherapies derived from these.
- The selection of which psychotherapy to use depends on local availability, practitioner experience, illness factors, and patient choice.

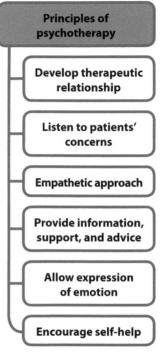

Fig. 15.1.1: Principles of psychotherapy.

Cognitive behavioral therapy (CBT)

- The theory/method of CBT was developed by **Aaron Beck** in the 1960s.
- Indications: Mild–moderate depressive illness, eating disorders, anxiety disorders, BAD, depression, substance use disorders, schizophrenia, and other psychotic disorders as an adjunct to pharmacotherapy, as well as chronic medical conditions (such as fibromyalgia, chronic fatigue syndrome) or chronic pain.
  NOTE: CBT is an active treatment requiring patient understanding and collaboration. Patients should be motivated to participate and be able to recognize, articulate, and link their thoughts and emotions.
- Rationale: Treatment is based on the idea that the disorder is not caused by life events, but by the way the patient views these events (*Fig. 15.1.2*). It is a short-term, collaborative therapy, focused on the 'here and now', the goals of which are symptom relief and the development of new skills to sustain recovery. Some people hold unhelpful core beliefs or 'silent assumptions' that they learn from early, traumatic life experiences. These people are more vulnerable to depression. When exposed to stress at a later date, these core beliefs are activated and they have **negative automatic thoughts** or **cognitive distortions** (*Fig. 15.1.3*).

- **Aim:** The aim of CBT is initially to help individuals to identify and challenge their automatic negative thoughts and then to modify any abnormal underlying core beliefs. The latter is important in reducing risk of relapse (*Fig. 15.1.2*).

- **Modes of delivery:** CBT can be delivered on an **individual** basis, in **groups**, or as **self-help** via **books** or **computer programs** (including online). It is usually fairly brief (12–20 sessions, with 1–2 sessions per week).

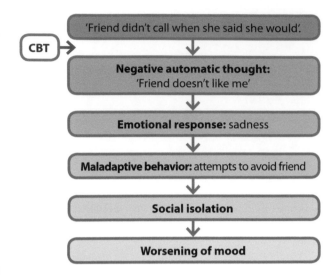

Fig.15.1.2: Thought process that CBT targets.

Selective abstraction

- Focusing on one minor aspect rather than the bigger picture, e.g. 'I have failed that exam because I got one question wrong.'

All or nothing thinking

- Thinking of things in all or nothing terms, e.g. 'If he doesn't see me today it means he hates me.'

Magnification/minimization

- Over- or under-estimating the importance of an event, e.g. 'He didn't talk to me at that meeting, so he must dislike me.'

Catastrophic thinking

- Anticipating the worst possible outcome of an event, e.g. 'I've got a headache. I think I have an underlying brain tumor.'

Overgeneralization

- If one thing is not going well, everything is going wrong, e.g. 'My friend didn't come to see me so she hates me.'

Arbitrary inference

- Coming to a conclusion in the absence of any evidence to support it, e.g. 'No one likes me.'

Fig. 15.1.3: Beck's cognitive distortions or thinking errors.

Behavioral therapies (*Table 15.1.1*)

- Behavioral therapies are based on the **learning theory**, and particularly **operant conditioning**. Operant conditioning states that behavior is reinforced if it has positive consequences for the individual, and it prevents any negative consequences.

Table 15.1.1: Behavioral therapies	
Relaxation training	This is particularly useful for those with **stress-related** and **anxiety disorders**. Here, the patient is asked to use techniques causing muscle relaxation during times of stress or anxiety. The patient also learns to put themselves in situations that they find relaxing, such as walking in the countryside.
Systemic desensitization	This is often used for **phobic anxiety disorders**. In this therapy, an individual is **gradually exposed** to a hierarchy of anxiety-producing situations (*Fig. 15.1.4*).
Flooding	Unlike systemic desensitization, flooding therapy involves the patient rapidly being exposed to the phobic object without any attempt to reduce anxiety beforehand. They are required to continue exposure until the associated anxiety diminishes. It is not a technique commonly used.
Exposure and response prevention (ERP)	This therapy can be used for a variety of anxiety disorders but is particularly useful for **OCD** and **phobias**. Patients are repeatedly exposed to the situation which causes them anxiety (e.g. exposure to dirt) and are prevented from performing the compulsive actions which lessen that anxiety (e.g. washing their hands). After initial anxiety on exposure, the levels of anxiety gradually habituate and decline.
Behavioral activation	This therapy is used for **depressive illness**. The rationale behind it is that patients avoid doing certain things as they feel they will not enjoy them or fear failure in completing them. Behavioral activation involves making realistic and achievable plans to carry out activities and then gradually increasing the amount of activity.

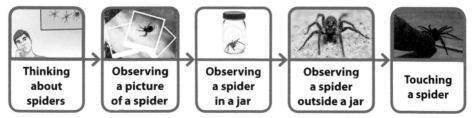

| Thinking about spiders | Observing a picture of a spider | Observing a spider in a jar | Observing a spider outside a jar | Touching a spider |

Fig. 15.1.4: An example of systemic desensitization.

Psychodynamic therapy

- Psychodynamic theories were developed by **Freud**, **Jung**, and **Klein**.
- **Indications:** Dissociative disorders, somatoform disorders, psychosexual disorders, certain personality disorders, chronic dysthymia, recurrent depression.

- **Rationale:** It is based upon the idea that **childhood experiences, past unresolved conflicts,** and **previous relationships** significantly influence an individual's current situation. It is based on psychoanalytic principles.
- **Aim:** The **unconscious** is explored using **free association** (the client says whatever comes to their mind) and the therapist then interprets these statements. Conflicts and defense mechanisms (e.g. denial, projection) are explored and the client subsequently develops insight in order to change their maladaptive behavior.
- There is much emphasis on the relationship between the therapist and patient. Therapies can be offered on an individual, couples, group, or residential community basis.
- Key therapeutic tools:
  1. **Transference:** The patient re-experiences the strong emotions from early important relationships, in their relationship with the therapist. When the current emotions are positive it is said to be positive transference and vice versa for negative emotions.
  2. **Counter-transference:** The therapist is affected by powerful emotions felt by the patient during therapy and reflects what the patient is feeling.
- **Mode of delivery:** Psychoanalysis is an intense therapy that usually involves between one and five 50-minute sessions per week, possibly for a number of years. This is a much longer duration than in CBT.

Other psychosocial interventions

Psychoeducation

- **Psychoeducation (PE)** is the **delivery of information** to people in order to help them **understand** and **cope** with their mental illness.
- It is usual to inform the patient of: 1) the **name and nature** of their illness; 2) likely **causes** of the illness, in their particular case; 3) what the **health services can do to help them**; and 4) what they can do to **help themselves** (self-help). PE may take place individually or in groups, and will usually take the person's own strengths and coping strategies into account.

Counseling

- Counseling is a form of **relieving distress** and is undertaken by means of active **dialogue** between the counselor and the client. It is less technically complicated than other forms of psychotherapy and can range from sympathetic listening to active advice on problem solving.
- **Indications:** Adjustment disorder; mild depressive illness; normal and pathological grief; childhood sexual abuse; other forms of trauma (e.g. rape, postpartum depression, pregnancy loss and stillbirth); substance misuse; chronic medical conditions; and prior to decision making, e.g. genetic testing or HIV testing.
- **Rationale:** Behavior and emotional life are shaped by **previous experience**, the **current environment**, and the **relationships** that individuals have. People have the tendency towards positive change and fulfilment which can be halted by 'life problems'. A collaborative relationship with a counselor is one method of addressing these issues.
- **Aim:** To help the client or patient find their own solutions to problems, while being supported to do so and being guided by appropriate advice.

Supportive psychotherapy

- Is used to describe the psychological support given by mental health professionals to patients with **chronic** and **disabling mental illnesses.**

- It does not aim to produce change, but rather to **help people cope with adversity** or unsolved problems over a sustained period.
- Key elements include active **listening**, providing **reassurance**, providing **explanation** of the patient's illness, providing **guidance** and possible **solutions** to difficulties they are faced with, as well as enabling the patient to express themselves in a safe environment.

Problem-solving therapy

- Consists of a structured combination of **counseling** and **CBT**. It facilitates individuals to learn to deal actively with their life problems by selecting an option for tackling each one, trialing out solutions and reviewing their effect.
- Indications are **mild anxiety** and **depressive disorders**.

Other

Interpersonal therapy (IPT)

- IPT is used to treat **depression** and **eating disorders**.
- The focus is on an **interpersonal problem** such as a complicated bereavement, relationship difficulties or interpersonal deficit, adopting techniques from different psychotherapies. The therapy focuses on the difficulties that arise in relationships and the impact on the individual.
- It has some overlap with CBT and psychodynamic therapy and deals with four interpersonal problems **(grief at the loss of relationships, role disputes within relationships, managing changes in relationships**, and **interpersonal deficits)** which may be causing difficulty in initiating or maintaining relationships.

OSCE tips: Psychotherapy indications	
Adverse life events	PE, counseling, relaxation training.
Depression	PE, counseling, CBT, psychodynamic therapy, IPT, behavioral activation.
PTSD	PE, CBT (trauma focused).
Schizophrenia	PE, CBT, supportive, family therapy.
Eating disorders	PE, CBT, IPT, family therapy, CAT.
Anxiety disorders	PE, CBT, behavioral therapies.
Substance misuse	PE, CBT, motivational interviewing, group therapy.
Borderline personality disorder	PE, DBT, psychodynamic therapy, CAT.

Dialectical behavioral therapy (DBT)

- DBT is used for individuals with **borderline PD, depression, and suicidal and self-harm behaviors**.
- The therapy adopts components of **CBT** and also provides **group skills training** to provide the individual with **alternative coping strategies** (rather than deliberate self-harm) when faced with emotional instability. There are four modules taught in DBT:
  - Mindfulness: Moment to moment awareness of one's feelings.
  - Interpersonal effectiveness: Decrease interpersonal chaos and create boundaries.

- Distress tolerance: Learn how to get through difficult situations without making it worse.
- Emotion regulation: Accept emotions, decrease emotional suffering, and learn not to act only on emotional state.

DBT is often done in a group format but can also be done individually. Sessions are usually 45 minutes and a full course of DBT usually takes around 6 months. Coaching calls in between sessions are often employed.

Format of psychotherapies

In addition to the orientation of the therapy, treatment can be offered in different formats. Therapy may be presented on an **individual, couple, family,** or **group basis** (see *Table 15.1.2*).

Table 15.1.2: Different formats of psychotherapy	
Individual therapy	It is the **most common** format of psychotherapy. It involves confidential interaction between the client and provider, **permitting maximum disclosure**. The majority of evidence for practicing psychotherapy involves individual therapy.
Couples therapy	Allows both partners to overcome **relationship difficulties** with the aid of the therapist. Specific issues may be addressed such as sexual relations and parenting. It is also a valuable adjuvant therapy for **psychiatric disorders** such as **depression** and **substance misuse**. Usually used when relationship problems are maintaining a psychiatric disorder.
Family therapy	Involves family members being seen together. It focuses on the family system and its ability to help both family problems and individual mental illness. Family therapy attempts to correct impaired communication and dysfunctional relationships as a means of helping the entire family including the patient with the disorder. It is particularly useful for **schizophrenia, depression, bipolar affective disorder**, and **conduct disorder**.
Group therapy	Group therapy offers supportive networks for individuals who suffer from similar difficulties. Group therapy can involve cognitive, psychodynamic, and supportive therapies. It is often used for **bereavement, substance misuse**, and **chronic conditions**.

Antidepressants

Introduction to antidepressants

- Antidepressants are drugs used for the treatment of **moderate** to **severe depressive episodes**.
- They are also used for a range of other conditions including **anxiety** and **panic attacks**, **obsessive–compulsive disorder (OCD)**, **chronic pain**, **eating disorders**, and **post-traumatic stress disorder (PTSD)**.
- Antidepressants were first developed in the **1950s and 1960s**.
- Most current antidepressants work (see *Section 3.2*, Depressive disorder) by enhancing the activity of the **monoamine neurotransmitters**, norepinephrine (NE) and serotonin (5-HT) (*Fig. 15.2.1*).
- There are over 30 antidepressants available today and there are six main groups (see *Table 15.2.1*).

Table 15.2.1: Classes of antidepressants

Abbreviation	Full name
SSRI	Selective Serotonin Reuptake Inhibitor
SNRI	Serotonin and Norepinephrine Reuptake Inhibitor
TCA	Tricyclic Antidepressant
MAOI	Monoamine Oxidase Inhibitor
NMDA antagonists	*N*-Methyl-D-Aspartate antagonists
5-HT2A	Serotonin 5-HT2 receptor antagonist

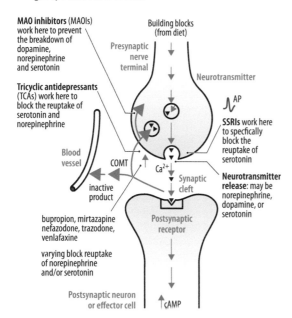

MAO inhibitors (MAOIs) work here to prevent the breakdown of dopamine, norepinephrine and serotonin

Tricyclic antidepressants (TCAs) work here to block the reuptake of serotonin and norepinephrine

Building blocks (from diet)

Presynaptic nerve terminal

Neurotransmitter

AP

SSRIs work here to specfically block the reuptake of serotonin

Blood vessel

COMT

Ca²⁺

inactive product

Synaptic cleft

Neurotransmitter release: may be norepinephrine, dopamine, or serotonin

bupropion, mirtazapine nefazodone, trazodone, venlafaxine

Postsynaptic receptor

varying block reuptake of norepinephrine and/or serotonin

Postsynaptic neuron or effector cell

↑cAMP

Fig. 15.2.1: The mechanism of action of SSRIs, TCAs, and MAOIs.

OSCE tips 1: Responding too well to antidepressants!

Be cognizant of those patients who have a rapid and exaggerated response to antidepressants, as all antidepressants can switch people with bipolar affective disorder from a depressive to a manic state. Indeed, bipolar affective disorder may be undiagnosed if the previous manic episode has not been picked up in the history or if they are yet to suffer from the manic episode.

- **SSRIs** tend to be well tolerated, easy to use, and fairly safe in overdose. Therefore, they are generally considered **first-line** for depression (see *Table 15.2.2*).
- Most antidepressants take **4–8 weeks** at a therapeutic dose before the maximum benefits are seen.
  - Newer antidepressants such as esketamine and brexanolone may show benefits in hours to days.
- SNRIs, mirtazapine, NMDA antagonists, and 5-HT2As antagonists are discussed in *Table 15.2.3*.

Selective serotonin reuptake inhibitors (SSRIs) (*Table 15.2.2*)

Table 15.2.2: SSRI treatment	
Examples	Citalopram, escitalopram, fluoxetine, paroxetine, sertraline, fluvoxamine.
Indications	**Depression** (all SSRIs), **panic disorder** (citalopram, escitalopram, paroxetine), **social phobia** (escitalopram, paroxetine), **bulimia nervosa** (fluoxetine), OCD (most SSRIs), PTSD (paroxetine, sertraline), GAD (paroxetine). **NOTE:** Fluvoxamine is not regularly prescribed as it is a cytochrome P450 enzyme inhibitor and therefore commonly interacts with other medications, potentiating their effects.
Mechanism of action	They work by inhibiting the reuptake of serotonin from the synaptic cleft into presynaptic neurons and therefore SSRIs **increase the concentration of serotonin** in the synaptic cleft.
Side effects (GI side effects & STRESS)	**Gastrointestinal:** nausea, dyspepsia, bloating, flatulence, diarrhea and constipation. **S**weating, **T**remor, **R**ashes, **E**xtrapyramidal side effects (uncommon), **S**exual dysfunction (loss of libido, delayed orgasm), **S**omnolence, 'Stopping SSRI' symptoms (discontinuation syndrome) – GI symptoms, 'chills', insomnia, hypomania, anxiety, and restlessness.
Contraindications and cautions	**Cautions:** History of mania, epilepsy, acute angle-closure glaucoma, diabetes mellitus (monitor glycemic control after initiation), concomitant use with drugs that cause bleeding, GI bleeding (or history of GI bleeding), hepatic/renal impairment, pregnancy and breastfeeding, young adults (possible ↑ suicide risk), suicidal ideation. **Contraindications:** Mania.
Dosage	**Sertraline** (50–200 mg/day), **fluoxetine** (20–60 mg/day), **citalopram** (20–40 mg/day), **escitalopram** (10–20 mg/day), **paroxetine** (20–60 mg/day).
Route	Oral.

OSCE tips 2: Choosing the right antidepressant

There are a number of factors which influence the type of antidepressant prescribed to a patient:

1. **Overall safety profile:** Most guidelines suggest SSRIs as first choice because of their safety profile in overdose as well as their effectiveness. Bupropion, mirtazapine, and SNRIs are also reasonable first choices.
2. **Patient preference:** After discussing side effects of each antidepressant, it is appropriate and important to involve the patient in the decision making.
3. **Prior treatment:** If a patient has had benefit from a previously used antidepressant, that same one should be used, provided no contraindications have developed; equally if an antidepressant has already been tried and not benefited, another one should be trialed.
4. **Type and severity of depression:** SSRIs are usually indicated for all severities of depression and when there is mixed anxiety and depression. In SSRI-resistant cases, SNRIs should be tried. When insomnia is present or weight gain is desired, mirtazapine can be given.
5. **Suicidal ideation:** Avoid drugs that are lethal in overdose such as TCAs and MAOIs (see *Key facts 2*). SSRIs should still be used with caution and appropriate review (see *DO* and *DO NOT* boxes).
6. **Age and co-morbidities:** SSRIs are usually the safest in elderly. Sertraline is the safest drug post-MI. See *Table 15.2.2* for all other cautions and contraindications.
7. **Drug–drug interactions: MAOIs contraindicated**. Avoid SSRIs in those on blood-thinning agents such as warfarin, heparin, and the newer anticoagulant agents (e.g. rivaroxaban, apixaban and dabigatran), as well as NSAIDs. See *BNF* if in doubt.
8. **Pregnancy and breastfeeding:** All antidepressants should be used with caution and if required, the lowest effective dose should be used. Sertraline and fluoxetine are the safest during pregnancy along with some TCAs such as amitriptyline.
9. **History of mania:** All antidepressants have the potential to trigger a manic episode but avoid TCAs and SNRIs which may be more problematic.

Key facts 1: Serotonin syndrome

- The **serotonin syndrome** is a **rare** but **life-threatening complication** of increased serotonin activity, usually rapidly occurring within minutes of taking the medication.
- It is most commonly caused by **MAOIs** combined with any serotonergic agent, including SSRIs, SNRIs, TCAs, triptans, meperidine, and other serotonergic agents.
- Clinical features include:
  1. **Cognitive effects** → headache, agitation, hypomania, confusion, hallucinations, and coma.
  2. **Autonomic effects** → shivering, sweating, hyperthermia, hypertension, and tachycardia.
  3. **Somatic effects** → myoclonus (muscle twitching), hyperreflexia, and tremor.
- Management involves stopping the offending drug and supportive measures.

Table 15.2.3: Overview of SNRIs, mirtazapine, NARIs and 5-HT2As (NOTE: All of the following medications are given via the oral route, except ketamine(s))

Group	Examples and doses	Indication	Mechanism of action	Side effects	Cautions
Serotonin and norepinephrine reuptake inhibitors (SNRIs)	Venlafaxine (75 mg/day in divided doses), duloxetine (60–120 mg/day)	Second or third line in the treatment of **depression** and **anxiety disorders**. SNRIs have a more rapid onset of action and are more effective than SSRIs (for major depression).	SNRIs work by preventing the reuptake of norepinephrine and serotonin but do not block cholinergic receptors and therefore do not have as many anti-cholinergic side effects as TCAs.	Nausea, dry mouth, headache, dizziness, sexual dysfunction, hypertension.	**Cautions** → similar to SSRIs. **Contraindications** → venlafaxine is associated with high risk of cardiac arrhythmia, uncontrolled hypertension, or if patient is on MAOIs.
Mixed norepinephrine serotonin specific antidepressant	Mirtazapine (15–45 mg/day)	Often used for **depressed patients** who would benefit from weight gain and who suffer from **insomnia**, e.g. geriatric patients. Low sexual side effects.	Mirtazapine has a weak norepinephrine reuptake inhibiting effect, has anti-histaminergic properties and is an α1 and α2 blocker. It therefore ↑ appetite and is a sedative.	↑ Appetite, weight gain, dry mouth, postural hypotension, edema, drowsiness, fatigue, tremor, dizziness, abnormal dreams, confusion, anxiety, somnolence.	Elderly, cardiac disorders, hypotension, urinary retention, susceptibility to angle-closure glaucoma, diabetes, psychoses (may aggravate psychotic symptoms).
NMDA receptor antagonists	Ketamine (IV 0.5 mg/kg), esketamine (56–84 mg intranasal)	Treatment-resistant depression, suicidality.	NMDA receptor antagonist.	Nausea, dissociation, addiction, hypertension, tachycardia, psychosis.	History of drug addiction, bipolar disorder, psychosis, uropathy.
5-HT2 antagonists	Trazodone (150–600 mg/day in divided doses)	**Depressive illness,** particularly where **sedation** is required. Anxiety and insomnia. Low sexual side effects.	A serotonin receptor antagonist.	Minimal anticholinergic side effects and relatively low cardiotoxicity compared with TCAs. May cause sedation, GI side effects, orthostatic hypotension, priapism.	History of orthostatic hypotension, priapism, on other sedating drugs.

Selective serotonin reuptake inhibitors

DO:	DO NOT:
• Prescribe SSRIs **first-line for moderate to severe depression** unless contraindicated. • Be cautious when prescribing to children and adolescents – **fluoxetine** is the drug of choice in this age group. • Prescribe **sertraline post myocardial infarction** as there is more evidence for its safe use in this situation over other antidepressants. • Review patients after **2 weeks** of prescribing SSRIs – patients **<30 years** of age or at ↑ **risk of suicide** should be reviewed after **1 week**. • Warn patients about side effects – GI and sexual side effects being the most common. • Counsel patients to be vigilant for ↑ **anxiety** and **agitation** after starting an SSRI.	• Co-prescribe MAOIs and NSAIDs, but if you have to prescribe an NSAID, prescribe a **proton pump inhibitor** too. • Co-prescribe **heparin/warfarin**. • Stop SSRIs suddenly – if stopping an SSRI, the dose should be gradually reduced over a **4 week period** (this is not necessary with fluoxetine). • Prescribe **citalopram** in congenital **long QT syndrome**, known pre-existing QT interval prolongation, or in conjunction with other medicines that prolong the QT interval, as they are associated with dose-dependent QT interval prolongation.

Serotonin and norepinephrine reuptake inhibitors (Table 15.2.3)

OSCE tips 3: SNRIs and cardiac disease

SNRIs should be used with caution in patients with advanced cardiac disease and uncontrolled hypertension. Blood pressure measurement should be taken before starting venlafaxine and should be monitored regularly thereafter.

Tricyclic antidepressants (TCAs) (Table 15.2.4)

Table 15.2.4: TCA treatment (*BNF 2015*)

Examples	Amitriptyline, clomipramine, doxepin, imipramine, nortriptyline, trimipramine.
Indications	Depressive illness, insomnia, nocturnal enuresis in children, insomnia, anxiety disorders, neuropathic pain (not FDA-approved), migraine prophylaxis (not FDA-approved).
Mechanism of action	TCAs work by inhibiting the reuptake of norepinephrine and serotonin in the synaptic cleft. They also have affinity for cholinergic receptors and 5-HT2 receptors and these contribute to side effects.
Side effects	**Anticholinergic:** dry mouth, constipation, urinary retention, blurred vision, confusion. **Cardiovascular:** arrhythmias, postural hypotension, tachycardia, syncope, sweating. **Hypersensitivity reactions:** urticarial, photosensitivity. **Psychiatric:** hypomania/mania, confusion or delirium (especially in elderly). **Metabolic:** ↑ appetite and weight gain, changes in blood glucose levels. **Endocrine:** testicular enlargement, gynecomastia, galactorrhea. **Neurological:** convulsions, movement disorders and dyskinesias, dysarthria, paresthesia, taste disturbances, tinnitus. **Others:** headache, sexual dysfunction, and tremor.

Table 15.2.4: TCA treatment (*BNF 2015*) *(continued)*

Contraindications and cautions	**Cautions** → cardiac disease, history of epilepsy, pregnancy, breast-feeding, elderly, hepatic impairment, thyroid disease, pheochromocytoma, history of mania, psychoses (may aggravate psychotic symptoms), susceptibility to angle-closure glaucoma, history of urinary retention, concurrent electroconvulsive therapy; drowsiness may affect performance of skilled tasks (e.g. driving); effects of alcohol enhanced. **Contraindications** → acutely suicidal patients, recent myocardial infarction, arrhythmias (particularly heart block), mania, severe liver disease, agranulocytosis.
Dosage	**Amitriptyline** (50–200 mg/day), **doxepin** (30–300 mg/day, up to 100 mg as single dose), **imipramine** (50–200mg/day, up to 100 mg as single dose), **clomipramine** (30–250 mg/day in divided doses or as a single dose at bedtime).
Route	Oral (tablet/solution).

Monoamine oxidase inhibitors (MAOIs) (*Table 15.2.5*)

Table 15.2.5: MAOI treatment

Examples	• Irreversible: **Phenelzine**, isocarboxide, transdermal selegiline.
Indications	• Third-line for depression: atypical or treatment-resistant depression. **NOTE:** Its use is substantially limited by toxicity, interaction with food and inferior efficacy compared to SSRIs and TCAs (see *Key facts 2*). • Social phobia.
Mechanism of action	• MAOIs inactivate monoamine oxidase enzymes that oxidize the monoamine neurotransmitters dopamine, noradrenaline, serotonin (5-HT), and tyramine. • There are two main forms of MAO enzymes: MAO-A and MAO-B. Selegiline MAOIs bind selectively to MAO-A, therefore nullifying the need for dietary restrictions at lower doses.
Side effects	**Cardiovascular** (postural hypotension, arrhythmias), **neuropsychiatric** (drowsiness/insomnia, headache), **GI** (↑ appetite, weight gain), **sexual** (anorgasmia), **hepatic** (↑ LFTs), **hypertensive reactions** with tyramine-containing foods (see *Key facts 2*).
Contraindications and cautions	**Cautions** → Suicidal patients, thyrotoxicosis, hepatic impairment, in bipolar disorders (may provoke manic episodes), pregnancy and breast-feeding. **Contraindications** → acute confusional states, pheochromocytoma, any serotonergic drug (see *Key facts 1*), high tyramine foods (see below).
Dosage	See *BNF*.
Route	Oral.

Key facts 2: Limited use of MAOIs!

- MAOIs also metabolize **tyramine**; therefore, eating tyramine-rich foods such as aged **cheese**, **pickled herring**, **liver** (of beef or chicken), and some **red wine** can cause **hypertensive crisis**. These foods should be avoided when taking MAOIs.
- Clinical features of the **hypertensive crisis: headache**, **palpitations**, fever, **convulsions**, and **coma**.
- MAOIs also interact with other drugs including any serotonergic drug (SSRIs, SNRIs), some opiates (meperidine), sympathomimetics (OTC cold preparation, stimulants).

Antipsychotics

Types of antipsychotics

- The first of the antipsychotics (also known as neuroleptics), **chlorpromazine**, was introduced in **1951** for anesthetic premedication and was noted to reduce delusions and hallucinations in schizophrenia.
- A distinction is made between typical (first generation) and atypical (second generation) antipsychotics (see *Table 15.3.1*). The difference between these groups is primarily the extent to which they cause **extrapyramidal side effects** (EPSE).
- **Atypical (2nd generation) antipsychotics** should be used **first-line** in patients with **schizophrenia**. The main advantage of the atypical agents is a significant reduction in extrapyramidal side effects, though these agents are more commonly associated with metabolic side effects.
- The efficacy of different antipsychotics is similar, therefore the choice of drug is often determined by the side effect profile and price. An exception is **clozapine**. Clozapine is the only antipsychotic that has been found to be superior in efficacy to other antipsychotics and is therefore indicated for **treatment-resistant schizophrenia**.

Indications for antipsychotics

- Antipsychotics are indicated for patients suffering from psychotic symptoms such as delusions and hallucinations. They are the **mainstay of treatment for schizophrenia** (*Fig. 15.3.1*). They are much less effective for **negative** or **cognitive symptoms** of schizophrenia.
- They can also be used for other conditions when they present with positive psychotic symptoms (e.g. delusions and hallucinations) such as **depression, mania, delusional disorders, acute and transient psychotic disorders, delirium**, and **dementia**, as well as those with **violent** or **dangerously impulsive behavior** and **psychomotor agitation**.
  - Antipsychotics are first line treatments for bipolar disorder, mania, depression, and maintenance treatment. They are also FDA-approved in the augmentation of antidepressant response in unipolar depression.
  - Aripiprazole and risperidone are approved for irritability in autism spectrum disorders.
- Clozapine is used as a **third-line treatment** for schizophrenia and it is the only antipsychotic that has evidence that it is more effective than other antipsychotics.
- Clozapine should generally only be prescribed after *failing to respond to two other antipsychotics* (**treatment-resistant schizophrenia**).

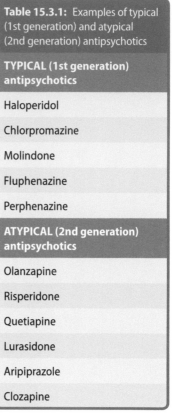

Table 15.3.1: Examples of typical (1st generation) and atypical (2nd generation) antipsychotics

TYPICAL (1st generation) antipsychotics
Haloperidol
Chlorpromazine
Molindone
Fluphenazine
Perphenazine

ATYPICAL (2nd generation) antipsychotics
Olanzapine
Risperidone
Quetiapine
Lurasidone
Aripiprazole
Clozapine

Mechanism of action

- Antipsychotics have actions on numerous **receptors** in the brain (*Fig. 15.3.2*).

- 1st generation antipsychotics treat psychosis by **blocking dopamine-2 (D2) receptors** in the brain (*Fig. 15.3.3*). The mechanism of action of 2nd generation antipsychotics varies, but unlike 1st generation antipsychotics, they have more **serotonergic effects (5HT-2 antagonism)**.

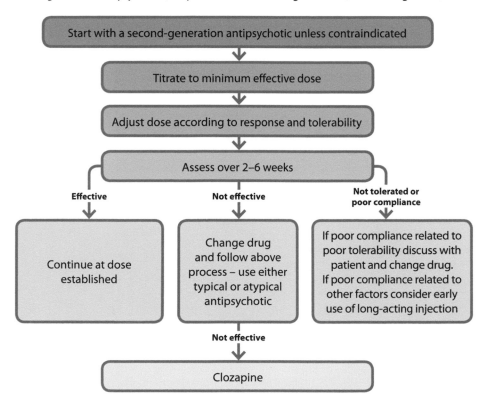

Fig. 15.3.1: Treatment of first-episode schizophrenia (adapted from *The Maudsley Prescribing Guidelines in Psychiatry*, 2015).

Anti-dopaminergic

- All antipsychotics work on **D2/D3** receptors to **reduce dopamine transmission**.
- **1st generation antipsychotics** usually have a **higher affinity**.

Serotonergic

- Mostly **2nd generation antipsychotics**.
- Thought to improve affective symptoms and modestly improve negative symptoms.
- Responsible for **metabolic side effects** (see *Mechanism of action*).

Anti-histaminergic, anti-adrenergic, anti-cholinergic

- Blocking of these receptors is responsible for many side effects (see *Mechanism of action*).

Fig. 15.3.2: The receptors that antipsychotics act upon.

- One of the main properties of antipsychotics is that they **block dopamine receptors**, in particular **D2 receptors**. However, they also have an affinity for **muscarinic, 5HT, histaminergic**, and **adrenergic** receptors, which explains their side effect profile:

  - **Extrapyramidal side effects** are more common in typical antipsychotics (see *Key facts 1*).

  - **Anti-muscarinic** ('can't see, can't wee, can't spit, can't s**t') – blurred vision (**can't see**), urinary retention (**can't wee**), dry mouth (**can't spit**), constipation (**can't s**t**).

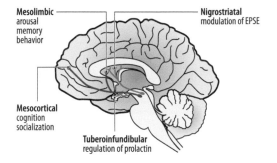

Fig. 15.3.3: Antipsychotics work on the **mesolimbic** and **mesocortical dopamine pathways** to inhibit positive and negative symptoms of schizophrenia, respectively. Antipsychotics cause EPSE via the **nigrostriatal pathway** and endocrine side effects via the **tuberoinfundibular pathway**.

  - **Anti-histaminergic:** sedation and weight gain.

  - **Anti-adrenergic:** postural hypotension, tachycardia, and ejaculatory failure.

  - **Endocrine/metabolic:** ↑ **prolactin** (sexual dysfunction, reduced bone mineral density, menstrual disturbances, breast enlargement, and galactorrhea), impaired glucose tolerance, hypercholesterolemia.

  - **Neuroleptic malignant syndrome** (see *Key facts 2*).

  - **Prolonged QT interval:** QT interval prolongation is a particular concern with pimozide and haloperidol. There is a higher probability in any antipsychotic drug (or combination of drugs) with doses exceeding the recommended maximum. Cases of sudden death have occurred through fatal arrhythmias (e.g. torsades de pointes).

- **Clozapine** has the specific side effects of **hypersalivation** (patients may wake up with their pillows soaked with saliva) and **agranulocytosis** requiring special monitoring (see *Table 15.3.2*). Clozapine may also cause syncope and lower the seizure threshold.

NOTE: Typical antipsychotics are more likely to cause EPSE and hyperprolactinemia but atypical antipsychotics are more likely to cause anticholinergic and metabolic side effects.

Key facts 1: Extrapyramidal side effects (**PAD-T**)

Extrapyramidal side effects (EPSE) are a major problem especially amongst typical (first generation) antipsychotics. There are four main types of EPSE:
1. **Parkinsonism:** Bradykinesia, ↑ rigidity, coarse tremor, masked facies (expressionless face), shuffling gait. This typically takes **weeks or months** to occur (*Fig. 15.3.4*).
2. **Akathisia:** Unpleasant feeling of restlessness. Occurs in the **first months** of treatment. It is managed by reducing the dose of antipsychotic and temporarily giving propranolol.
3. **Dystonia:** Acute painful contractions (spasms) of muscles in the neck, jaw, and eyes (oculogyric crisis). This can occur within **days** (*Fig. 15.3.4*).
4. **Tardive dyskinesia: Late onset (years)** of choreoathetoid movement (abnormal, involuntary movements). May occur in up to 20% of patients and may be irreversible. Most commonly presents as oral-buccal chewing, tongue protrusion, and smacking of the lips (*Fig. 15.3.4*).

Key facts 2: Neuroleptic malignant syndrome

- **Definition:** Neuroleptic malignant syndrome (NMS) is a rare but life-threatening condition seen in patients taking antipsychotic medications. It may also occur with dopaminergic drugs (such as levodopa) for Parkinson's disease, usually when the drug is suddenly stopped or the dose reduced.
- **Epidemiology:** Carries a mortality of up to 10%. It is more common in young male patients.
- **Clinical features:** Onset usually in first 10 days of treatment or after increasing dose. Presents with pyrexia, muscular rigidity, confusion, fluctuating consciousness, and autonomic instability (e.g. tachycardia, fluctuating blood pressure). May have delirium.
- **Investigations:** CK (↑ creatinine kinase is usual), CBC (leukocytosis may be seen), LFTs (deranged).
- **Management:** Stop antipsychotic, monitor vital signs, IV fluids to prevent renal failure, cooling, dantrolene (muscle relaxant) may be useful in select cases, bromocriptine (a dopamine agonist) may be used, consider benzodiazepines.
- **Complications:** Pulmonary embolism, renal failure, shock.

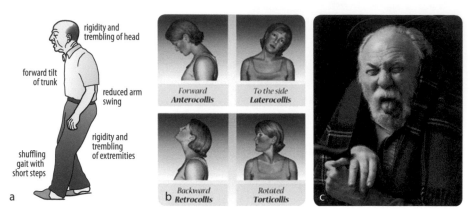

Fig. 15.3.4: (a) Parkinsonian features; (b) Dystonia; (c) Tardive dyskinesia.

Cautions and contraindications

- **Cautions:** Cardiovascular disease (an ECG may be required), Parkinson's disease (may be exacerbated by antipsychotics), epilepsy (and other conditions predisposing to seizures), depression, myasthenia gravis, prostatic hypertrophy, susceptibility to angle-closure glaucoma, severe respiratory disease, history of jaundice, blood dyscrasias (perform blood counts if unexplained infection or fever develops).

- **Contraindications:** History of NMS, comatose states, CNS depression, pheochromocytoma.

Monitoring (Table 15.3.2)

Table 15.3.2: Antipsychotic monitoring	
Investigation	*BNF* **advice**
CBC, BUN/Cr, and LFTs	Monitoring is required at the **start** of therapy with antipsychotic drugs, and then **annually** thereafter. **Clozapine** requires **absolute neutrophil counts** monitoring **weekly** for the **first 6 months** then every 2 weeks for months 6–12, and then **monthly** as part of the clozapine patient monitoring service.
Fasting blood glucose	Should be measured at **baseline**, at **4–6 months**, and then **yearly**. Patients taking **clozapine** or **olanzapine** should have fasting blood glucose tested at **baseline**, after **one month's** treatment, then every **4–6 months**.
Blood lipids	Should be measured at **baseline**, at **3 months** then **yearly** to detect antipsychotic-induced changes.
ECG	**Before** initiating antipsychotic drugs, an ECG may be required, particularly if physical examination identifies cardiovascular risk factors, if there is a personal history of cardiovascular disease, or if the patient is being admitted as an inpatient. ECG monitoring is advised for **haloperidol** and mandatory for **pimozide**. Check in particular for prolonged QT interval.

Table 15.3.2: Antipsychotic monitoring *(continued)*

Investigation	*BNF* advice
Blood pressure	Monitoring is advised **before** starting therapy and frequently during dose titration of antipsychotic drugs. Orthostatic hypotension more common with low potency 1st generation drugs (e.g. chlorpromazine) and clozapine.
Prolactin	It is advisable to monitor prolactin concentration at the **start** of therapy, at **6 months**, and then yearly. Needed less with aripiprazole and clozapine.
Weight	Including waist size and BMI (if possible). Should be measured at **baseline**, **frequently for 3 months** then **yearly** to detect antipsychotic-induced changes.
Physical health	Patients with schizophrenia should have physical health monitoring (including cardiovascular disease risk assessment) at least **once per year**.
Creatine phosphokinase	Baseline CK. Then measure if neuroleptic malignant syndrome is suspected.

OSCE tips: Stopping antipsychotics

- It should be recommended to patients for antipsychotics to be continued for at least 1–2 years following an episode of psychosis and some recommend continuing for 5 years to prevent relapse.
- Patients tend not to adhere to this advice and stop taking antipsychotics much before this. It is therefore essential to take appropriate measures to improve compliance.
- If stopping antipsychotics, it is important to advise patients to taper their medication over a period of approximately 3 weeks as opposed to stopping suddenly. The relapse rate in the first 6 months after abrupt withdrawal is double that seen after gradual withdrawal.

Route and dose

- The mode of administration of antipsychotics is usually **oral**.
- Some of the antipsychotics can also be given by short-acting **intramuscular (IM) injection**.
- Some antipsychotics can be given as **long-acting injections every 1–3 months** (see *Key facts 3*).
- The patient should be started on the lowest possible dose and then the dose should be titrated to the lowest dose known to be effective. Dose increases should then take place only after 1 or 2 weeks of assessment during which the patient shows poor or no response. Typical doses of 1st and 2nd generation antipsychotics are listed in *Table 15.3.3*.

Key facts 3: Long-acting injectable antipsychotic drugs

- These are **long-acting**, **slow release** medications given **intramuscularly** every **1–3 months**.
- There are numerous 1st generation antipsychotic injectables such as **haloperidol** and **fluphenazine**, and several 2nd generation drugs (**risperidone**, **olanzapine** and **aripiprazole**).
- Long-acting injections **bypass first-pass metabolism**.
- They are used to **improve adherence** with medication for patients who may find it difficult to take oral medication regularly.

Table 15.3.3: Doses for 1st generation vs. 2nd generation antipsychotics

1st generation antipsychotics

Name	Route	
	Oral	Intramuscular
Haloperidol	2–20 mg	2–12 mg (short-acting injection). A long-acting Haldol depot is also available 50–300 mg (every 4 weeks)
Chlorpromazine	75–300 mg but up to 1 g daily may be required	IM short-acting is available but rarely used
Fluphenazine	n/a	25 mg (every 2 weeks)

2nd generation antipsychotics

Name	Route	
	Oral	Intramuscular
Olanzapine	5–20 mg	150–300 mg (every 2–4 weeks)
Risperidone	2–16 mg	25–50 mg (every 2 weeks)
Quetiapine	50–750 mg	n/a
Lurasidone	40–120 mg	n/a
Aripiprazole	10–30 mg	400 mg (monthly)
Clozapine	200–900 mg	n/a

Key facts 4: 1st generation antipsychotics vs. 2nd generation antipsychotics	
1st generation antipsychotics	**2nd generation antipsychotics**
Have more **extrapyramidal side effects**	Have fewer **extrapyramidal side effects**
Less **tolerability**	Overall greater **tolerability**
↓ Efficacy against **depressive** and **negative** symptoms	↑ Efficacy against **depressive** and **cognitive** symptoms
Metabolic syndrome less likely	**Metabolic syndrome** more likely
Weight gain less likely	**Weight gain** more likely
Less associated with **type 2 diabetes**	More associated with **type 2 diabetes**
Less associated with **CVA in the elderly**	More associated with **CVA in the elderly**
More likely to cause **tardive dyskinesia**	Less likely to cause **tardive dyskinesia**
More likely to cause **high prolactin** levels	Less likely to cause **high prolactin** levels (aripiprazole, clozapine)

Antipsychotic medication	
DO:	**DO NOT:**
• Discuss the benefit and side effect profile with each patient before starting antipsychotics. • Start the patient on the lowest possible dose and then the dose should be titrated. • Perform **ECG** and **bloods** before starting on antipsychotic (see *Table 15.3.2*). • Monitor and record the following regularly: **efficacy**, **side effects**, **adherence**, **physical health**, **nutritional status**, rationale for **continuing**, **changing**, **or stopping medication**. • Consider offering **depot/long-lasting injectable** antipsychotic medication to avoid non-adherence (intentional or unintentional). • Offer **clozapine** to people who have not responded adequately to at least two different antipsychotic medications.	• Use a loading dose of antipsychotic medication. • Routinely initiate regular combined antipsychotic medication (except for short periods, e.g. when changing medication). • Stop the antipsychotics in between schizophrenic episodes. • Prescribe antipsychotics without thought in patients with a significant cardiovascular history. • Stop antipsychotics abruptly.

Introduction to mood stabilizers

- **Mood stabilizers** are drugs that are used to **prevent depression** and **mania** in **bipolar affective disorder** and **schizoaffective disorder**.
- **Lithium** was the first to be used in the treatment of bipolar disorder in the early 1950s.
- Other mood stabilizers were initially introduced as **anti-epileptic drugs** but later found to have therapeutic effects in patients with bipolar disorder (**sodium valproate, carbamazepine, and lamotrigine**).
- **2nd generation antipsychotics** have a rapid onset of action compared to the mood stabilizers and so can be used in an **acute manic episode** (*Fig. 15.4.1*). They are also used to prevent episodes of mania and are the only drugs approved to treat **bipolar depression**. They are also used in maintenance treatment.

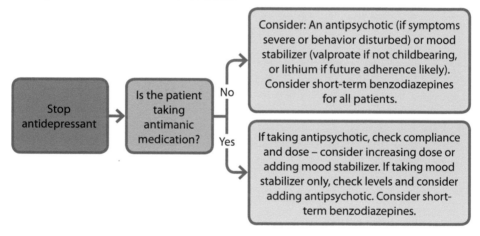

Fig. 15.4.1: Treatment of acute mania or hypomania.

Lithium

See *Section 3.3*, Bipolar affective disorder, and *Table 15.4.1*.

Table 15.4.1: Lithium treatment	
Indications	First-line prophylaxis (maintenance Rx) in **bipolar affective disorder**. Also effective in an **acute manic episode** (if a 2nd generation antipsychotic is ineffective) and as an adjunctive treatment for **depression**.
Mechanism of action	Lithium is an element in the body that is handled in a similar way to sodium. There is some evidence that bipolar patients have an ↑ intracellular concentration of sodium and calcium, and that lithium can ↓ these. With lithium, a decreased activity of sodium-dependent intracellular secondary messenger systems has been shown, as well as modulation of dopamine and serotonin neurotransmitter pathways, ↓ activity of protein kinase C, and ↓ turnover of arachidonic acid. Lithium may also have neuroprotective effects mediated through its effects on *N*-methyl-ᴅ-aspartate (NMDA).

Table 15.4.1: Lithium treatment *(continued)*

Side effects (GI & 'LITHIUM')	**GI disturbances, Leukocytosis, Impaired renal function, Tremor** (fine)/ **Teratogenic, Thirst** (polydipsia), **Hypothyroidism/Hair loss, Increased weight and fluid retention, Urine** ↑ (polyuria), **Metallic taste.** *In toxicity* ('**TOXIC**'): **Tremor** (coarse), **Oliguric renal failure, AtaXia, Increased reflexes, Convulsions/Coma/Consciousness** ↓. **NOTE:** Normal therapeutic levels of lithium are **0.5–1.2 mmol/L**. Toxic levels are **>1.5 mmol/L** (lithium has a narrow therapeutic window).
Contraindications and cautions	Avoid in **renal failure, pregnancy** (teratogenic), and **breastfeeding**. Caution with **QT prolongation** (including concomitant use of drugs that ↑ QT interval), **epilepsy** (↓ seizure threshold), **diuretic therapy**. Lithium is contraindicated in **untreated hypothyroidism, Addison's** disease, and **Brugada syndrome** (heart disease with ↑ risk of sudden cardiac death).
Monitoring	• *Before lithium treatment* is started **BUN/Cr** and **eGFR** (lithium has renal excretion and may be nephrotoxic), **TFTs, pregnancy status**, and baseline **ECG** should be checked. Drug levels should be closely monitored and patients should be informed of potential side effects and toxicity. • **Lithium levels** should be monitored **12 hours** following the first dose, then **weekly** until **therapeutic level (0.4–1.0 mmol/L)** has been stable for **4 weeks**. Once stable check every **3 months**. • **BUN/Cr** should be checked every **6 months**. • **TFTs** should be checked every **12 months**.
Dosage	Usually given as lithium carbonate. Must be given for at least **18 months** for clear benefit. Starting dose **400 mg** at night. Titrate dose **(400–1200 mg/day)** to keep plasma levels between **0.5** and **1.2 mmol/L**.
Route	Oral.

Lithium therapy

DO:	DO NOT:
• Check **lithium levels (12 hours post dose)**, at least **every 3–6 months** and during any intercurrent illness (can ↑ causing toxicity). • At each consultation, ask about any signs of toxicity or **signs of hypothyroidism**. • Check **thyroid function, BUN/Cr, calcium**, and **creatinine** every **6–12 months**. • Inform patients: of **potential toxicity** and symptoms of this; the need for **contraceptives** in women of child-bearing age; the need for **regular fluid intake**; the need for compliance in taking medication; of the dangers of crash diets; to **avoid NSAIDs**; not to exceed more than 1 drink of alcohol per day; that it takes **3–6 months** to be established on lithium, and that **lithium cards** are available from pharmacists.	• Prescribe if you are unfamiliar with the drug. • Give lithium to women who **plan to become pregnant**. Lithium is **teratogenic** and can cause **congenital heart defects** (Ebstein's anomaly). • Give in **severe renal failure**. • **Prescribe NSAIDs, diuretics** (particularly thiazides), or **ACE inhibitors** without careful thought. • Prescribe lithium if you feel that adherence to treatment will be a problem. • **Withdraw lithium abruptly**. Abrupt withdrawal (either because of poor compliance or rapid change in dose) can precipitate relapse. Withdraw lithium slowly over several weeks, monitoring for signs of relapse.

Key facts: Management of lithium toxicity

- Lithium toxicity is a **medical emergency** which can lead to **seizures**, **coma**, and **death**.
- Lithium toxicity is enhanced by the 4 Ds: **D**ehydration, **D**rugs (ACE inhibitors, NSAIDs), **D**iuretics (thiazide), **D**epletion of sodium.
- If signs of toxicity are identified, lithium should be **stopped immediately**.
- A **high intake of fluid** should be provided including **intravenous sodium chloride** therapy, to stimulate **osmotic diuresis**. In the most severe cases, **renal dialysis** may be needed.

Sodium valproate (Table 15.4.2)

Table 15.4.2: Sodium valproate (valproic acid) treatment

Indications	Comparable efficacy to lithium as a mood stabilizer. If lithium (and a 2nd generation antipsychotic) is ineffective or unsuitable in acute mania. Used in combination with lithium for rapid cycling bipolar affective disorder.
Mechanism of action	Valproate is a simple branched-chain fatty acid. It is thought to inhibit the catabolism of GABA, ↓ turnover of arachidonic acid and activate extracellular signal-regulated kinase. This alters synaptic plasticity, interferes with intracellular signaling, promotes brain-derived neurotrophic factor (BDNF) expression and ↓ levels of protein kinase C.
Side effects (GI & VALPROATE)	**GI disturbances**, **V**ery fat (↑ **weight**), lowered **A**ggression, **L**FTs ↑, **P**latelets low (thrombocytopenia), **R**eversible hair loss (in 10%), **O**edema (peripheral), **A**taxia, **T**remor/**T**iredness/**T**eratogenic, **E**mesis.
Contraindications	Avoid in **pregnancy** (can cause neural tube defects in the fetus and result in **spina bifida and lowered infant IQ**), **hepatic dysfunction**, and **porphyria**.
Monitoring	**CBC** (to check platelets) before therapy and before any surgery. Monitor **LFTs** and **prothrombin time (PT)** before therapy and during **first 6 months. Pregnancy test** and **weight/BMI** before commencing. Check LFTs, CBC and weight again after 6 months then annually.
Dosage	Dose started at **250–500 mg** daily, and subsequently titrated upwards.
Route	Oral. IV only used for epilepsy.

Carbamazepine (Table 15.4.3)

Table 15.4.3: Carbamazepine treatment

Indications	Mania (**not first-line**), prophylaxis of bipolar affective disorder unresponsive to lithium. Alcohol withdrawal.
Mechanism of action	Carbamazepine blocks voltage-dependent sodium channels, and therefore inhibits repetitive neuronal firing. It ↓ glutamate release and ↓ turnover of dopamine and norepinephrine.
Side effects	**GI disturbances, dermatitis, dizziness, hyponatremia, blood disorders**, e.g. leukopenia, aplastic anemia, thrombocytopenia.

Table 15.4.3: Carbamazepine treatment *(continued)*

Contraindications	Caution in **cardiac disease** and **blood disorders**. Contraindicated in **AV conduction abnormalities** and **acute porphyria**. Avoid in **pregnancy** (can cause neural tube defects in the fetus). MAOIs are contraindicated. **NOTE:** Is a **potent CYP450 3A4 enzyme inducer** so many drugs will be metabolized faster. These include oral contraceptives, some antipsychotics, calcium channel blockers, some HIV meds, etc.
Monitoring	Check CBC. Measure **plasma carbamazepine levels** if signs of toxicity. **LFTs** and electrolytes (hyponatremia). Baseline measure of weight is desirable.
Dosage	Start at **400 mg daily** in **divided doses**. Build up (max 1.6 g/day).
Route	Oral.

OSCE tips: Mood stabilizer counseling

Mood stabilizers are dangerous drugs in that they have many side effects, can reach toxic levels, and interact with numerous other drugs. A simple and effective tip for providing information on mood stabilizers is to offer your patient an **information leaflet** providing details of what to avoid, side effects, and what to do if features of toxicity arise. This is a potential additional mark that the examiner will award for your communication and for aiding patient understanding.

Lamotrigine *(Table 15.4.4)*

Table 15.4.4: Lamotrigine treatment

Indications	Used as a maintenance treatment to prevent episodes of depression and mania. It is less teratogenic than the other mood stabilizers and therefore usually the drug of choice in women of child-bearing age. Lamotrigine does not treat or prevent manic episodes.
Mechanism of action	Lamotrigine is thought to work by inhibition of sodium and calcium channels in presynaptic neurons and subsequent stabilization of the neuronal membrane.
Side effects	**GI disturbances**, **rash** (in around 10% of patients), **headache** and **tremor**. Risk of **Stevens–Johnson syndrome** (SJS) in 0.04%.
Contraindications	A combination of **lamotrigine** and **valproate** may increase the risk of SJS and requires slower titration of the valproate.

Table 15.4.4:	Lamotrigine treatment *(continued)*
Monitoring	**LFTs**, **CBC** and **electrolytes** prior to starting. Do not routinely measure plasma lamotrigine levels unless there is evidence of ineffectiveness, poor adherence or toxicity. **NOTE:** Inform patients to see doctor if signs of hypersensitivity, e.g. severe rash, fever, lymphadenopathy (antiepileptic hypersensitivity syndrome).
Dosage	Must be initiated very gradually beginning at **12.5–25 mg daily**. **NOTE:** Avoid abrupt withdrawal (unless serious SJS rash).
Route	Oral.

NOTE: Medication side effects are commonly asked about in exams and if stuck, remember: any drug that is consumed orally always has the potential to cause GI disturbances!

Introduction to anxiolytics and hypnotics

- **Anxiolytics** (previously called minor tranquilizers) are any drugs that are used for a variety of anxiety disorders. They are called **hypnotics** if they are used to induce sleep.

- **Benzodiazepines** (BZD) used to be the main drug choice for anxiety disorders, but with increasing knowledge that these drugs cause **dependency** and **withdrawal effects**, the *first-line* drugs for anxiety disorders are **antidepressants**, notably SSRIs.

- Other drugs that can be used as anxiolytics are **barbiturates** (not used any more due to side effect profile and toxicity in overdose), **buspirone, gabapentin, pregabalin, antihistamines (hydroxyzine), beta-blockers** and **antipsychotics**.

- Hypnotics are used to improve sleep but are generally used short term.

- The following drugs can be used as hypnotics: **Benzodiazepines**, low dose **amitriptyline**, trazodone, quetiapine, mirtazapine, suvorexant, so-called **Z** drugs: **Zopiclone**, **Zolpidem**, and **Zaleplon**.

Benzodiazepines (*Table 15.5.1*)

Table 15.5.1: Benzodiazepine treatment

Examples	**Long-acting** (>24 hours duration of action): diazepam, chlordiazepoxide, clonazepam, flurazepam. **Short-acting** (<12 hours duration of action): lorazepam, oxazepam, temazepam, midazolam, triazolam.
Indications (in psychiatry)	(1) **Insomnia** (short-term use). (2) **Anxiety disorders** including panic disorder and phobic anxiety disorder. They are indicated for short-term (2–4 weeks) relief if the anxiety disorder is severe, disabling, or causing the patient unacceptable stress. (3) **Delirium tremens** and **alcohol detoxification:** Chlordiazepoxide is commonly used, starting with a dose that is high enough to control withdrawal symptoms and then reducing over approximately a week. (4) **Acute psychosis:** Adjunctive to antipsychotics for sedation. (5) **Depression:** Adjunctive to treat associated anxiety and insomnia.
Mechanism of action	BZDs enhance the effect of the **inhibitory** neurotransmitter **gamma-aminobutyric acid (GABA)** by increasing the **frequency** of chloride channels via the benzodiazepine-binding site of the **GABA-A receptor**. These receptors are located throughout the cortex and limbic system in the brain and function to inhibit neuronal activity.
Side effects	Drowsiness and light-headedness the next day, confusion and ataxia (especially in the elderly), amnesia, dependence; paradoxical increase in aggression, muscle weakness, respiratory depression. See *BNF* for full list of side effects.
Cautions and contraindications	Respiratory depression and hepatic impairment (where they can precipitate coma). See *BNF* for full list.
Dosage	**Diazepam:** 2–5 mg OD or BD (PO). **Lorazepam:** 0.5–4 mg QDS (PO, IV or IM). Max. dose 4 mg/24 hours. See *BNF* for doses of other benzodiazepines.
Route	**PO** (most common); **IM, IV,** and **PR** benzodiazepine preparations are used mainly for non-compliant patients and status epilepticus.

Key facts 1: Overdose of benzodiazepines and management

- Benzodiazepines can be dangerous in overdose (particularly in combination with other CNS depressants such as alcohol). Clinical features of benzodiazepine overdose include: **ataxia**, **dysarthria**, **nystagmus**, **coma**, **respiratory depression**.
- As with all emergencies, an **ABCDE** approach should be adopted and **IV flumazenil** should be given as the specific antidote for BZD poisoning.

Key facts 2: Benzodiazepine withdrawal syndrome

May develop at any time up to **3 weeks** after stopping a long-acting benzodiazepine, but may occur within a day in the case of a short-acting one. Effects include **insomnia**, **anxiety**, **loss of appetite**, **tremor**, **muscle twitching**, **sweating**, **tinnitus**, **perceptual disturbances**, and **seizures** (rarely).

Other anxiolytics/hypnotics (Table 15.5.2)

Table 15.5.2: Anxiolytics other than BZDs	
Antidepressants	Antidepressants are approved for a variety of anxiety disorders. **SSRIs** and **SNRIs** are first-line and are particularly useful for **OCD, GAD, social anxiety and panic disorder**. Unlike BZDs their optimal effectiveness is delayed. They are not addictive and therefore can be used long term.
Propranolol	Beta-blockers (antagonists), notably **propranolol** at a starting dose of 10–40 mg can be used in anxiety disorder for reducing somatic symptoms such as tachycardia, palpitations, and tremor. Contraindicated in asthma, COPD, bronchospasm, heart block, marked hypotension, and acute left ventricular failure.
Buspirone	Buspirone is a **non-sedating** anxiolytic that can be used for **GAD**. It works as a 5HT-1A partial agonist. It does not cause dependence, but its anxiolytic effect develops more slowly. Side effects include nausea, headache, light-headedness, and dizziness.
Barbiturates	Examples include **phenobarbital**, **secobarbital**, **amobarbital sodium**. Like benzodiazepines they act on GABA-A receptors. They were used as antiepileptics as well as anxiolytic medication. Due to their side effect profile and their toxicity in overdose they have now mainly been replaced by BZDs, and are no longer used.
Pregabalin	Pregabalin and gabapentin do not act directly on GABA-A, but rather are inhibitors of glutamate, norepinephrine, and substance-P. They are anticonvulsants and are approved to be used in **GAD**, and are also used for neuropathic pain. Side effects include dizziness, drowsiness, blurred vision, diplopia, confusion, and vivid dreams.

Table 15.5.2: Anxiolytics other than BZDs *(continued)*

The 'Z' drugs	Include **zopiclone**, **zolpidem**, and **zaleplon**. They work like BZDs by enhancing GABA transmission but are mainly used as hypnotics as they have shorter half-lives, reduced risk of tolerance and dependence and reduced psychomotor and hangover effects as compared to BZDs.
Antipsychotics	Antipsychotics are potent anxiolytics. However, their side effect profile does not make them suitable to be used as anxiolytics in their own right.

Anxiolytics and hypnotics

DO:	DO NOT:
• **Wean** patients off benzodiazepines as sudden cessation can cause benzodiazepine withdrawal syndrome. • Warn patients that hypnotics and anxiolytics may **impair judgement** and **increase reaction time**, and so affect their ability to drive or operate machinery. • Use benzodiazepines for insomnia only when it is **severe**, **disabling**, or causing the patient **extreme distress**. This should only be for a short period of time. • Warn patients that consuming alcohol can enhance sedative effects of hypnotics and sometimes cause dangerous respiratory depression.	• Prescribe in patients with a history of alcohol or other abuse. • Routinely prescribe benzodiazepines **long term**. They should not generally be prescribed for more than **2–4 weeks** (however, some patients may use benzodiazepines and hypnotics safely long term (zolpidem and eszopiclone are approved for chronic use). • Use benzodiazepines to treat short-term 'mild' anxiety. • **Withdraw** anxiolytics **abruptly**. • Forget alternatives – **antidepressants** have secondary anxiolytic effects and are safer for long-term use.

Electroconvulsive therapy (ECT)

Definition

Electroconvulsive therapy (ECT) involves the passage of a **small electrical current** through the brain with a view to inducing a **modified epileptic seizure** which is **therapeutic**.

Background

- ECT was developed in the **late 1930s** by Ugo **Cerletti** and Lucio **Bini**, building on earlier work by **Ladislas Meduna**.
- It was initially used **without general anesthetic** or **muscle relaxants.**
- The mechanism of action is not fully understood. ECT affects **multiple CNS components** including hormones, nerve growth factors, neurotransmitters, and the blood–brain barrier.
- Evidence supporting ECT includes the **Assessment Report**[1] which analyzed **90 randomized controlled trials**. This found real ECT to be more effective than placebo ECT. It also reported *no* evidence to suggest mortality is greater with ECT versus any other minor procedure with the use of general anesthetic.

What it involves

- ECT is only performed by **psychiatrists** under controlled conditions. A thorough **pre-anesthetic assessment** (with physical examination, blood tests, ECG, and chest radiograph) is required to ensure patient safety.

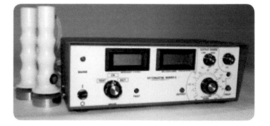

- An **electric current** is applied (via **electrodes**) to the patient's skull, aiming to induce a seizure for at least **30 seconds**. (An ECT machine is shown in *Fig. 15.6.1.*)

Fig. 15.6.1: ECT machine.

- The procedure occurs under **general anesthetic**.
- A **muscle relaxant** (e.g. succinylcholine) is given by the **anesthetist** which **limits the motor effects** of the seizure.
- One electrode can be placed on each side of the head (**bilateral** ECT) or both electrodes on the **non-dominant cerebral hemisphere** alone (**unilateral** ECT).
- **Bilateral** ECT has been shown to be **more effective** but with **more cognitive side effects**.
- Unilateral is considered if **cognitive side effects** were suffered with previous ECT, and in the **elderly**.
- Physiologically, there are **EEG changes** which are monitored (*Fig. 15.6.2*). The **pulse** and **BP** ↑ and **cerebral blood flow** ↑ **by 200%**.
- The patient usually requires around **6–12 treatment sessions**, delivered 3 times a week.

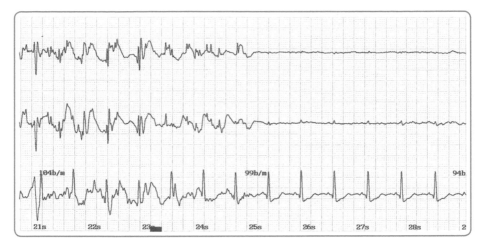

Fig. 15.6.2: EEG trace during ECT, showing initial seizure activity and termination of the seizure.

- The **seizure threshold** is the minimum electrical stimulus required to induce a seizure and it is used in calculating the electrical current dose. Several drugs affect this threshold:

   Drugs which ↑ seizure threshold: Anesthetic drugs, anticonvulsants, benzodiazepines, barbiturates.

   Drugs which ↓ seizure threshold: Antipsychotics, antidepressants (TCAs, SSRIs, MAOIs), lithium.

Indications

The main indications for ECT are 'ECT' (**Euphoric Catatonic Tearful**):

1. **Prolonged or severe mania** (Euphoric).
2. **Catatonia** (Catatonic).
3. **Severe depression** (Tearful):
   - Treatment-resistant depression.
   - Imminent suicide risk.
   - Life-threatening depression, e.g. when the patient refuses to eat or drink.
   - Psychotic features.

Key facts 1: Consent
<ul><li>ECT is a procedure where **written, informed consent** is vital.</li><li>For most patients, an independent second opinion should be obtained to determine suitability for ECT.</li></ul>

NOTE: (1) **Severe depression** is the **most common indication** for the use of ECT.
(2) The use in schizophrenia is controversial, with critics claiming that it is harmful and that it invades patient autonomy.

Side effects (Table 15.6.1)

Table 15.6.1: Side effects of ECT	
SHORT-TERM side effects ('CC DAMS')	**LONG-TERM side effects**
Cardiac arrhythmias, Confusion	**Anterograde and retrograde amnesia** – the deficit is greater in those who receive bilateral ECT versus unilateral ECT.
Dental and **oral trauma**	
Anesthetic risks → laryngospasm, sore throat, N+V	
Muscular aches and **headaches**	
Short-term memory impairment, Status epilepticus	

NOTE: ECT may precipitate a manic episode in patients with bipolar affective disorder.

Relative contraindications ('MARS')

- **MI** (<3 months ago), **Major unstable vertebral fracture**.
- **Aneurysm** (cerebral).
- **Raised ICP**, e.g. intracranial bleed, space-occupying lesion (the **only absolute contraindication**).
- **Stroke** <1 month ago, a history of **Status epilepticus**, **Severe anesthetic risk** (e.g. severe cardiovascular or respiratory disease).

Key facts 2: ECT and mortality

The mortality rate from the use of anesthesia is higher than from the ECT itself. The number of deaths resulting from ECT is estimated to be **1 per 10 000 patients**.

NOTE: The risks associated with ECT may be enhanced during **pregnancy**, in **older people**, and in **children**. Therefore clinicians should exercise particular caution in these groups.

[1] The School of Health and Related Research, University of Sheffield and Nuffield Institute for Health, University of Leeds, ECT for Depressive Illness, Schizophrenia, Catatonia and Mania, May 2002.

15.7 Transcranial magnetic stimulation (TMS)

Definition

Transcranial magnetic stimulation is a non-invasive neuromodulation device (*Fig. 15.7.1*) that uses magnetic fields to stimulate or inhibit neuronal firing.

Background

- Modern TMS was introduced by Anthony Barker and colleagues in 1985 as a way of non-invasively mapping the brain.
- In the mid-1990s TMS began to be actively studied in the treatment of major depression.
- The use of TMS is currently being studied in a variety of mental disorders.

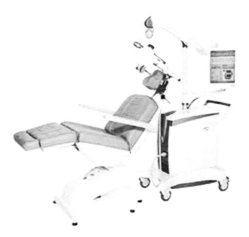

Fig. 15.7.1: A Neuronetics TMS device.

What it involves

- TMS involves the application of a magnetic coil to the scalp.
- The two most common coils are the figure 8 and H coils. The figure 8 coil allows focused superficial stimulation, while the H coil allows more diffuse but deeper stimulation.
- At higher frequencies (>10 Hz) magnetic pulses stimulate underlying cortical tissue, while lower frequencies are inhibitory.
- The standard brain targets are the dorsolateral pre-frontal cortex for depression and the medial frontal and supplementary motor area for OCD.
- TMS treatments usually last 10–40 mins and are done 5 days/week for 4–6 weeks.
- TMS does not require general anesthesia and is usually done on an outpatient basis.

Indications

- Currently, the FDA has approved TMS for the treatment of major depression and OCD in which medications have been poorly tolerated or are incompletely effective.
- TMS does not appear to be as effective as ECT in the treatment of depression so is typically not used in psychotic depression, catatonia, and or imminently life-threatening depression.
- Other potential psychiatric indications under study include PTSD, bipolar depression, negative symptoms of schizophrenia, auditory hallucinations in psychotic disorders, cognitive decline in early Alzheimer's, and learning disorders, among other potential indications.
- The only non-psychiatric indication currently approved by the FDA is migraine headache. TMS is currently being studied in the treatment of pain disorders, Parkinson's disease, and other indications.

Side effects

- TMS tends to be well tolerated, with the most common side effects being headache and scalp sensitivity under the coil.
- Other common side effects include tingling, spasms or twitching of the face and scalp, and light-headedness.
- Less common side effects include temporary visual changes, temporary hearing loss, and mania. Higher frequency TMS is associated with the risk of inducing seizures in <1% of patients.

Contraindications

- The only clear contraindication is having ferrous metal in the brain (e.g. an older aneurysm clip or stents, bullet fragments, deep brain stimulation (DBS) leads, cochlear implants, etc.) or skull. The magnetic coil could move ferromagnetic metal in close proximity.
- Caution should be used in patients with a history of head trauma, recent stroke, facial or scalp tattoos, acute alcohol withdrawal, or anyone at greater risk for a seizure.

15.8 Vagus nerve stimulation (VNS)

Definition

Vagus nerve stimulation (VNS) is the use of a device to indirectly stimulate the brain via the vagus nerve (see *Fig. 15.8.1*).

Background

- VNS was originally developed for the treatment of refractory epilepsy.
- VNS is thought to work by sending regular electric impulses to the brain via the vagus nerve and this appears to reduce the frequency of seizures.
- Some epileptic patients noted an improvement in mood and depressive symptoms independent of an improvement of their seizure disorder.
- Multicenter trials suggested an improvement in depression in about 30–40% of patients unresponsive to other strategies.

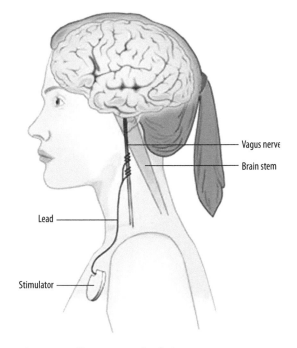

Fig. 15.8.1: Vagus nerve stimulation.

What it involves

- VNS is a surgically implanted (under general or regional anesthesia) pacemaker type device that includes a battery implanted under the left clavicle and a wire attached to left vagus nerve (see *Fig. 15.8.1*).
- Electrical stimulation occurs around the clock (typically 30 sec on/5 min off) with the stimulation ascending in one direction towards the brain. Thus parasympathetic symptoms are avoided.
- Improvement is very gradual and may take 1–2 years to see maximum improvement.

Indications

- VNS is FDA-approved for the treatment of chronic and recurrent, either unipolar or bipolar, disorder, resistant to at least 4 medication trials.
- VNS was previously approved in the treatment of medication-resistant epilepsy.
- Other potential indications under study include eating disorders, anxiety disorders, and substance use disorders.

Side effects

- Common side effects include hoarseness, voice alteration, cough, and paresthesias.
- Surgical complications can include pain, infection, and vocal cord paralysis.
- Less common side effects can include difficulty swallowing, worsening of sleep apnea, shortness of breath, and headaches.

Contraindications

- The two primary contraindications are patients who have had a left or bilateral cervical vagotomy or require diathermy (high intensity heat therapy to the tissues in proximity to the leads or generator).

Chapter 16

Mental health law and forensic psychiatry

16.1   Mental health and the law   218
16.2   Forensic psychiatry   221

Mental health and the law

Consent and capacity

- A fundamental principle of medical care is that for treatment to be given to the patient, consent should be gained, i.e. the patient has a right to decide for themselves which treatment to undergo and which treatments to refuse.
- Consent can be **implied** (the patient does not object to, and cooperates with the procedure, e.g. sticking their arm out when approached with a blood pressure cuff) or **expressed** (verbal or written permission is explicitly asked for and recorded, often on a consent form).
- **Mental capacity** is defined as one's ability to **make decisions**. Capacity can involve consent about **personal welfare, healthcare**, and **financial decisions**.
- Mental capacity is **time specific** and **decision specific**:
  1. *Time specific*: Person may lack capacity at one point in time but may have capacity at another point in time. If the lack of capacity is likely to be temporary, e.g. delirium, it may be possible to delay the decision until the person has recovered.
  2. *Decision specific*: May have capacity to consent for one decision but not for another (e.g. may have capacity to consent for a simple endoscopy but not for a more complex surgical procedure which poses greater risks, such as a hemicolectomy).
- The nature of psychiatric disorders means that patients may refuse treatment. Situations where treatment can take place without consent can be divided into three broad areas:
  1. A medical emergency exists and the patient is incapacitated.
  2. The patient is under a mental health conservatorship that includes medical decisions.
  3. Treatment authorized by a **court**.

> **OSCE tips:** When to suspect a lack of capacity: **'CARD'**
>
> - Cognitive impairment, e.g. dementia.
> - Abnormal behavior.
> - Refusing treatment.
> - Delirium.

Durable power of attorney

- This allows a person with capacity to appoint an **individual** (usually a relative or close friend) to make future decisions on their behalf if they lose capacity.
- There are **two types** of durable power of attorney:
  1. **Property and affairs** deals with property and financial affairs.
  2. **Personal welfare** deals with decisions about healthcare, living conditions, and location.

Advance directive (*Fig. 16.1.1*)

- **Advance care planning** is a process that allows patients to make decisions about their future care. It takes the form of making an **advance statement** or an **advance decision** to refuse treatment, or appointing a **durable power of attorney**.
- An **advance directive** is **a legal document** with a **specific refusal of treatment** in a predefined future situation (where the person would have lost capacity) that is signed by the patient and witnessed. Advance

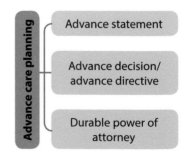

Fig. 16.1.1: Advance care planning.

decisions permit a person to **refuse treatment but *not* demand it**. They do not allow patients to refuse basic care needs such as food and drink by mouth or basic hygiene. Persons writing an advance decision should have capacity at the point of writing it.

- An **advance statement** (made **verbally** or **written**) allows the patients to make **general statements** about their **wishes and preferences** for the future, if they were to lose capacity.

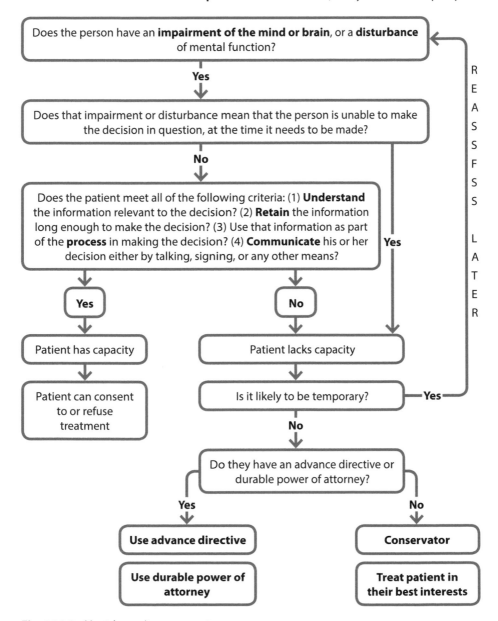

Fig. 16.1.2: Mental capacity assessment.

Involuntary detainment (psychiatric holds)

A psychiatric hold is the involuntary civil commitment of a patient with a mental disorder. Specific civil commitment statutes vary somewhat from state to state. Involuntary civil commitment of psychiatric patients may be necessary to protect both the patient and society from the consequences of a serious mental illness.

- A hold may allow for the involuntary hospitalization for purposes of psychiatric observation for a limited time period (up to 72 hours).
- Psychiatric holds do not typically allow for the administration of treatment other than emergency psychiatric medications against the will of the patient.
- A psychiatric hold may be initiated by a mental health professional, a police officer, an ER physician, or other professional designated by a particular county or municipality.
- Judicial oversight (a hearing) is typically necessary to extend the hold for up to 14 days. The hold may be released at any time a designated mental health professional (usually a licensed psychiatrist or psychologist) deems the patient no longer holdable.

Basis for an involuntary hold on the basis of a psychiatric disorder

1. Imminent danger to self (may include deliberate self harm, misuse of medications, suicide risk, etc.).
2. Imminent danger to others (may include viable threats, assault, stalking, etc.).
3. Grave disability, defined as the inability to provide for food, clothing, and/or shelter on the basis of a psychiatric disorder.

- A hold may be extended by a judge or hearing officer for a specified period (usually 14 days) if evidence indicates that the patient remains holdable by the above criteria after 72 hours.
- For patients who remain gravely disabled, the court may be petitioned to have the patient conserved (see below).
- For patients who remain a danger to others on the basis of a psychiatric disorder, most states allow the possibility of extended involuntary detainment with judicial oversight (for periods of 3–6 months).
- Some treatments can't be given without consent unless certain criteria are met. These treatments include **ECT**.
- A person may lack capacity to make a decision for a variety of reasons, e.g. psychosis, substance abuse, dementia, delirium, intellectual disability, neurological disorder.

Mental health conservatorship

A **conservatorship** is a court case in which a judge appoints a responsible person (called the 'conservator') to care for another adult (called the 'conservatee') who cannot care for himself or herself or manage his or her own finances or medical decisions.

- **Psychiatric conservatorships can be temporary (30 days) or more continuous (renewed annually).**
- **Conservatorships can be limited (i.e. just around financial decisions) or more general including living arrangement, psychiatric treatment, medical decisions, etc.**
- **Psychiatric patients typically must be demonstrated to be gravely disabled on the basis of a major psychiatric disorder in order to be conserved.**

Forensic psychiatry

What is forensic psychiatry?

- **Forensic psychiatry** is a branch of psychiatry that deals with the **assessment and treatment** of **mentally disordered offenders**. It deals with the interface between psychiatry and the criminal justice system.

- There is a significantly **higher prevalence** of mental illness among **prisoners** as compared to the general population. More than **70%** of prisoners have a mental disorder.

- Forensic mental health services may support a patient:

  - Who was unwell at the time of committing the offense.

  - In prison for an offense unrelated to a mental health problem, who becomes unwell whilst in prison.

  - With mental health problems in the community who has a significant history of risk issues or poses significant risk to others.

- The forensic psychiatrist has many roles which include:

  - Psychiatric assessment (and if appropriate, treatment and rehabilitation) of offenders charged with a serious crime.

  - Providing treatment for convicted prisoners charged with a serious crime.

  - Assessment and treatment of non-offenders with difficult or dangerous behavior in a secure setting (see *Table 16.2.1*).

  - Giving advice to other psychiatrists encountering forensic issues.

- See *Fig. 16.2.1* and *Key facts 2* for specific psychiatric conditions associated with crime.

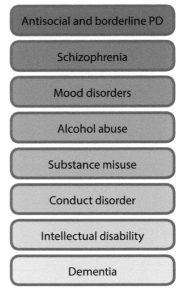

Antisocial and borderline PD

Schizophrenia

Mood disorders

Alcohol abuse

Substance misuse

Conduct disorder

Intellectual disability

Dementia

Fig. 16.2.1: Conditions associated with crime.

Table 16.2.1: Psychiatric care levels	
Setting	**Description**
Locked acute ward	Locked units in psychiatric or general hospital provide acute care for patients who need a more secure facility. Most patients are on a psychiatric hold as a danger to self, danger to others, or gravely disabled. Length of stay is usually days to weeks.
Open acute ward	General inpatient units for voluntary patients in community or psychiatric hospitals. Length of stay is days to weeks.
Subacute care	A step below acute inpatient care. Usually locked units for patients on a conservatorship. Lengths of stay usually weeks to months.
Board and care	Open long-term living facilities for patients with chronic mental illness. Board and care homes may provide support around administering medications and some activities of daily living that may include bathing, meals, and transportation. Length of stay usually years.

Court proceedings

- There are two main considerations in court proceedings. These are **fitness to stand trial** and **criminal responsibility** (see *Key facts 1*).
- Fitness to stand trial is the capacity for an offender to mount a defense against his or her charges. A jury determines whether the charged can:
  - **Understand the nature of the charges** and the meaning of guilty and non-guilty pleas.
  - **Challenge jurors.**
  - **Communicate with their lawyer.**
  - **Follow court proceedings** and the evidence presented before the court.

Key facts 1: *Mens rea* (guilty mind)

It should be determined whether the convicted understood the nature of the unlawful act and what their intentions were. If they fully intended to commit the act and were aware of the ramifications, this is known as *mens rea*. There are a number of circumstances in which a defendant may lack *mens rea*:

- **Age:** By default, children under the age of 10 are typically deemed incapable of criminal intent. Those between the ages of 10 and 14 are not criminally responsible unless the prosecution can prove otherwise. After the age of 14–16, individuals may be legally responsible for their actions in most states.
- **Severe mental illness or intellectual disability:** a mental or intellectual disability may be so profound that the patient is unfit to stand trial. This defense could be used if a patient with schizophrenia commits a murder as a direct result of his/her mental health problems.
- **Automatism:** An act committed without presence of mind (e.g. during sleepwalking).

Predictors of violent behavior

The minority of violent crime is committed by people with major psychiatric disorders. However, mental health issues can predispose some individuals to violent acts. Substance abuse and antisocial personality have the highest association with violent acts. Some patients with acute paranoid delusions in a manic or schizophrenic state may also be prone to violence. Likewise, some patients with more severe intellectual deficits may also be at risk for committing violence. Risk factors for violence can be divided into demographic and personal (see *Table 16.2.2*).

Table 16.2.2: Risk factors for violence

Demographic	Personal
• Male. • Young age. • Low socioeconomic status. • Lack of social support (lack of friends, relationship issues). • Access to weapons or other means of violence.	• Past history of violent behavior. • Substance misuse and alcohol abuse. • Major psychiatric illness (*Fig. 16.2.1*). • Difficult upbringing, e.g. childhood abuse. • Impulsivity and risk taking. • Cruelty to animals, fire setting.

Key facts 2: Specific associations between a psychiatric condition and the offense

- **Depression:** Shoplifting, homicide, and infanticide (in postpartum depression).
- **Mania:** Violence (usually minor), reckless driving, inappropriate sexual behavior.
- **Schizophrenia** and **personality disorder:** Violent acts (e.g. assault, murder).
- **Learning disability:** Sexual offenses, arson.
- **Dementia:** Violence, inappropriate sexual behavior (e.g. indecent exposure).
- **Alcohol** and **substance misuse:** Violence (assault), driving offenses.

OSCE tips: Features to look out for in the MSE that may indicate impending violence

- Expressed violent intentions or direct threats.
- Paranoid delusions, delusions of control, or morbid jealousy.
- Second person auditory (command) hallucinations encouraging patient to commit violent act.
- Disinhibited behavior or irritable mood.

Chapter 17

Common OSCE scenarios

Outline of chapter

This section is most suited for group study in the weeks leading up to your OSCE examinations. The section includes:

1. **Student briefing:** Contains the candidate instructions and time allowance.
2. **Simulated patient briefing:** Includes the directions and instructions for the simulated patient.
3. **Checklist:** This contains a checklist of tasks and competencies which the candidate is expected to complete within the station, along with point schemes. There are also a number of potential questions which an examiner may have for a candidate.

These scenarios and point schemes will vary between universities and these should be used to aid your revision. You will need to familiarize yourself with the examination structure within your own institution.

Student briefing

Station 1

You are a resident working in a primary care setting. Mrs Cook has come to see you because she has been feeling very tired and low in mood. Please take a history. You have 10 minutes.

Station 2

You are a resident in the ER. A 24-year-old man has been brought in by his family because he has been acting 'very strangely' and they are very concerned about his recent behavior. Please take a history and perform a mental state examination. You have 20 minutes.

Station 3

You are a resident in the ER. The police have brought in a 30-year-old woman who was found playing guitar in the middle of the night in her next door neighbor's garden. Please take a history and perform a mental state examination. You have 20 minutes.

Station 4

You are a resident in the ER. You have come to see Miss West who has been brought in by her partner because she took an overdose of acetaminophen following an argument. She is now medically stabilized. Please take a psychiatric history focusing particularly on the risk, in order to be able to make a clear management plan. You have 10 minutes.

Station 5

You are a resident working in Primary Care. Mr Anderson has been brought in by his wife because she believes his drinking has become out of control. Please take a history from Mr Anderson. You have 10 minutes.

Simulated patient briefing

Station 1

Patient's details

Patient's name: Michelle Cook

Patient's age: 37 years

Patient's occupation: Unemployed

Presenting complaint

- You have come to see your PCP because you have been feeling very tired and low in mood. This has been going on for 3 months.
- You find it difficult to fall asleep and strangely wake up earlier in the morning than usual and are then unable to fall asleep again. You used to wake at 7am, and now find yourself wide awake at 4am, despite feeling extremely tired all of the time. You do not sleep during the day.
- You also lack enjoyment in the things you used to enjoy, which was going out with friends and going for walks.
- All of these symptoms started to develop when you lost your job as a financial advisor, 4 months ago. You are currently unemployed.
- You have also found that your relationship with your husband has diminished as he feels frustrated by your lack of interest in everything, including having sex.
- You have lost your appetite and have noticed that your clothes have become looser, although you haven't measured your weight recently.
- You feel worthless as a mother and as a wife, and feel guilty for the way that you feel.
- You have no thoughts of self-harm or suicide as you would never put your two children through that.
- You do not have any psychotic symptoms.
- There is no past history of any psychiatric or mental health conditions.

Past medical history and drug history

No medical history of note. No regular medication, and you have never used illicit drugs. NKDA.

Social history

- You do not smoke or drink alcohol and have never taken any illicit drugs.
- You live at home with your husband and two children.

Ideas, concerns, and expectations

- You know that a problem exists but are not sure what it could be.
- You are concerned that the children are also suffering because you think you are an unfit mother.
- You are hoping for some form of counseling.

Diagnosis

Moderate to severe depression.

Differentials

- Other depressive disorders, e.g. persistent depression disorder, seasonal affective disorder.
- Bipolar affective disorder.
- Organic disorder, e.g. hypothyroidism.

Station 2

Patient's details

Patient's name: Jermaine Powell

Patient age: 24 years

Patient's occupation: Restaurant waiter

Presenting complaint

- When asked why you are here you are not sure and say that you are fine.
- You appear slightly restless and appear to be responding to voices that are talking about you.
- You can hear voices that are commenting on what you are doing. There are two voices which you do not recognize. This has been very distressing for you. The voices are not talking directly to you. The voices started when you were at home only, but now you hear them wherever you go. You can hear them in the hospital. You do not understand how this is happening.
- For approximately 2 weeks, you feel that the police and FBI are after you because you have access to top secret information. They are trying to access your thoughts and you sometimes feel that your thoughts are not your own. You are very defensive if questioned about whether this is actually true because your family and friends have not believed you and you are already very upset about this and do not trust anyone.
- You are in control of your actions, thoughts, and behaviors (passivity phenomenon) if asked about this.
- You do not have any formal thought disorder or disorders of speech.
- You do not feel depressed and you are not elated in mood.

Ideas, concerns, and expectations

You have no insight that you could be suffering from a mental disorder. You are concerned that the police and FBI will torture you. You want to be left alone. You do not feel safe in the hospital.

Past medical history

Mild asthma.

Drug history

Salbutamol 100 µg inhaler, 2 puffs PRN.

Social history

- You live with your parents and one brother in rent-controlled public housing but you want to move out because your family are turning against you.
- You do not smoke cigarettes but smoke cannabis around once a week and have done so for several years. You have never been a heavy cannabis user. You do not use any other illicit drugs, or legal highs.
- You drink alcohol occasionally.

Family history

None significant.

Diagnosis

Acute psychotic episode.

Differentials

- Schizophrenia
- Drug-induced psychosis
- Psychosis secondary to a mood disorder
- Schizoaffective disorder
- Organic disorder, e.g. space-occupying lesion
- Delusional disorder.

Station 3

Patient's details

Patient's name: Sandy Williams

Patient's age: 30 years

Patient's occupation: Musician

Presenting complaint

- Your speech is fast and you seem restless and fidgety. You find it difficult to sit still, and spend time pacing during the interview. You also have more eye contact than normal and make flirtatious comments from time to time.
- You do not see anything wrong with playing guitar in your next door neighbor's garden.
- You have been feeling 'over the moon' for the last few weeks and think that everyone else is boring and needs cheering up. You are extremely happy.
- You haven't been having much sleep but still find that you have lots of energy. At most you have had 1–2 hours a night.
- You have been having sex with lots of men recently but have not told your husband. You describe your husband as 'frigid'.
- You have also spent lots of money on things such as clothes and alcohol. You have spent approximately $4000 in the last week.
- You do not have any grandiose delusions.

Ideas, concerns, and expectations

You have no insight. You have no concerns as you have never felt better. You want to be left alone.

Past medical history

You suffered from depression 2 months ago.

Drug history

Fluoxetine 20 mg OD over the last 2 months.

Social history

- You live alone after your husband left you 3 days ago for cheating on him. You have no children.
- You do not smoke but drink moderate amounts of alcohol.
- You have never taken any illicit drugs.

Family history

Your mother suffers from bipolar affective disorder.

Diagnosis

Bipolar affective disorder: current episode mania without psychosis.

Differential diagnoses

- Manic episode
- Cyclothymia
- Organic disorder.

Station 4

Patient's details

Patient's name: Amy West

Patient's age: 26 years

Patient's occupation: Bar tender

Presenting complaint

- You took 15 acetaminophen tablets in the moments after an argument with your boyfriend. You got extremely scared shortly after you had consumed the tablets and told your boyfriend. You both then immediately went to the hospital.
- The reason you took the tablets was to take your own life to get back at your boyfriend, but you regretted this impulsive act shortly after you consumed the tablets.
- You have never done anything like this before.
- You no longer want to kill yourself but still feel down and depressed about your life. You have no diagnosed psychiatric illness.
- You have never planned to harm or kill yourself and have never written a suicide note.
- You have been feeling quite low in mood for 2 months now and this started ever since your dog, who you were very close to, died. You also feel more tired than before and have not had sex for over a month because your sexual drive has diminished. You feel very lonely because your boyfriend is busy most of the time balancing two jobs, and your family live far away. You haven't told any of your friends because you think that they have their own stress to deal with.
- You are not getting any enjoyment from life, and haven't had an appetite recently.

Ideas, concerns, and expectations

You realize that you might be suffering from depression. You are concerned that you will get worse, to a point that you won't want to live any more, but you are willing to accept help. You do not have any current thoughts about ending your life. You want to get well.

Past medical history

None significant.

Drug history

None significant.

Family history

Your mother suffered from depression.

Social history

You live in an apartment with your boyfriend and are currently unemployed. You smoke 15 cigarettes a day and consume 14 alcoholic drinks a week. You do not take illicit drugs.

Diagnosis

Moderate depressive disorder.

Attempted suicide with low risk of follow-up suicide, and no ongoing thoughts to end her life.

Differential diagnosis

- Adjustment disorder
- Acute stress reaction
- Organic cause of depression
- Borderline personality disorder – very unlikely given the information.

Station 5

Patient's details

Patient's name: James Anderson

Patient's age: 50 years

Patient's occupation: Mechanic

Presenting complaint

- You have been persuaded by your wife to come in because you have been drinking more than usual.
- You have been drinking high amounts of alcohol for a number of years. Your drinking began getting out of control 5 years ago. You have drunk daily over the last 3 years, and this has gradually increased. You put this down to stress because of financial difficulties.
- You consume about one 700 ml bottle of vodka (40% alcohol by volume) a day now.
- 6 months ago you were drinking about half this amount.
- You feel shaky and agitated when you don't drink alcohol and drink to prevent this from happening, even if it is first thing in the morning. You often need a drink first thing in the morning in bed, to allow you to get up.
- You are aware of the harmful effects of alcohol but still choose to continue drinking. You admit that you have lost control of your drinking, and are drinking more and more to get the same effect.
- You have tried cutting down in the past but have failed to maintain this.
- Your mood has been low but you have no other symptoms of depression.
- Your entire life now revolves around drinking alcohol.
- You have no problems with your memory.

Ideas, concerns, and expectations

You are aware that you are an 'alcoholic'.

Past medical history

- Acute pancreatitis (2 years ago).
- You have been told that your 'liver blood tests are abnormal'.

Drug history

Omeprazole 20 mg OD for reflux.

Social history

- You live with your wife and have one child aged 20 who does not live with you.
- You are a self-employed mechanic and your business seems to be having significant financial problems as a result of your drinking.
- You do not smoke and do not take illicit drugs.

Diagnosis

Alcohol dependence syndrome.

Point schemes

For each station we have developed a checklist, identifying the core aspects of the history and mental state that would need to be covered. At the end of each point sheet there are a series of questions that the examiner might ask the student. For each competency the examiner will have to identify whether the student has met this in their interaction with the patient, or simulated patient. We have also identified a number of questions that could be asked in a viva situation. Across different universities there will be different point schemes or competency lists. We have given an indication of what would be expected for a given clinical scenario.

Station 1

Competency level	Yes	Partial	No
Introduction			
Appropriate introduction and checks patient's name			
Explains the purpose of the interview and gains consent			
Presenting complaint and history of presenting complaint			
Starts with an open question and listens without interrupting			
Establishes the onset and course of the low mood			
Enquires about precipitating factors such as stress, life events, current social situation			
Asks about the other core symptoms of depression: anhedonia and lack of energy			
Asks about biological symptoms of depression: difficulty sleeping, weight loss, loss of appetite, loss of libido			
Asks about cognitive symptoms of depression, e.g. guilt, lack of concentration, hopelessness, negative views of the future and those around them			

Competency level	Yes	Partial	No
Explores possibility of organic symptoms by asking about symptoms of thyroid dysfunction, anemia, etc.			
Explores possibility of psychotic depression by asking about delusions and hallucinations			
Explores the patient's ideas, concerns, and expectations – what does the patient want?			
Risk assessment			
Thoughts about self-harm, suicide, thoughts of harming others			
Past psychiatric history			
Past medical history			
Drug history including allergies			
Relevant family history			
Social history			
Asks about housing circumstances, dependants, occupation			
Asks about alcohol, smoking and substance misuse history			
Communication skills			
Appropriate questioning style (mix of open and closed questions)			
Organized approach to history taking			
Examiner to ask the candidate: What are your differential diagnoses?			
Appropriate differentials: moderate or severe depression, bipolar affective disorder, adjustment disorder, thyroid dysfunction or other organic causes			
Examiner to ask the candidate: What are the causes of depression?			
Candidate provides an organized answer with biological as well as psychosocial causes			
Examiner to ask the candidate: What is an appropriate management plan for the patient?			
Gives an organized answer using the bio-psychosocial model. Antidepressants with SSRI first-line, psychotherapies most notably CBT, social support groups, etc. Lifestyle changes, exercise, healthy diet, consider activity scheduling – voluntary work, adult education, etc.			

Station 2

Competency level	Yes	Partial	No
Introduction			
Appropriate introduction and checks patient's name			
Explains the purpose of the interview and gains consent			
Presenting complaint and history of presenting complaint			
Starts with an open question and listens without interrupting			
Enquires about precipitating factors such as stress, life events that may have led up to this			
Identifies and tests the patient's delusions by asking whether they think their thoughts are unusual			
Screens for other delusional beliefs – persecution, reference, grandiose			
Explores hallucinations in different modalities. Identifies the third person auditory hallucinations in the form of a running commentary			
Asks appropriate follow-up questions regarding the hallucinations, e.g. in what person, how many voices, content of voices			
Asks about thought interference (thought insertion, withdrawal and broadcast)			
Asks about passivity phenomenon			
Enquires about current mood, and a history of depressive and manic episodes. When checking current mood, asks about anhedonia and energy			
Checks the patient's cognition			
Enquires about previous episodes of mental health problems			
Explores the patient's ideas, concerns, and expectations			
Risk assessment			
Thoughts about self-harm, suicide, thoughts of harming others			
Past psychiatric history			
Past medical history			
Drug history including allergies			
Relevant family history			
Social history			

Competency level	Yes	Partial	No
Asks about housing circumstances, dependants, occupation			
Asks about alcohol, smoking and substance misuse history			
Communication skills			
Appropriate questioning style (mix of open and closed questions)			
Organized approach to history taking			
Examiner to ask the candidate: What are the differential diagnoses?			
Appropriate differentials: acute psychotic episode, schizophrenia, drug-induced psychosis, psychosis secondary to a mood disorder, delusional disorder, schizoaffective disorder			
Examiner to ask the candidate: What are Schneider's first rank symptoms?			
Thought interference (thought insertion, withdrawal and broadcast), third person auditory hallucinations, delusional perception, and passivity phenomenon			

Station 3

Competency level	Yes	Partial	No
Introduction			
Appropriate introduction and checks patient's name			
Explains the purpose of the interview and gains consent			
Presenting complaint and history of presenting complaint			
Starts with an open question and listens without interrupting			
Enquires about onset, timing, and course of the symptoms			
Asks about current mood			
Asks about increased energy and lack of sleep			
Asks about increased libido			
Asks about racing thoughts			
Asks about grandiose delusions			
Asks about passivity phenomenon			

Competency level	Yes	Partial	No
Asks about other types of delusional beliefs			
Asks about hallucinations in a variety of modalities			
Asks appropriate questions to check cognition			
Enquires about previous episodes of mania			
Enquires about previous episodes and treatment for depression			
Explores the patient's ideas, concerns, and expectations			
Risk assessment			
Thoughts about self-harm, suicide, thoughts of harming others			
Past psychiatric history			
Past medical history			
Drug history including allergies			
Relevant family history			
Social history			
Asks about housing circumstances, dependants, occupation			
Asks about alcohol, smoking and substance misuse history			
Communication skills			
Appropriate questioning style (mix of open and closed questions)			
Organized approach to history taking			
Examiner to ask the candidate: What are the differential diagnoses?			
Appropriate differentials: bipolar affective disorder current episode mania or hypomania, acute manic episode without psychosis, drug-induced mania, organic disease, cyclothymia			
Examiner to ask the candidate: What is formal thought disorder?			
Candidate recognizes that it refers to abnormalities of the way thoughts are linked together. Candidate gives examples of different types of formal thought disorder, e.g. derailment of thought, tangential thinking, word salad, circumstantiality, thought blocking and neologism			
Examiner to ask the candidate: What is the difference between mania and hypomania?			
Hypomanic episodes must last for several days and do not usually require hospitalization. Hypomania does not involve psychotic features such as grandiose delusions. In mania, symptoms are more severe to the point that the individual's everyday life is significantly impaired and psychotic features may be present			

Station 4

Competency level	Yes	Partial	No
Introduction			
Appropriate introduction and checks patient's name			
Explains the purpose of the interview and gains consent			
Risk assessment			
Starts with an open question and listens without interrupting			
Enquires about onset, timing, and course of the mood symptoms			
Asks about precipitating factors for the overdose			
Identifies the steps leading up to the overdose, and then the steps to getting help and coming to hospital			
Asks about current suicidal ideation			
Asks about planning for the suicide attempt			
Asks whether a letter was written beforehand			
Asks about final acts such as writing a will, sorting out finances, etc.			
Asks about attempts to avoid discovery			
Asks about previous suicide attempts			
Asks about self-harm previously			
Explores any current mood disorder symptoms			
Explores history of psychiatric illness, e.g. depression			
Explores other risk factors of suicide			
Explores protective factors			
Explores risk to others			
Explores the patient's ideas, concerns, and expectations			
Past medical history			
Drug history including allergies			
Relevant family history			
Social history			
Asks about housing circumstances, dependants, occupation			

Competency level	Yes	Partial	No
Asks about alcohol, smoking, and substance misuse history			
Communication skills			
Appropriate questioning style (mix of open and closed questions)			
Organized approach to history taking			
Examiner to ask the candidate: What is the appropriate management plan for this patient?			
Candidate identifies that the patient wishes to seek help. The patient and partner can be seen to discuss going home with support. The patient should be seen by the Crisis Team and have a complete psychosocial assessment including a risk assessment. The patient can possibly be home treated. Assessment for depression is needed with a discussion about a bio-psychosocial approach to the management of this.			
Examiner to ask the candidate: What are the risk factors for suicide?			
Candidate gives a number of risk factors (five or more – see *Section 12.2*, Suicide and risk assessment). An extra point is given for a structured answer, e.g. divided into clinical and socio-demographic.			
Examiner to ask the candidate: What are the protective factors for suicide, in general, and in this situation?			
Candidate gives a number of protective factors (five or more – see *Section 12.2*, Suicide and risk assessment).			

Station 5

Competency level	Yes	Partial	No
Introduction			
Appropriate introduction and checks patient's name			
Explains the purpose of the interview and gains consent			
Presenting complaint			
Starts with an open question and listens without interrupting			
Establishes the onset and current level of use of alcohol			
Enquires about precipitating factors such as stress, life events, etc.			
Establishes current amount of alcohol consumed in drinks			
Explores increased tolerance to alcohol			

Competency level	Yes	Partial	No
Explores withdrawal effects			
Explores compulsive need to drink			
Explores use despite knowledge of harm			
Explores difficulties in control over alcohol			
Explores the importance of alcohol/primacy of alcohol in his life			
Explores narrowed repertoire of drinking			
Asks about mood symptoms			
Asks about delusional beliefs and any visual or auditory hallucinations			
Explores any cognitive symptoms			
Explores the patient's ideas, concerns, and expectations			
Risk assessment			
Thoughts about self-harm, suicide, thoughts of harming others			
Past medical history			
Drug history including allergies			
Relevant family history			
Social history			
Asks about housing circumstances, dependants, occupation			
Asks about smoking and substance misuse history			
Communication skills			
Appropriate questioning style (mix of open and closed questions)			
Organized approach to history taking			
Examiner to ask the student: Does the patient have alcohol dependence syndrome, and if so, why?			
Candidate identifies that the patient has alcohol dependence syndrome and gives evidence to back this up			

Competency level	Yes	Partial	No
Examiner to ask the student: What drug is used for alcohol detoxification and how is this prescribed? What other medication could be appropriate?			
Candidate identifies that a benzodiazepine is used, e.g. chlordiazepoxide and this is given as a tapering dose orally, over approximately 7 days. Candidate also identifies the importance of vitamin B replacement, orally with thiamine, or possibly with IV vitamin B replacement. Identifies the importance of this to prevent Wernicke's encephalopathy/Korsakoff's psychosis			
Examiner to ask the candidate: What are the long-term solutions to alcohol misuse for this patient?			
Candidate gives an organized answer giving both pharmacological (disulfiram, acamprosate, naltrexone) and psychosocial (motivational interviewing and support groups such as Alcoholics Anonymous) management options			

Chapter 18

Board-style questions

1. **A 24-year-old patient presents to the ER. During the mental state examination he describes hearing the voices of three individuals outside his flat. He has never been able to see these individuals. The three individuals talk about him, and the patient has heard them plotting to kill him. On several occasions he heard a presenter on the radio talk to him, mention his name, and threaten to kill him.**
   What symptoms are described in the scenario?
   A. Pseudo-hallucinations and delusions of reference.
   B. Auditory hallucinations and thought broadcasting.
   C. Auditory hallucinations and thought insertion.
   D. Auditory hallucinations and delusions of reference.
   E. Command auditory hallucinations and persecutory delusions.

2. **A 56-year-old woman presents to her PCP with a 3-week history of low mood. She is waking up at 4am, and is unable to get back to sleep. She is averaging only 4 hours of sleep a night. In addition, she has lost her appetite and is not interested in food. She feels very tired and is having a hard time concentrating. She used to enjoy walking her dog and going to the gym, but hasn't felt like doing this. Six weeks ago her mother who she was very close to passed away after a long illness. She feels guilty about not having spent more time with her.**
   What is the most appropriate diagnosis?
   A. Adjustment disorder.
   B. Bereavement reaction.
   C. Major depressive episode.
   D. Psychotic depressive episode.
   E. Bipolar affective disorder.

3. **A 22-year-old man presents to the ER. He has been taken there by friends from university who are concerned about his behavior. He has not been sleeping for the last 7 days. He is talking extremely quickly and it is difficult to follow his conversation. He tells the ER resident that his blood has healing powers, and offers to use this to help staff in the department. He appears elated in mood.**
   What is the most appropriate diagnosis?
   A. Bipolar I affective disorder, manic state.
   B. Bipolar affective disorder, hypomanic state.
   C. Mixed state.
   D. Hypomania with psychotic features.
   E. Mania without psychosis.

4. **A 16-year-old male is taken to his PCP by his mother. He has been socially withdrawn for 2 weeks and has been very frightened. He confides in the PCP that for the last 2 weeks he has been concerned that his neighbors are talking about him. He can hear them outside his bedroom. He is worried that they can see everything that he does, as they talk about everything he does in the house.**

He believes that there must be cameras in the house, and he has been looking for these over the last 2 weeks. His mood is currently euthymic. He has smoked cannabis in the past. The last occasion was 3 weeks ago with some friends.

What is the most appropriate diagnosis?

A. Schizophreniform disorder.
B. Delusional disorder.
C. Bipolar II disorder.
D. Schizoaffective disorder.
E. Severe depressive episode with psychosis.

5. A 50-year-old with known paranoid schizophrenia reported that on the way to see his sister he suddenly had a desire to go to a fast food restaurant. He had never eaten there before. He believes that the thought about going to a fast food restaurant is not his own. He becomes worried that it may be a trap where some harm will come to him if he goes to the fast food restaurant.

What is the symptom described above?

A. Delusion of reference.
B. Persecutory delusion.
C. Thought broadcast.
D. Thought insertion.
E. Thought withdrawal.

6. A 26-year-old woman presents to her PCP. She is extremely worried about a presentation she is due to give at work in the coming weeks. She has never felt comfortable giving presentations. She also states that she does not like going out and eating in public, and worries that she may vomit. She describes herself as quiet and shy and lacking in confidence around others. When she gets worried she complains that she blushes excessively, starts to feel hot and sweaty, and shakes. This can last for 10 to 30 minutes depending on the situation. In the past she has always found a reason not to give presentations.

What is the most likely diagnosis?

A. Generalized anxiety disorder.
B. Panic disorder with agoraphobia.
C. Panic disorder without agoraphobia.
D. Social (phobia) anxiety disorder.
E. Vomiting phobia.

7. A 47-year-old man presents to the PCP complaining of recurrent episodes of chest pain. These episodes can happen at any time of the day or night, and the pain is not made worse on exertion. He explains that when the chest pain starts he becomes convinced that he will die. He has called an ambulance and been to the ER on five occasions over the last month. When the chest pain starts he complains of breathlessness, chest tightness, tingling in his fingers, and a feeling of being lightheaded. He has worried that he will pass out. These episodes can last for up to an hour. When seen in the ER he has had blood tests and an ECG, and there has

been no evidence of a cardiac cause for his problems. Between episodes he feels well, and has no other physical or mental health concerns. The last three episodes all occurred when he was out shopping, and he has avoided going back to the supermarket, in case it happens again. He has continued to go to work.

What would be the appropriate treatment?

A. Cognitive behavioral therapy.

B. Further investigations including ECG.

C. Refer on for psychiatric review within a community mental health team.

D. Short course of benzodiazepines, and advice to stop avoiding situations causing anxiety.

E. Watch and wait and see again in 2–4 weeks in primary care.

8. An 18-year-old man is brought to see his PCP by his parents. They are concerned about his behavior. It takes him 2 hours to get ready in the morning. He has a very set routine, including cleaning the bathroom, and then washing himself. He explains he has to clean himself in a particular way, and finishes by washing his hands 11 times. The cleaning routine takes him about 2 hours. If he is interrupted he has to start the routine from the very beginning. The skin on his hands is very dry and scaly. He gets very frustrated by his cleaning, and wishes he didn't have to do this. He accepts that he is not dirty or contaminated. If he tries to resist he becomes distressed and describes multiple unpleasant physical symptoms of anxiety. He continues to worry that he is dirty, and washes his hands throughout the day. When he gets home, he has to take off his clothes immediately and put these in the washing machine before showering again. He has tried to make his parents do the same thing in case they are contaminated, but they have so far refused. The PCP thinks he has an obsessive–compulsive disorder.

Which of the following is most important when making this diagnosis?

A. Asking about a family history of obsessive–compulsive disorder.

B. Checking that the patient believes the thoughts are his own.

C. Checking the core and other symptoms of depression.

D. Checking the patient's insight into his presentation.

E. The symptoms need to have been present for 1 week.

9. A 21-year-old complains that since a car accident where he was driving, he has not been able to get back in a car, either as a driver or as a passenger. No one was seriously hurt in the accident, although his car was totaled. When he goes to get in a car he complains of multiple symptoms of anxiety. The accident happened 3 months ago, and the problems are not getting any easier. The man has read about post-traumatic stress disorder and wonders if he has this.

What features (other than those described above) would you need to check to clarify this diagnosis?

A. Flashbacks to the accident, insomnia, startle reaction.

B. Flashbacks to the accident, low mood, and nightmares.

C. Flashbacks to the accident, nightmares, insomnia, and anhedonia.

D. Flashbacks to the accident, startle reaction, and nightmares.

E. Flashbacks to the accident, startle reaction, low mood, insomnia.

10. **A 35-year-old woman presents to her PCP with a 3-month history of gradually worsening low mood, anhedonia, and being easily fatigued. She has been off work for 1 week, as she has struggled to get out of bed. She appears unkempt and is quietly spoken. Her speech is not very spontaneous, but she does answer questions when asked. She feels that she is a bad person and is being punished for letting her partner down. Her partner has brought her to the doctor for help. She is struggling to eat and has lost over 20 lbs in weight. She does manage to sleep, but wakes up repeatedly during the night. She needs to be encouraged to shower. She denies any active suicidal thoughts but states she deserves to be dead. She cannot concentrate for very long, and during the brief consultation, a lot of the history has to come from the partner. She has no history of mental or physical health problems.**
    What is the most appropriate treatment?
    A. Offer an antipsychotic for her beliefs about needing to be punished.
    B. Offer sertraline (an SSRI).
    C. Offer imipramine (a TCA).
    D. Refer for urgent CBT treatment in primary care.
    E. Watch and wait and see in clinic in 2 weeks' time.

11. **A 33-year-old man is being seen by a psychiatrist in clinic. He has had three previous admissions with mania. On two of these occasions he was found by the police naked in public, trying to gain access to the White House. On these two occasions he stated that he was the President, and needed to make a speech. The last admission for mania was approximately 1 year ago. He understands that he has bipolar affective disorder. He presents in clinic today with a 3-week history of low mood. He has never had an episode of depression before. He rates his mood as 0 out of 10, and is extremely tearful. He has multiple symptoms of depression and is diagnosed with severe depression. He is referred to the home treatment team as he has some passive suicidal thoughts. He is currently taking lithium which has treated his mania.**
    What would be the most appropriate treatment?
    A. Duloxetine (SNRI).
    B. Quetiapine (antipsychotic).
    C. Imipramine (TCA).
    D. Sertraline (SSRI).
    E. Sertraline (SSRI) and cognitive behavioral therapy (CBT).

12. **A 33-year-old man presents to the ER. He is brought there by his wife. He has a 4-week history of a severe depressive disorder. He has been depressed once before 3 years ago, and during that episode he tried to hang himself. Over the last 6 months his antidepressants have been reduced and stopped. He is again presenting with low mood, rating his mood as 0 out of 10. He feels hopeless about the future. On questioning he states that he wishes he were dead and has bought a rope and has planned to hang himself. He cannot see any other way out of his current situation. He also states that he has bankrupted his family, and he**

deserves to die. His wife states that this is not the case. During his last episode of depression he was treated for a depression with psychosis with antidepressants and antipsychotics. He believes he will die whatever is done, and that no one can help him. His wife is extremely distressed. She is also the main care provider for their 3 children, aged 6 years, 3 years, and 6 months. He is not interested in an inpatient stay but would consider other treatment. He wishes to go home.

As the ER resident you make a referral to the on-call psychiatry team. What do you feel would be an appropriate treatment?

A. Place a psychiatric hold as a danger to self and admit to a locked unit for observation.

B. Admission to an open psychiatry unit for assessment and treatment.

C. Discharge home, with a letter to the PCP to refer on for psychiatry support, and advice about starting antidepressants.

D. Discharge home with a prescription for antidepressants and antipsychotics and a follow up appointment in psychiatry outpatients.

E. Discharge home with a referral to the local community mental health team for outpatient follow-up and support.

13. A 23-year-old woman presents to the ER having vomited fresh red blood. During the history she reports that she has been making herself vomit on a regular basis for the last 5 years. She is worried about putting on weight and is concerned that she is fat. Her height is 5'2" (1.6 m), and she weighs 123 lbs (53 kg). She describes periods of time where she eats large quantities of food, followed by episodes of induced vomiting. She also abuses laxatives on a daily basis and exercises excessively. She is clear that she needs to lose at least 10 lbs (5 kg) before she will be happy with her weight. She has very low self-esteem, and eats for comfort.

What is the most likely diagnosis?

A. Anorexia nervosa.

B. Atypical anorexia nervosa.

C. Bulimia nervosa.

D. Eating disorder not otherwise specified.

E. Overeating associated with other psychological disturbances.

14. A 16-year-old girl is brought into the ophthamologist by her mother. The patient reports that she suddenly lost her vision approximately 2 weeks ago. Her mother reports that it has been a difficult time for the family as there was a home invasion in which the patient's father was killed. Both the patient and mother witnessed the murder. Ophthalmologic exam including pupillary reflexes, mirror test, and tests for optokinetic nystagmus are all normal.

What is the most likely diagnosis?

A. Factitious disorder

B. Malingering.

C. Conversion disorder.

D. Somatic symptom disorder.

E. Retinal detachment.

15. **A 49-year-old man presents repeatedly to see his PCP. He is complaining of abdominal pain, which is intermittent. This is central in nature and is referred through to his back. Occasionally the pain is associated with a feeling of being bloated and intermittent diarrhea. There is no blood or mucus when he goes to the bathroom. He has had a number of investigations for this, but to date, there are no positive clinical findings.**

    If we presume that there is no physical cause for this presentation, what is the most likely diagnosis?
    A. Somatic delusional disorder.
    B. Factitious disorder.
    C. Illness anxiety disorder.
    D. Malingering.
    E. Somatic symptom disorder.

16. **A 36-year-old man is brought to the ER. He has been in the department four times before in the last 6 months, and it is known that he has a severe alcohol use disorder with a history of complicated withdrawal. There is a concern that he has developed Wernicke's encephalopathy.**

    What are the signs and symptoms of this disorder?
    A. Ataxia, clouding of consciousness, disorientation to time, peripheral neuropathy.
    B. Ophthalmoplegia, nystagmus, ataxia, clouding of consciousness.
    C. Ophthalmoplegia, nystagmus, clouding of consciousness, short-term memory loss.
    D. Ophthalmoplegia, nystagmus, ataxia, disorientation to time.
    E. Nystagmus, ataxia, short-term memory loss, peripheral neuropathy.

17. **A 47-year-old patient is admitted to a medical assessment unit with hematemesis. He is known to drink 2 bottles of whiskey each day and has been drinking this heavily for about 12 months. Within 4 hours of admission he begins to sweat and shake.**

    What treatment is appropriate for his alcohol problems?
    A. Gradually reducing doses of benzodiazepines over 5–7 days with oral thiamine and vitamin B.
    B. Gradually reducing doses of benzodiazepines over 5–7 days with thiamine injections.
    C. Low dose benzodiazepines for 1–2 days with oral thiamine and vitamin B.
    D. Low dose benzodiazepines for 1–2 days with thiamine injections.
    E. Low dose benzodiazepines for 5–7 days with thiamine injections.

18. **A 21-year-old intravenous heroin user is admitted with a groin abscess. He has been injecting and smoking heroin since the age of 15 on a daily basis. He rapidly starts to demonstrate symptoms of heroin withdrawal.**

    Apart from withdrawal, what other features make up the dependence syndrome?
    A. Compulsion to take the substance, evidence of tolerance, spending significant amounts on the substance, continuing to take the substance despite evidence of harm.
    B. Compulsion to take the substance, evidence of tolerance, neglect of alternative pleasures, continuing to take the substance despite evidence of harm, inability to control substance use.

C.   Compulsion to take the substance, evidence of tolerance, neglect of alternative pleasures, continuing to take the substance despite evidence of harm, spending significant amounts on the substance.

D.   Compulsion to take the substance, evidence of tolerance, neglect of alternative pleasures, spending significant amounts on the substance.

E.   Compulsion to take the substance, evidence of tolerance, spending significant amounts on the substance, inability to control substance misuse.

19. **A 50-year-old man is found collapsed in a public place. During the admission it is clear that he has no friends or family, and has been living alone since his early twenties. He has lost contact with his family, and has no wish for social contact. He has worked for nearly 30 years in a warehouse. He appears cold and detached, and does not report that he has any particular interests. He watches television, and occasionally goes cycling. He is dressed appropriately but takes little interest in his appearance. There is no history of any psychotic or affective symptoms. His collapse was caused by an undiagnosed medical condition. He has not seen his PCP in the last 10 years.**
What could the diagnosis be in this situation?
A.   Autism spectrum disorder.
B.   Paranoid personality disorder.
C.   Schizophrenia.
D.   Schizoid personality disorder.
E.   Social phobia.

20. **A 20-year-old man is seen in the ER. He has a fracture to his 5th metacarpal on the left hand. He has been in an altercation with two other youths. He is impatient to be seen and staff report that he has been intimidating. When he is told he has to wait he loses his temper and the security guards are called. He has been seen in the ER before, and on reading this report it is clear he has a significant forensic history. He has been convicted of assault and battery on numerous occasions. He has a history of poly-substance misuse and drinks alcohol heavily on a social basis. He was expelled from several schools because of his behavior, including assaults on teachers and staff. He has a history of self-harm through cutting, dating back to early teens. When seen he reports he got into a fight at a bar because he didn't like how the two youths looked. He blamed them for the fight, as he states they shouldn't have been in the bar. He wants to leave to see his girlfriend. They have been together 2 months, and she is 6 weeks pregnant. She had been with him at the bar, and had threatened to leave him when the fight started. The police arrive in the department to see him about the fight. He is rude and dismissive about the police, and doesn't appear to be worried about the situation.**
In DSM-5 terms, what is the most likely diagnosis?
A.   Antisocial personality disorder.
B.   Borderline personality disorder.
C.   Histrionic personality disorder.

D.   Schizoid personality disorder.

E.   Paranoid personality disorder.

21. **A 23-year-old woman presents to the ER with a self-inflicted cut to her left arm. She is well known to the department with a 6-year history of regular self-harm through cutting. She tells staff she has had an argument with her mother and was distressed. She uses self-harm to help her manage and relieve tension and distress. She has presented to the ER on approximately 30 occasions in the last 12 months. She states that the cut was not an attempt to end her life. She requires 15 stitches, and asks to be discharged from hospital. She has no immediate thoughts to self-harm, but states that if the argument continues she may self-harm again to relieve tension. She is seen by the on-call psychiatrist in the ER. She is having weekly group psychotherapy and sees a consultant psychiatrist in the outpatient clinic every 6 weeks, and is due to be seen in 5 days' time.**

What would be an appropriate course of action?

A.   Consider admission to a psychiatric hospital.

B.   Discharge home and counsel about immediately stopping self-harm.

C.   Discharge home and prescribe a TCA.

D.   Discharge home with a letter to the psychiatrist and psychotherapist.

E.   Discharge home with a prescription of benzodiazepines as an alternative way of managing distress/tension.

22. **A 70-year-old man is admitted to the medical assessment unit. He has a 5-day history of coughing up green sputum, and being increasingly short of breath with oxygen saturations on air of 86%. He is not known to have COPD. His only other significant past medical history is a 1-year history of Alzheimer's disease. He has been living with his wife, and before admission was independent with his activities of daily living. During the first night in a bay with five patients he becomes agitated and appears extremely confused. He tells the doctor and staff to get out of his house. He is disoriented in time. He appears to be visually hallucinating.**

What would be the most appropriate treatment?

A.   Ensure he remains on oxygen and prescribe 10 mg haloperidol for his agitation and ask nursing staff to stay with him to provide reassurance.

B.   Ensure he remains on oxygen, move him to a well-lit side room, and prescribe 10 mg haloperidol for his agitation.

C.   Ensure he remains on oxygen, move him to a well-lit side room, ask nursing staff to talk slowly and calmly to him to provide reassurance.

D.   Ensure he remains on oxygen, move him to a side room to avoid distress to other patients, and prescribe benzodiazepines for his agitation.

E.   Ensure he remains on oxygen, prescribe benzodiazepines for his agitation and ask nursing staff to stay with him to provide reassurance.

23. **An 85-year-old woman presents to her PCP. She reports that she is losing items in her house and is concerned about her short-term memory. She complains that she is becoming increasingly forgetful. On formal testing she struggles with orientation**

to time and short-term memory. She scores 23 out of 30 on the Mini-Mental State Examination. Family report that her memory has deteriorated over the last 12 months. She has never smoked. She has a history of hypertension, but no other significant medical or family history. Her physical examination is unremarkable. She recalls an incident one night several weeks ago when she thought she heard something in her garden. It was 4am, and she got up and looked out of her bedroom window. She thinks she might have seen someone lurking in a bush, but she is not sure. She recalls going downstairs and turning the outside light on, but no-one was there. She admits to drinking one bottle of white wine (11%, 750 ml) each week.

If she does have an early dementia what is the most likely diagnosis?

A. Alcoholic dementia.

B. Alzheimer's disease.

C. Frontal lobe dementia.

D. Lewy body dementia.

E. Vascular dementia.

24. A 21-year-old woman is being cared for in an intellectual disability home. She has had difficulties since birth, including some motor problems. She is able to express her basic needs, and needs support with all aspects of personal care. Her IQ is tested and found to be 45. She has poorly controlled epilepsy with regular tonic–clonic seizures.

How would you classify her intellectual disability?

A. Mild intellectual disability.

B. Moderate intellectual disability.

C. Autism spectrum disorder, moderate.

D. Profound intellectual disability.

E. Severe intellectual disability.

25. A 17-year-old man is brought to the PCP by his mother. While his mother has no major concerns, there have been ongoing problems with his behavior reported by his school. He has always struggled to make friends easily, and has been in a few fights at school when other students have objected to comments he has made. He struggles to understand other people's motivations, and has a limited range of interests. He cannot show or feign interest in other hobbies, or people. He is interested in a particular comic which he has collected for the last 5 years. He always carries some of these with him, and unless distracted will start reading these. He has done well in school in some subjects that he is interested in, getting 3 As, 2 Bs, 3 Cs and 2 Ds. The school find that he is very inflexible, and struggles with any change. He has no close friends.

What could be your preferred diagnosis to explore?

A. Autism spectrum disorder (mild).

B. Depressive disorder.

C. Schizoid personality disorder.

D. Prodromal phase of a psychotic disorder.

E. Obsessive personality disorder.

26. **An 18-year-old man presents with a first episode of psychosis. He has third person auditory hallucinations in the form of a running commentary, and has persecutory delusions. He has been threatening towards people he believes are trying to kill him and he is admitted to hospital. There is no history of substance misuse. He is started on oral risperidone.**
What lab studies would be appropriate before starting antipsychotics?
    A. ECG and blood glucose.
    B. ECG, blood glucose, and lipids.
    C. Complete blood count and an ECG.
    D. Complete blood count, blood glucose, and lipids.
    E. Complete blood count, urea and electrolytes, and liver function tests.

27. **A 27-year-old woman with a treatment-resistant depression is advised and agreed to start on lithium carbonate. She is also prescribed venlafaxine and mirtazapine. After 3 months her mood improves on this combination.**
What regular blood tests are needed while on this new medication?
    A. Complete blood count, thyroid function tests, and lithium levels.
    B. Complete blood count, BUN/Cr and electrolytes, and liver function tests.
    C. Liver function tests, thyroid function tests, and lithium levels.
    D. BUN/Cr and electrolytes, liver function tests, thyroid function tests, and lithium levels.
    E. BUN/Cr and electrolytes, thyroid function tests, and lithium levels.

28. **A 49-year-old man is being prepared for ECT for treatment-resistant depression. He is not eating and drinking without prompting as a result of severe depression. He has not responded to oral antidepressants. He has agreed to have ECT, as this has been effective for him in a previous episode of severe depression. He has a number of lab studies to prepare him for the general anesthetic.**
What would be an absolute contraindication for proceeding with this treatment?
    A. A recent myocardial infarction.
    B. Cardiac arrhythmia.
    C. Cerebral aneurysm.
    D. High anesthetic risk.
    E. Raised intracranial pressure.

29. **A 23-year-old man is in hospital for the third time. The three admissions have had a similar picture. He becomes convinced that his neighbors have installed cameras in his flat and are watching everything he is doing. He hears the neighbors talking about him and commenting on his actions. On each occasion he has been threatening towards the neighbors. On the first admission he did not respond to oral olanzapine, but did get somewhat better on quetiapine and was discharged home. He was re-admitted 4 weeks later. During the second admission it was clear that he was not improving on quetiapine and he was changed to a 2nd generation long-acting antipsychotic, and some of his symptoms improved, although he remained paranoid. He was discharged on the**

depot which he accepted, but he became increasingly unwell despite maximum doses of the depot injection. This was changed to a different 2nd generation long-acting antipsychotic injection which he was on for 4 months before the third admission. He has repeatedly been offered cognitive behavioral therapy for psychosis but does not want to proceed with this.

What is the next appropriate step in treatment?

A. Trial of cognitive behavioral therapy while in hospital.
B. Trial of a depot 1st generation antipsychotic such as haloperidol.
C. Trial of a different 2nd generation antipsychotic such as risperidone.
D. Trial of an oral 1st generation antipsychotic such as haloperidol.
E. Trial of oral clozapine.

30. A 31-year-old woman presents to her PCP. She has a long history of a poorly controlled generalized anxiety disorder with a recurrent depressive disorder. She is currently prescribed sertraline (an SSRI) for depression and anxiety, sodium valproate (as a mood stabilizer), pregabalin (an anti-epileptic used in her situation for anxiety), lorazepam (an anxiolytic), and propranolol (a beta-blocker sometimes used in anxiety). She describes an overwhelming desire to take one of these drugs, and admits to buying it over the internet, as well as taking those prescribed by her PCP. When she doesn't take this substance she sweats, shakes, and feels physically unwell. She has noticed that in the year that she has been taking this drug she has needed larger doses to make her feel better, and treat her anxiety symptoms.

Which of the following drugs is she describing and is causing these problems?

A. Lorazepam.
B. Pregabalin.
C. Propranolol.
D. Sertraline.
E. Sodium valproate.

31. A patient presents to the ER. They have been brought by their parents concerned about their mental health. You are the resident in the department. There is one consultant and a team of ER nursing staff and health care assistants. There are also three security guards in the department. The patient is a 22-year-old man who has taken a significant overdose. He reports that there are people outside the department who have been following him for 3 days. He can hear them now talking about him. They have made threats to kill him and they told him to take the overdose to end his life. There is no evidence of a mood disorder (depression or bipolar). He still believes he needs to 'sacrifice himself.' He accepts physical treatment for his overdose but repeatedly states he wants to leave the ER to end his life. The on-call psychiatrist is assessing another patient and will not be available for 1 hour.

What actions can you and the team in the ER take?

A. Ask the nurses to detain him on a psychiatric hold, which allows his detention for up to 6 hours.

B.   You could ask security to prevent him from leaving until the psychiatrist arrives.
C.   Legally you have to allow him to leave the department and ask his parents to keep him under close observation.
D.   The psychiatric social worker can detain him on a psychiatric hold which allows his detention for up to 12 hours.
E.   You, as the medicine resident, can detain him on a psychiatric hold which allows his detention for up to 72 hours.

32.   **A 30-year-old woman is in labor. She has a significant needle phobia. During the delivery there are complications, and she requires a cesarean section to save her life and the life of her baby. She initially consents to the operation. In theater she subsequently refuses to have the procedure. She has a panic attack when anyone approaches her with a needle, and states she cannot have the procedure. She is extremely distressed by the situation and has multiple symptoms of anxiety. Her husband tells the treating team to perform the cesarean section. A mental capacity assessment is performed.**
What do you think should happen?
A.   She is deemed to have capacity and no action is taken.
B.   She is deemed to have capacity but the procedure must legally happen to save her baby.
C.   She is deemed to lack capacity and in her best interests and in the best interests of the baby the operation should proceed to save her.
D.   She is deemed to lack capacity and in her best interests the operation should proceed to save her.
E.   She is deemed to lack capacity and therefore her husband can make decisions for her as next of kin, and therefore the operation should proceed.

33.   **A 69-year-old woman is admitted to the ER. She is struggling to communicate. She is extremely low in mood, and has been getting worse over the last 6 months since her husband died. She has no physical health problems. She has no enjoyment from life and describes feeling exhausted. She states her husband died suddenly in a car accident. She states that she is responsible for the car accident, although she was not there at the time. She took a large overdose of various medications earlier today with the intention to end her life. Her daughter visited today, found her, and alerted the ambulance services. Her daughter reports that her mother has lost a lot of weight, has not been looking after herself or the house, and has been struggling to sleep. The patient wishes to leave hospital and be allowed to die at home. The medication taken includes a lethal dose of acetaminophen. The patient does not want the overdose treated medically. She feels that she has no future without her husband. She previously enjoyed spending time with her grandchildren, gardening, socializing with friends, and holidays, none of which she has done for 4 months. Her daughter insists that her mother is treated and is the legal next of kin with a durable power of attorney.**
You perform a capacity assessment. What are your options?

A. Admit her to a medical ward and try to persuade her to have treatment. If you cannot persuade her to have treatment for the overdose, offer palliative care on the ward.

B. Allow her to leave hospital and die at home as these are her wishes.

C. As the daughter is next of kin you can act on her wishes in this difficult situation.

D. In her best interests treat the overdose and organize aftercare.

E. Arrange (with the ER personnel or consulting psychiatrist) to have her placed on a psychiatric hold as a danger to self and treat the overdose when detained as a medical emergency under the daughter's durable power of attorney.

34. **A 75-year-old woman has been in a residential home specializing in dementia for the past 3 years. She has a known diagnosis of Alzheimer's disease and her current Mini-Mental State Examination is 8 out of 30. Her husband died 3 years ago prompting the admission to the home, but she is visited by her children and grandchildren. Until recently there have been no management issues in the home. Over the last 3 months she has not engaged in any activities that she used to. She has been less talkative, and has been lashing out at staff when they try to support her with her activities of daily living. She has been wandering in the home and has been tearful on occasions. She has been increasingly difficult for staff to manage. There has not been a marked deterioration in her memory. She is struggling to sleep and from the early hours of the morning is wandering the home, and is aggressive to staff when they try to get her back into bed. Her PCP has seen her and examined her physically. There are no new clinical findings. All of her routine bloods and urinalysis are normal. She is known to have hypertension and type 2 diabetes, but both of these are well controlled. She is a lifelong non-smoker and drinks alcohol very occasionally. Her family are continuing to visit but are clearly distressed. Her daughter is also concerned that in the last 3 months her mother has not been eating well and has lost a substantial amount of weight. She is currently only prescribed donepezil for Alzheimer's, and is on no other psychiatric medication. She has been on this for 4 years.**

She is seen by a geriatric psychiatrist. What might be an appropriate pharmacological treatment?

A. A low dose of an oral antipsychotic to calm her when agitated and distressed, but not on a regular basis.

B. An oral benzodiazepine to treat her agitation.

C. A selective serotonin reuptake inhibitor.

D. Changing her anti-Alzheimer's medication to a different one.

E. Night-time sedation such as zopiclone to help her to sleep.

35. **A 45-year-old patient is seen in a psychiatric clinic. He talks about the 'omnimicrotask' but is unable to describe this in detail. He is known to have schizophrenia. When asked a question he repeats the last syllable of the last word in the sentence repeatedly.**

What two symptoms are described above?

A. Neologisms, circumstantiality.

B.   Neologisms, knight's move thinking.
C.   Neologisms, perseveration.
D.   Perseveration, circumstantiality.
E.   Perseveration, dysarthria.

36. **A 14-year-old boy with a mild learning disability is seen by his new PCP. He is attending a special school. He has an autism spectrum disorder, an elongated face, large protruding ears, macro-orchidism, and social anxiety. The PCP does not have access to the previous medical records.**
What syndrome is most likely?
A.   Autism syndrome.
B.   Down's syndrome.
C.   Fragile X syndrome.
D.   Klinefelter's syndrome.
E.   Prader–Willi syndrome.

37. **A 27-year-old woman with schizophrenia is prescribed a depot antipsychotic injection once a month, due to repeated admissions with non-compliance to oral medication. She has now been on this medication for 9 months. She responds well to the treatment and her psychotic symptoms are well controlled. She presents to see her psychiatrist. She reports that she has not had a menstrual cycle for 6 months, whereas before she had regular periods. She also reports that she is getting a milky discharge from her breasts. The psychiatrist suspects the depot is causing these symptoms and requests a blood test to confirm.**
Which dopaminergic pathway is implicated in the side effects above?
A.   Basal forebrain cholinergic.
B.   Mesocortical.
C.   Mesolimbic.
D.   Nigrostriatal.
E.   Tuberoinfundibular.

38. **An 83-year-old single man is seen in the memory clinic by a consultant psychiatrist. He has been struggling at home for 6 months and has had a deteriorating memory. He is accompanied by his son to the clinic. He has no other medical conditions relevant to the memory problems but does have rheumatoid arthritis. The CT brain scan demonstrates marked hippocampal atrophy and his MMSE is 20 out of 30 on the last two clinic visits. He is fiercely independent and does not want to consider any day groups. He has accepted a small package of care. He is struggling to wash and dress in the morning, and is having difficulty making hot drinks. An OT from the community mental health team sees him at home and believes some of his problems relate to his rheumatoid arthritis. He cannot get in and out of the bath, but does not want the bath turned into a shower. He sees his PCP on a regular basis for the monitoring of his arthritis.**

He has appointments with the rheumatologist several times a year, and has had intermittent input from the physical therapists both in the community and in outpatient settings.

Which professional would be best placed to coordinate his care?

A. Primary care practitioner.
B. Occupational therapist.
C. Physical therapist.
D. Psychiatrist.
E. Rheumatologist.

39. A 37-year-old man with a history of bipolar depression is brought in to the ER after being found by family in an obtunded state. On examination, he is found to have a bilateral tremor, hyperreflexia tachycardia with a heart rate of 115, a blood pressure of 200/120, an elevated temperature and downbeat nystagmus. The most effective treatment for this overdose is:

A. Lavage with charcoal.
B. Dialysis.
C. A beta-blocker and baclofen.
D. A cooling blanket and thiazide diuretic.
E. Leave to work through system.

40. An army veteran who served two tours of duty in Afghanistan complains of intrusive memories of a combat situation in which he witnessed several of his platoon members and a number of civilians, including small children, killed by gunfire. He has intrusive memories and nightmares about this experience. He often hears the voices of children screaming, just as had occurred in the combat situation. He is hypervigilant whenever he leaves the house and gets anxious in unfamiliar places. He frequently feels on edge. The most effective treatment for this condition is:

A. An SSRI.
B. An antipsychotic.
C. A benzodiazepine.
D. A mood stabilizer.
E. CBT.

Glossary of terms

Acute intoxication: Physiological and psychological response due to the administration of a psychoactive substance.

Affect: Refers to the transient flow of emotion in response to a particular stimulus, i.e. the immediate expression of emotions.

Agnosia: Impaired recognition of sensory stimuli not attributed to sensory loss or language disturbance. May be a feature of dementia.

Akathisia: Unpleasant feeling of restlessness. May be a side effect of antipsychotics.

Amenorrhea: The absence of menstruation. May be a feature of anorexia nervosa.

Amnesia: A deficit in memory. A feature of organic disorders such as dementia and delirium. Anterograde amnesia is diminished ability to form new memories and retrograde amnesia involves loss of memories of events that have occurred in the past.

Anergia: A lack of energy (core feature of depression).

Anhedonia: A lack of interest in things which were previously enjoyable to the patient.

Anticipatory anxiety: Anxiety at the prospect of encountering the feared situation.

Anxiety: An unpleasant emotional state involving subjective fear and somatic symptoms.

Apathy: Lack of interest, enthusiasm, or concern.

Apraxia: Inability to carry out previously learned purposeful movements despite normal coordination and strength. May be a feature of dementia.

Autonomic arousal: A general state of physiological arousal associated with what is commonly referred to as the 'fight or flight syndrome'. Mediated by the sympathetic nervous system with features including sweating, dry mouth, and tachycardia.

Beck's triad: A feature of depressive disorder with negative feelings about the self, the world and the future.

Bereavement: Reaction in response to loss of a loved one which may be normal or abnormal.

Bingeing: A feature of bulimia nervosa where patients overeat.

Blunted affect: Reduced expression of emotion.

Body mass index (BMI): A measure of weight relative to height. Calculated as weight (kg) $\div$ [height (m)]^2.

Briquet's syndrome: Multiple, recurrent, and frequently changing physical symptoms not explained by a physical illness (also known as somatization or somatic symptoms disorder).

Capgras' syndrome: Delusion that a familiar person has been replaced by an exact duplicate.

Catatonia: Abnormality of tone, posture, or movement arising from a disturbed mental state, typically schizophrenia. Can be excessive or decreased motor activity.

Circumstantiality: Thinking progresses slowly as a result of many unnecessary digressions but it eventually returns to original point.

Clang association: Ideas related only by similar or rhyming sounds rather than meaning.

Cognition: Consists of consciousness, orientation, attention, concentration, and memory.

Cognitive behavioral therapy: A psychotherapy used to help individuals identify and challenge their negative thoughts and then to modify any abnormal underlying core beliefs.

Compulsions: Repetitive, purposeful behaviors or mental acts that a person feels driven into performing.

Confabulation: Gaps in memory which are unconsciously filled with false memories.

Conversion: Distressing events are transformed into physical symptoms. A feature of dissociative disorder.

Cotard's syndrome (nihilism): Delusion that everything is non-existent including themselves.

Counter-transference: In psychodynamic therapy, refers to the therapist's emotions and attitudes towards the patient.

de Clérambault's syndrome: Delusion that an exalted or famous person is in love with them.

Déjà vu: The illusion that an event or experience has already been experienced in the past.

Deliberate self-harm: Refers to an intentional act of self-poisoning or self-injury.

Delirium: An acute, transient, global organic disorder of central nervous system functioning resulting in impaired consciousness and attention.

Delirium tremens: A withdrawal delirium after alcohol cessation, characterized by cognitive impairment, delusions, hallucinations, and autonomic arousal.

Delusion: A fixed false belief, which is firmly held, despite evidence to the contrary and out of keeping with the individual's social, religious, educational, and cultural background.

Delusional perception: A new delusion that forms in response to a real perception without any logical sense. It is one of Schneider's first rank symptoms of schizophrenia.

Dementia: A syndrome of generalized decline of memory, intellect, and personality, without impairment of consciousness, leading to functional impairment.

Dependence syndrome: Prolonged, compulsive substance use leading to addiction, tolerance, and the potential for withdrawal syndromes.

Depersonalization: Feeling of detachment from the normal sense of self.

Depot: Long-acting, slow release medications given intramuscularly to improve adherence (e.g. certain antipsychotics).

Depression: A mood disorder characterized by a persistent low mood, loss of pleasure, and/or lack of energy.

Derealization: The feeling that surroundings or people are experienced as unreal.

Disinhibition: A lack of restraint manifested in disregard for social conventions, impulsivity, and poor judgement.

Dissociation: A process of 'separating off' certain memories from normal consciousness (feature of dissociative disorder).

Diurnal mood variation: The patient's low mood is more pronounced during certain times of the day (usually in the morning).

Dizygotic twins: Twins formed after fertilization of two separate eggs.

Dopamine hypothesis: States that schizophrenia is secondary to over-activity of the mesolimbic dopamine pathways in the brain.

DSM-5: Published by the American Psychiatric Association and used in the diagnosis and classification of mental disorders.

Dysarthria: A disorder in articulating speech.

Dysmorphophobia: Excessive preoccupation with barely noticeable or imagined defects in their physical appearance.

Dysphasia: Disorder in language (e.g. problems finding words).

Dysthymia: Depressive state for at least 2 years, which does not meet the criteria for a mild, moderate or severe depressive disorder (now named persistent depressive disorder in DSM-5).

Dystonia: Acute painful contractions (spasms) of muscles. May be a side effect of antipsychotic use.

Echolalia: Repetition of words. May be a feature of autism.

Elated mood: Elevation of mood.

Electroencephalogram (EEG): A measure of the electrical activity of the brain – gives information about the state of the patient's brain and their level of consciousness.

Enuresis: Involuntary voiding of urine in children who should have established bladder control. Can be linked to psychosocial stressors and organic causes must be excluded.

Erotomania: See *de Clérambault's syndrome*.

Euphoria: An exaggerated feeling of wellbeing – commonly associated with substance misuse.

Euthymic: An objective description of normal mood.

Executive function: Higher functions include planning, organization, problem solving, abstract thinking, and decision making, which may be lost in dementia.

Exposure and response prevention: A technique in which a patient is repeatedly exposed to a situation which causes them anxiety and they are prevented from performing the actions which lessen that anxiety – commonly used in OCD.

Extrapyramidal side effects: Potential problem with taking antipsychotics. Includes parkinsonism, akathisia, dystonia, and tardive dyskinesia.

Flight of ideas: Speech difficult to understand as it switches rapidly from one loosely connected idea to another.

Folie à deux: A syndrome in which a delusional belief is transmitted from one individual to another such that they share the delusion.

Formal thought disorder: Abnormality of the way that thoughts are linked together.

Free association: Articulation of all thoughts that come to the mind. This is used in psychodynamic therapy.

Graduated exposure: A technique in the treatment of phobias where one is exposed to a feared stimulus in a controlled manner with the end purpose of eradicating the fear.

Grandiosity: Inflated ideas about oneself. A feature of mania.

Hallucination: A false perception in the absence of an external stimulus.

Hyperarousal: An exaggerated response to normal stimuli (e.g. sound); a feature of PTSD.

ICD-10: International classification of diseases is the standard diagnostic tool for clinical purposes, published by the World Health Organization.

Illness anxiety (hypochondriacal) disorder: Misinterpretation of normal bodily sensations, leading to a non-delusional preoccupation of having a serious physical disease.

Illusion: A false mental image produced by the misinterpretation of an external stimulus.

Insight: The extent to which the patient understands the nature of their condition.

Kleptomania: Inability to refrain from stealing, a differential diagnosis for OCD.

Knight's move thinking: A form of loosening of association where there is discourse consisting of a sequence of unrelated ideas.

Korsakoff's psychosis: Profound short-term memory loss characterized by confabulation, disorientation to time, and personality change.

Labile mood: Refers to a fluctuating mood state.

Libido: Refers to sexual drive. May be reduced in depression.

Loosening of associations: A type of formal thought disorder involving the loss of the normal structure of thinking.

Malingering: Patient seeks advantageous consequences of being diagnosed with a medical condition. For instance, evading criminal prosecution or receiving benefits.

Mental capacity: The ability to take in information, process it in a structured way, weigh up the options, arrive at a decision, and then communicate one's thoughts coherently.

Monoamine hypothesis: A deficiency in monoamine neurotransmitters causes depression.

Monozygotic twins: Two individuals with the same genetic makeup after a single egg was fertilized and split early in embryonic development.

Mood: Refers to a patient's sustained, subjective, experienced emotion over a period of time.

Multidisciplinary team (MDT): A group of professionals working together to ensure optimal patient management for their condition, with the patient at the center of their treatment.

Munchausen's syndrome (factitious disorder): The individual wishes to adopt the 'sick role' in order to receive the care of a patient, for internal emotional gain.

Negative symptoms: Are deficits in association with schizophrenia and include apathy, blunting of affect, poverty of thought and speech, social isolation, and poor self-care.

Neologism: Words or phrases devised by the patient which have no ordinary meaning.

Neuroleptic malignant syndrome: Rare but life-threatening condition seen in patients taking antipsychotic medications, characterized by pyrexia, muscle rigidity, and autonomic instability.

Neurosis: Collective term for psychiatric disorders characterized by distress, that are non-organic, have a discrete onset, and where delusions and hallucinations are absent.

Night terrors: Episode where individual (commonly a child) awakes suddenly from sleep, screaming in extreme distress and unresponsive to the efforts of others to console them.

Obsession: Unwanted, persistent, intrusive thoughts, images, or urges that repeatedly enter the individual's mind in a stereotyped form.

Operant conditioning: States that consequences of actions (positive or negative) will affect future behavior.

Othello syndrome: Delusion that their partner is being unfaithful without having any proof.

Overvalued idea (preoccupation): An isolated, preoccupying, strongly held belief derived through normal mental processes, which dominates a person's life and affects their actions.

Paraphrenia: Late onset schizophrenia. Positive symptoms occur in the absence of negative symptoms.

Passivity phenomenon: Belief that thoughts, sensations, and actions being controlled by an external force.

Perseveration: Uncontrollable and often inappropriate repetition of a particular response (e.g. word or phrase).

Pervasive developmental disorder: A group of disorders characterized by delays in the development of socialization and communication skills (e.g. autism).

Phobia: An intense, irrational fear of an object, situation, place, or person that is recognized as excessive (out of proportion to the threat) or unreasonable.

Positive symptoms: In relation to schizophrenia are active symptoms such as delusions, hallucinations, and formal thought disorder.

Postpartum depression: Onset of depression after having a baby. Usually develops within 3 months of delivery and at its most extreme, patient can have intrusive thoughts of harming the baby.

Postpartum psychosis: Development of psychotic symptoms in the postpartum period (usually occurs within 4 weeks).

Poverty of speech: Reduced speech. May be a feature of depression or dementia.

Premorbid personality: Personality or character prior to the onset of psychiatric illness.

Pressure of speech: Speech is abnormally fast as if there are too many ideas to verbalize at a given moment in time. May be a feature of mania.

Prion disease: A prion is a particle that does not contain DNA or RNA. Known to cause fatal diseases of the brain with spongiform degeneration. CJD is an example.

Prodrome: A symptom or group of symptoms indicating the onset of a disease.

Pseudodementia: Poor concentration and impaired memory are common in depression in the elderly population. May represent a progressive dementia unmasked by depression.

Pseudohallucination: As with hallucination but recognized by the individual as unreal.

Psychomotor agitation: Excessive activity or restlessness.

Psychomotor retardation: Slowing of movements or speech.

Psychosis: A mental state in which reality is greatly distorted.

Purging: Compensatory weight loss behaviors in bulimia nervosa, e.g. self-induced vomiting.

Rapid cycling: A category of bipolar disorder with a poor prognosis.

Risk assessment: In a psychiatric context it is assessing the risk of self-harm, suicide, and/or risk to others.

Rumination: Repetitively mulling over the same thoughts to the extent that other mental activity is impaired. A feature of PTSD.

Russell's sign: Calluses on the back of the hand indicative of self-induced vomiting and therefore a feature of bulimia nervosa.

Schizoaffective disorder: Characterized by both symptoms of schizophrenia and a history of mood disorder (depression, mania, or hypomania) in which the psychotic symptoms are not limited to just the mood episodes.

Schizophrenia: Characterized by hallucinations, delusions, and thought disorders which lead to functional impairment.

Schneider's first rank symptoms: If present, are strongly suggestive of schizophrenia (delusional perception, auditory hallucinations, thought interference, passivity phenomenon).

Serotonin syndrome: A rare but life-threatening complication of increased serotonin activity (e.g. with MAOI + a serotonergic medication). Ranges from mild to severe and life-threatening. Characterized by diaphoresis, increased reflexes, tremor, elevated body temperature, autonomic instability, coma, and potentially death.

Sick role: Refers to sickness and the rights and obligations of those affected. In somatic symptom disorders this role may be adopted for personal gain.

Social learning theory: Behavior is learned based on observation and imitation.

Somatic symptoms: Symptoms relating to the physical body (e.g. palpitations, dyspnea).

Stress-vulnerability model: Predicts that schizophrenia occurs due to environmental factors interacting with a genetic predisposition.

Suicidal ideation: Recurrent thoughts about taking one's own life.

Suicide: A fatal act of self-harm initiated with the intention of ending one's own life.

Sundowning: In delirium, cognition often fluctuates and is more impaired at night compared to in the day, a feature referred to as sundowning. Thought to be related to decreased sensory input, fatigue, and other factors.

Tangentiality: Diversion from original train of thought but no return to it.

Tardive dyskinesia: Late onset spontaneous, involuntary movements of the lips, tongue, fingers, toes, that may be a result of antipsychotic use.

Thought blocking: Sudden cessation to flow of thoughts.

Thought broadcast: The belief that thoughts are audible to others or being broadcast (e.g. on television, radio) to the public.

Thought insertion: Belief that thoughts are being put into the mind from an outside agency.

Thought withdrawal: Belief that thoughts are being extracted from the mind by external agency.

Tics: Repeated, sudden, involuntary, irregular movements involving a group of muscles.

Tolerance: Need for increasing quantity of substance to produce desired effects.

Transference: In the context of psychodynamic psychotherapy, refers to the patient's relationship with the therapist in connection to previous relationships held with others.

Wernicke's encephalopathy: An acute encephalopathy which may be seen in chronic alcoholism, due to thiamine deficiency, presenting with delirium, nystagmus, ophthalmoplegia, and ataxia.

Withdrawal syndrome: Physical or psychological effects from cessation of a substance after prolonged, repeated or high use.

Word salad: Speech that is reduced to senseless repetition of sounds or phrases.

Yerkes–Dodson law: States that anxiety can be beneficial up to a plateau of optimal functioning.

Appendix A

Answers to board-style questions

1. **Answer: D**
   The three individuals are talking about him and therefore he is experiencing auditory hallucinations. The patient has also heard the radio presenter talking directly to him, and this would be a delusion of reference. In delusions of reference the patient would hear what anyone hears when listening to the radio, but derive a delusional meaning from this. Pseudo-hallucinations would be recognized by the individual as unreal but there is no evidence to suggest this. Thought insertion is the belief that others are inserting thought into the patient's mind that are not their own. Thought withdrawal refers to the belief that others are taking thoughts out of the patient's mind. A command auditory hallucination is a command to do something like hurt oneself.

2. **Answer: C**
   Although the trigger may be the death of her mother and some could argue that this is an adjustment disorder, she meets the criteria for a major depressive illness. However, following bereavement, or any life event, if the individual meets the criteria for a depressive disorder, this diagnosis and treatment should be followed. If the bereavement is an important factor, bereavement counseling may be an appropriate psychological intervention. Although she is only sleeping 4 hours, she is tired and has no other symptoms of mania or hypomania. There are no psychotic symptoms and no evidence of a psychotic depression.

3. **Answer: D**
   The presence of psychotic symptoms precludes hypomania or bipolar II disorder. His beliefs about his blood are probably grandiose delusions and therefore he would be classed as suffering from mania with psychosis (see *Fig. 3.3.2*). Mixed states refer to symptoms of depression and mania or hypomania simultaneously.

4. **Answer: A**
   He has only had the symptoms for 2 weeks so cannot yet be diagnosed with schizophrenia, despite having first rank symptoms (remember symptoms have to be present for at least 6 months). For schizoaffective disorder you need to meet the criteria for schizophrenia and a mood disorder. He is not suffering from a delusional disorder as in this disorder, patients present with delusions but no accompanying prominent hallucinations, but he has auditory hallucinations. No information has been given about mood symptoms to diagnose a severe depressive disorder.

5. **Answer: D**
   He is describing a thought being placed into his head that belongs to someone else (thought insertion). With thought withdrawal, patients believe their own thoughts are being taken away from them by someone else and in thought broadcast, patients believe that their thoughts are being heard out loud. He is clearly becoming paranoid about this being a trap, and he may have a secondary persecutory delusion.

6. **Answer: D**

    This is a classic description of social phobia, or fear of scrutiny by other people. To rule out agoraphobia you would want to know whether she struggles to go out. In social phobia individuals are able to function in crowds, but struggle in more intimate social situations, or when public speaking. Vomiting phobia or emetophobia is an intense, irrational fear of vomiting including fear of vomiting in a public place, fear of seeing vomit, or fear of seeing the action of vomiting. Generalized anxiety disorder is a chronic disorder in which the patient is in a constant state of high anxiety; conversely in this patient, her anxiety is attributable only to social events.

7. **Answer: A**

    The description in the scenario is for panic disorder, which is causing significant problems for the individual, and is beginning to lead to avoidance. Benzodiazepines should probably be avoided and are not going to treat the underlying condition. Antidepressants such as SSRIs or TCAs could be used, depending on patient choice, but are not given in the options. CBT is the most appropriate treatment from the list. CBT should be offered in primary care and a referral to see a psychiatrist is unwarranted at the present time. Further investigation to rule out an organic cause of anxiety (e.g. hyperthyroidism) is warranted, but further ECGs when this has been done in the Emergency Department are unlikely to reveal any new abnormalities.

8. **Answer: B**

    While it is important to check about a co-morbid history of depression, a family history and his insight, these will not help to confirm the diagnosis of OCD. However, the diagnostic guidelines for OCD do include checking that the patient recognizes the thoughts as his own. Individuals with OCD are often very frustrated that they know the thoughts are their own, know the thoughts are irrational, but struggle to resist these thoughts because of the unpleasant physical anxiety symptoms this causes.

9. **Answer: D**

    All of the symptoms listed are possible in PTSD. Patients will often have co-morbid depression with low mood, anhedonia, etc. However, flashbacks, which include repeated reliving of the accident, are common, as is a state of autonomic hyperarousal with an exaggerated startle reaction. He may be on edge walking on the sidewalk and you may see him being easily startled at road noises. Nightmares are also common, which can affect sleep.

10. **Answer: B**

    There is no past history and the description is of a woman with a severe depression, with a possible depressive psychosis. First-line treatment would be with an SSRI and not with tricyclic antidepressants. Given the patient is struggling to concentrate during a brief assessment with her PCP, she will not currently be an ideal candidate for CBT. An antipsychotic may be appropriate, although we would need more information; however, this again is not first-line. In this situation, watching and waiting would not be appropriate as she is at risk of remaining severely depressed or even becoming suicidal if not treated. This patient may need referral to secondary care, perhaps to home treatment, but that is not an option given.

11. **Answer: B**

    This man has bipolar affective disorder as he has had previous episodes of mania. It would therefore be best to avoid any of the antidepressants. Quetiapine is approved for bipolar depression and is therefore the most appropriate option from the list. CBT may be an appropriate longer-term treatment, but not in combination with an antidepressant. Antidepressants are less effective in bipolar disorder than in unipolar depression and they can also trigger manic or hypomanic episodes. With active suicidal thoughts you may wish to limit prescriptions to 1 week to limit access to more dangerous medications.

12. **Answer: A**

This is a challenging question. Discharge home may be appropriate with more information, but only with urgent (same-day) home treatment. However, this is potentially a high risk situation, and the options C, D, and E do not offer the level of support needed. All of the follow-up options will not be immediate and will take several weeks, during which time the patient and his wife will be left alone. That leaves the admission options. It can be argued that he is willing to accept treatment and so is suitable for less restrictive care. However, his unwillingness to accept hospitalization in the context of a severe depression, clear suicidal intent, and a distressed spouse suggest that he should not be sent home.

13. **Answer: C**

The patient has a normal BMI of 20.7. Although anorexics may sometimes binge and purge, the normal BMI goes strongly against this. Binge eating disorder alone would not explain the long history of purging. Remember that over 50% of individuals with an eating disorder do not meet the DSM-5 criteria for AN and BN and may be diagnosed with an eating disorder that is not specified. Also consider the physical consequences of repeated vomiting which can include biochemical and metabolic, as well as structural problems and esophageal tears. The cause of this woman's presentation is probably a Mallory–Weiss tear due to repeated vomiting.

14. **Answer: C**

The patient is experiencing a psychogenic blindness which is a type of **conversion disorder**. The patient witnessed a traumatic event, the death of her father, and the psychological compensation was to stop seeing anything. Psychogenic blindness is very rare and, like all conversion disorders, stems from a psychological conflict that manifests physically. Often, the physical symptom in a conversion disorder is neurological, such as paralysis or pseudo-seizures. Physical and laboratory examination reveals normal findings or findings that are not consistent with an organic illness. Most conversion disorders remit over time. Hypnosis and psychotherapies are effective treatments for a conversion disorder.

15. **Answer: E**

In this situation the patient is presenting with symptoms with no physical cause, which is probably a somatic symptom disorder. In illness anxiety (hypochondriacal) disorder the patient would present with a concern about a specific illness, e.g. Crohn's disease. There is no evidence of secondary gain which would point towards a diagnosis of malingering, and there is no evidence that the individual is consciously producing these symptoms, which would point towards factitious disorder.

16. **Answer: B**

Wernicke's encephalopathy is caused by a severe thiamine deficiency (vitamin B_1), and presents with a classical set of symptoms: delirium, nystagmus, ophthalmoplegia, and ataxia. It requires urgent treatment with parenteral thiamine to prevent progression to Korsakoff's psychosis. Korsakoff's psychosis is a profound (often irreversible) short-term memory loss characterized by confabulation (the unconscious filling of gaps in memory with imaginary events) and disorientation to time.

17. **Answer: B**

With the amount of alcohol being consumed, the patient will require a high dose of benzodiazepines (often chlordiazepoxide), gradually reducing over 5–7 days, depending on the local protocol. The patient may be vitamin B deficient, and to prevent Wernicke's encephalopathy, thiamine injections should be considered, as oral thiamine and vitamin B tablets may not be sufficient. These oral supplements should be considered long term after thiamine injections.

18. **Answer: B**
Remember that the six features of dependence syndrome can be recalled using the mnemonic **D**rug **P**roblems **W**ill **C**ontinue **T**o **H**arm: **D**esire/compulsion to consume substance, **P**reoccupation with substance (neglect of alternative pleasures), **W**ithdrawal effects, **C**ontrol impaired, **T**olerance increased, **H**armful effects known but continues to persist. A diagnosis of dependence syndrome can be made if at least three of these six factors are present together.

19. **Answer: D**
This is a classic description of an individual with a schizoid personality, who has no interest in friends or normal social contacts, including relationships. Without any history of positive symptoms of psychosis such as hallucinations, delusions, and thought disorder it would be difficult to say this is a case of paranoid schizophrenia. Individuals with a paranoid personality are suspicious, bear grudges, and usually have relationships, although these are often difficult to maintain because of the suspiciousness. There is no evidence at present to suspect an autistic spectrum disorder, and no evidence of a social phobia. Indeed, individuals with social phobia may struggle with relationships but find this frustrating and distressing.

20. **Answer: C**
A clear sociopathic picture, with an individual who appears to accept no responsibility for his behavior and actions, with problems dating back to adolescence. In the DSM-5 classification, this would be an antisocial personality disorder. Individuals with a paranoid personality are suspicious, bear grudges, and usually have relationships, although these are often difficult to maintain because of the suspiciousness. Self-harm is more common in emotionally unstable personality disorder (borderline subtype), but the rest of the history is more convincing for sociopathic difficulties.

21. **Answer: D**
In this situation there is no immediate severe risk. Self-harm will continue in the short and medium term as it is being used as a coping strategy. The most appropriate treatment is most likely the group psychotherapy. An admission to a psychiatric hospital is unlikely to improve the current situation, and may make the situation worse. Given that she is already seeing a psychiatrist and has an appointment in 5 days, it is most appropriate to contact them, and the psychotherapist. Decisions about other support should be left to the existing care team in discussion with the patient, and not be made in a crisis situation. It would be inappropriate to prescribe from the ER, and there may be a risk that this prescription could then be used to self-harm. Although it may be tempting to ask people to stop self-harming, this is a gross over-simplification of the behavior, and is unlikely to effect any change.

22. **Answer: C**
C is the best answer in the first instance. This is probably an acute confusional state (delirium) on a background of early dementia. This could be caused by the infection, hypoxia, or another cause. Ensure his oxygen saturations are adequate, and move him to a well-lit side room. Ensure that when nurses are in his room they only talk to him in a calm and clear manner. Benzodiazepines would not be appropriate, as these may lower his oxygen saturations by causing respiratory depression. Haloperidol may be appropriate, but it would not be the first action you take to manage the situation and may be used at very low dose if the environmental and nursing measures do not safely manage his agitation and he poses a risk to himself or others. Furthermore, 10 mg of haloperidol is a very large dose, and should not be used, especially in an individual who has not had antipsychotics before, and never in a patient of this age, in this situation. A dose of 0.5 mg haloperidol may be more appropriate.

23. **Answer: B**

    The picture of disorientation to time and short-term memory loss would suggest Alzheimer's. There are no features to suggest a frontal lobe dementia, such as worsening of social behavior, disinhibition (reduced control over one's behavior), apathy/restlessness, repetitive behavior, or changes in personality. Furthermore, memory is usually preserved in frontal lobe dementia in its early stages. The incident at night may be an illusion, and is not necessarily suggestive of a Lewy body dementia, which typically presents with visual hallucinations. One bottle of wine each week, spread across the week is approximately 4–5 drinks per week which is still under 1 drink/day and not likely to result in alcoholic dementia (unless she had been drinking much more than this for many years). The only vascular risk factor is hypertension, but the clinical picture is more suggestive of Alzheimer's.

24. **Answer: B**

    Mild intellectual disability: IQ 50–69
    Moderate intellectual disability: IQ 35–49
    Severe intellectual disability: IQ 20–34
    Profound intellectual disability: IQ difficult to measure but less than 20
    Pervasive developmental disorder: a descriptive term for conditions including autism.

25. **Answer: A**

    The best answer is A. He is presenting with inflexibility, communication problems, and a seeming lack of being able to understand other people, all of which may point to an autism spectrum disorder. It is best to avoid the diagnosis of a personality disorder in a 17-year-old, and we would need to know more before starting to think about a schizoid or obsessive personality. There is no evidence of psychosis such as hallucinations and delusions, but social withdrawal may represent a prodromal phase.

26. **Answer: B**

    B is the best answer from the list. An ECG is important as antipsychotics do have cardiac side effects including prolonged QTc interval which can predispose to torsades de pointes. Atypical antipsychotics cause metabolic syndrome and can lead to significant weight gain and therefore measurement of BMI, waist circumference and blood glucose and lipids at baseline, and then at regular intervals, is important.

27. **Answer: E**

    Lithium can be nephrotoxic and excreted via the kidneys and so BUN/Cr are measured at baseline and every 6 months. It is not metabolized by the liver, therefore liver function tests are not needed. Lithium levels are important as lithium works within a narrow therapeutic window (normal limit = 0.64–1.2 mmol/L), and if levels are high (>1.5 mmol/L) it can be extremely toxic, and can cause seizures, coma, and even death. Lithium also damages the thyroid and therefore TFTs need to be monitored at baseline and every year.

28. **Answer: E**

    The only absolute contraindication is E. The other four are relative contraindications, and a decision would have to be made about the risk of progressing with ECT versus the benefits of treatment. With options A–D, early discussion with the anesthetist and appropriate further investigations and interventions may be considered.

29. **Answer: E**

    Based on the symptoms described above, clozapine is the next appropriate step. Clozapine is approved as a third-line treatment for schizophrenia and it is the only antipsychotic that has evidence that it is more effective than other antipsychotics. It should only be prescribed after failing to respond to two other antipsychotics (treatment-resistant schizophrenia). There may be reasons why clozapine is not prescribed, which might include poor compliance with oral medication; however, it should be considered. If it is not appropriate an alternative antipsychotic will be needed. The choice of oral versus long-acting injectable will depend on compliance issues. Given that the patient has not wanted to consider CBT, unless he can be persuaded to agree to this he cannot be forced into having talking therapies, and in this situation, it is unlikely to be effective.

30. Answer: A

The patient is describing four symptoms of the dependence syndrome: a desire to take the substance, difficulties in controlling the substance-taking behavior (buying from the internet), withdrawal symptoms (sweats, shakes, and physically unwell) and tolerance (needing bigger doses to get the same effect). Certain drugs can cause a dependence syndrome, e.g. alcohol, opiates, and benzodiazepines. Lorazepam is a benzodiazepine and can rapidly cause a dependence syndrome.

31. Answer: B

The power to place a patient on a psychiatric hold varies from state to state. Generally, only certain medical personnel are designated by a county or municipality and given the power to institute a psychiatric hold (usually a licensed psychiatrist or psychologist). B is the best answer given that he appears to pose an immediate risk to himself as a result of his mental state and therefore it would be best to try to prevent him from leaving. If he does leave, C would still not be appropriate. Whilst you would want his parents to keep him under observation in this situation you would also contact the police to find him. The police could place a patient on a psychiatric hold if they feel the patient meets the criteria for a psychiatric hold in a public place, and take him to a place of safety for assessment.

32. Answer: D

When assessing capacity the first question you should ask yourself is 'Does the person have an impairment that limits capacity to reason about the risks and benefits of a given treatment?' A severe phobia in this situation is an impairment of the mind that could impact on her ability to weigh up a decision. In this situation it can be argued that the patient lacks capacity. If a decision is taken that she lacks capacity, her husband can be consulted, but he cannot make decisions for her unless he has a medical lasting power of attorney (power of attorney can be over medical matters or finances), which the scenario does not describe. B is not correct, as the unborn baby has no legal status until outside the womb.

33. Answer: D

The description in the scenario is of a patient with a severe depressive disorder. She has ideas, possibly delusions of guilt relating to her husband's death. These depressive cognitions may impact on her ability to weigh up a decision. Therefore, it can be argued that she lacks capacity, and in her best interests the overdose can be treated. Remember that psychiatric hold can only be used to provide observation of a psychiatric but not medical illness and therefore her lack of capacity is demonstrated to proceed with urgent care. In addition, her daughter's durable power of attorney may well allow treatment to proceed. She will, however, need psychiatric follow-up, which might include an admission and treatment for her mental health condition on a psychiatric hold as a danger to self.

34. Answer: C

The description may fit with a patient who has become depressed, is tearful, not engaging in activities, neglecting herself, has lost weight, and is struggling to sleep. Indeed, patients with Alzheimer's disease can also have non-cognitive symptoms of depression. A trial of an antidepressant would therefore be most appropriate. Options A, B and E will lead to sedation only and will not treat the underlying cause of depression. Changing her anti-dementia medication to another medication such as memantine may help with memory but is unlikely to have an effect on her depressive symptoms.

35. **Answer: C**

The 'omnimicrotask' may be an example of a neologism. These can be new words created by the patient, or an everyday word used in an unusual way by the patient. The repetition of words or phrases is an example of perseveration. Circumstantiality is where thinking and speech are filled with unnecessary trivial details. Knight's move thinking is a form of formal thought disorder where there do not appear to be links between ideas in speech. Dysarthria is a problem with the articulation of speech seen in many different disorders, e.g. stroke.

36. **Answer: C**

This is a classical description of fragile X syndrome. It will be important as you approach board exams to review all of your basic sciences, including genetics, as these conditions are easy to test, both in SBA and clinical examinations. Klinefelter's is 47 XXY, but intelligence is usually normal. Prader–Willi usually presents in childhood, with the best known feature being chronic and excessive hunger, leading to obesity, although incomplete sexual development is usually seen rather than the macro-orchidism described. Asperger's is a form of autism, and does not present with the other features.

37. **Answer: E**

The tuberoinfundibular pathway, when blocked, can cause raised prolactin levels, which in turn has a number of effects. This includes abnormal lactation, changes to menstrual cycle including amenorrhea, and sexual dysfunction. A–D are all dopaminergic pathways. Antipsychotics work on the mesolimbic and mesocortical dopamine pathways to inhibit positive and negative symptoms of schizophrenia, respectively. Antipsychotics cause EPSE via the nigrostriatal pathway. E is not a dopaminergic pathway as its name suggests. Again in board exams, basic sciences including neuroanatomy can be tested and this needs to be reviewed.

38. **Answer: B**

This question tests your knowledge of the roles and responsibilities of the multidisciplinary team. The OT may be best placed to coordinate his care from the list given. He needs adaptations to support him with his ADL at home. The psychiatrist may only see him every 6 months to monitor his Alzheimer's disease (hippocampal atrophy), and the rheumatologist likewise for the arthritis. The primary care practitioner would be next best placed to coordinate the community care options needed. The physical therapist does not currently have a role from the scenario described.

39. **Answer: B**

This is most likely to be a lithium overdose. The downbeat nystagmus in the context of autonomic hyperactivity is strongly suggestive of a lithium overdose in a bipolar patient. Symptomatic treatment for the blood pressure, heart rate, and hyperthermia will not prevent other complications of a lithium overdose including seizures and death. Lithium does not adhere to charcoal, so this strategy is also not likely to be useful. The most effective strategy for treating an acute lithium overdose is dialysis.

40. **Answer: A**

SSRIs are currently the only class of drugs FDA-approved for the treatment of PTSD. Multiple studies have concluded that benzodiazepines are not effective in the management of PTSD and may contribute to a worsening of symptoms. The patient hearing voices of children screaming is not a psychotic symptom but an intrusive memory and not likely to be helped by antipsychotics. The Department of Defense has concluded that antipsychotics do not generally appear useful in the treatment of PTSD. While mood stabilizers can sometimes help mood instability or impulsive anger in PTSD patients, they will not improve the core symptoms of PTSD in most patients.

Appendix B

Answers to self-assessment questions

3.2 Depressive disorder

1. Anhedonia (lack of enjoyment). *(1 point)*

2. Any four of the following: diurnal variation in mood *(1 point)*, early morning wakening *(1 point)*, loss of libido *(1 point)*, psychomotor retardation *(1 point)*, weight loss *(1 point)*, and loss of appetite *(1 point)*.

3. In a woman of this age, it is very important to rule out thyroid dysfunction as it can present very similarly *(1 point)*. It is therefore necessary to carry out thyroid function tests (TFTs) including TSH, free T_3 and T_4 *(1 point)*.

4. First-line antidepressants are selective serotonin reuptake inhibitors (SSRIs) *(1 point)*. An example can include any of the following *(1 point)*: citalopram, escitalopram, fluoxetine, paroxetine, sertraline, fluvoxamine.

5. Treatment-resistant depression *(1 point)*, suicidal ideation *(1 point)*, life-threatening depression, e.g. when the patient refuses to eat or drink *(1 point)*, catatonia *(1 point)*, psychotic symptoms *(1 point)*.

3.3 Bipolar affective disorder

1. Bipolar or bipolar affective disorder *(1 point)*.

2. Any six of the following *(1/2 point for each, total = 3 points)*: BAD I, BAD II, cyclothymia, schizoaffective disorder, borderline or narcissistic personality disorder, illicit drug ingestions (e.g. amphetamines, cocaine), or acute drug withdrawal. Non-psychiatric medical presentation including hyper-/hypothyroidism, Cushing's disease, cerebral tumor (e.g. frontal lobe lesion with disinhibition), stroke, and side effect of corticosteroid use.

3. Any three of the following *(1 point for each, total = 3 points)*: grandiosity/inflated self-esteem, decreased sleep, pressure of speech, flight of ideas, distractibility, psychomotor agitation, involvement in pleasurable activities without consequential thought, e.g. spending sprees.

4. Hypomania is mildly elevated mood present for four or more days. Mania is as with hypomania but to a greater extent *(1 point)*. Symptoms are present for >1 week, with more complete disruption of work and social activities. In mania, they may have grandiose ideas and excessive spending could lead to debts *(1 point)*. There may be sexual disinhibition and reduced sleep may lead to exhaustion in mania *(1 point)*. Insight may be preserved in hypomania *(1 point)*. Psychotic symptoms and the need for hospitalization further distinguish mania from hypomania.

5. Any three of the following: lithium *(1 point)*, valproate *(1 point)*, carbamazepine *(1 point)* and lamotrigine *(1 point)*. They are teratogenic and should therefore ideally be avoided in women of child bearing age or, if required, should be used with extreme caution and careful monitoring *(1 point)*.

4.2 Schizophrenia

1. Schizophrenia *(1 point)*. Any four of the following differential diagnoses *(1/2 point for each)*: schizophreniform disorder, brief psychotic disorder, schizoaffective disorder, delusional disorder, psychotic depression, mania with psychosis, drug-induced psychosis. It is unknown the length of time he has had the symptoms.

2. Delusional perception ('He states he saw lightning and is now convinced that the FBI is after him and that federal agents gather information about his whereabouts') *(1 point)*, thought interference ('He believes that they are trying to control his thoughts and movement') *(1 point)*, auditory hallucinations talking about the patient in the third person ('He also hears them outside his house talking about how they will murder him') *(1 point)*.

3. Any four of the following *(1 point for each, total = 4 points)*: Avolition (↓ motivation), asocial behavior, anhedonia, alogia (poverty of speech), blunted affect, cognitive deficits.

4. Any four of the following *(1 point for each, total = 4 points)*: CBC, ESR, TFTs, glucose, serum calcium, electrolytes and LFTs, cholesterol, vitamin B_{12} and folate, urine drug test, ECG, EEG or CT scan.

5. Any of the following 2nd generation (atypical) antipsychotics *(1 point)*: olanzapine, risperidone, quetiapine, lurasidone, aripiprazole. **NOTE:** Clozapine should not be given at this stage and would therefore be an incorrect answer. Any of the four following side effects *(1 point for each, total = 4 points)*: extrapyramidal side effects (e.g. parkinsonism), blurred vision, urinary retention, dry mouth, constipation, sedation, weight gain, postural hypotension, tachycardia, ejaculatory failure or sexual dysfunction, reduced bone mineral density, menstrual disturbances, breast enlargement, galactorrhea, impaired glucose tolerance, hypercholesterolemia, neuroleptic malignant syndrome, prolonged QT interval.

6. Any four of the following psychosocial interventions *(1 point for each, total = 4 points)*: CBT, psychoeducation, art therapy (e.g. music, dancing, drama), social skills training, social support groups, peer groups, supported employment programs.

5.2 Generalized anxiety disorder

1. 6 months *(1 point)*.

2. Any three of the following *(1 point for each, total = 3 points)*: CBC (for infection/anemia), TFTs (hyperthyroidism), glucose (hypoglycemia), ECG (may show sinus tachycardia).

3. Any six of the following *(1/2 point for each, total = 3 points)*: difficulty breathing, feeling of choking, nausea, abdominal distress, loose motions, hot flushes or cold chills, numbness or tingling, headache, muscle tension, aches or pains, restlessness, sensation of lump in throat (globus hystericus), difficulty swallowing (dysphagia).

4. The first-line drug treatment of choice is an SSRI *(1 point)*.

5. Any two of the following *(1 point for each, total = 2 points)*: psychoeducation, CBT, applied relaxation, self-help methods, social support.

5.3 Phobic anxiety disorders

1. Specific phobia to flying *(1 point)*.

2. Any two from *Fig. 5.3.1* *(1 point for each, total = 2 points)*.

3. Social anxiety disorder and agoraphobia *(1 point)*. Social anxiety disorder is a pointed fear or avoidance of social situations, or fear of acting in a way that will be embarrassing or humiliating *(1 point)*. Agoraphobia is a fear of public spaces or fear of entering a public space from which immediate escape would be difficult in the event of a panic attack *(1 point)*. **NOTE:** social anxiety disorder may occur with or without agoraphobia.

4. Self-help methods, CBT, SSRIs benzodiazepines (short term) *(1 point for each, total = 3 points)*.

5. Symptoms of GAD occur most of the time whereas features of phobic anxiety disorders occur in response to particular situations *(1 point)*. Commonly, agitation is an associated behavior of GAD whereas avoidance of the particular situation typically occurs in phobic anxiety disorders *(1 point)*. Concerning cognition, there is constant worry about everyday life events in patients with GAD whereas patients with phobic anxiety disorders only worry about or fear a particular situation *(1 point)*.

5.4 Panic disorder

1. A panic attack/panic disorder *(1 point)*.

2. Any three of the following *(1 point for each, total = 3 points)*: pheochromocytoma, hyperthyroidism, hypoglycemia, carcinoid syndrome, arrhythmias.

3. Symptoms in GAD present persistently, symptoms in panic disorder occur episodically and symptoms in phobic anxiety disorders occur in response to certain situations *(1 point)*. GAD is associated with agitation; panic disorder is associated with a feeling of wanting to escape; phobic anxiety disorders are associated with avoidance of the particular situation *(1 point)*. GAD patients commonly suffer from depression. Patients with panic disorder often have depression, agoraphobia and suffer from substance misuse. Those with phobic anxiety often suffer from substance misuse *(1 point)*.

4. SSRIs are first-line for panic disorder *(1 point)*.

6 Trauma and stressor-related disorders

1. Any six of the following *(1/2 point for each, total = 3 points)*: flashbacks, vivid memories, recurring dreams, distress when exposed to similar circumstances as stressor, avoiding reminders of trauma (e.g. associated people or locations), excessive rumination about the trauma, inability to recall aspects of the trauma, irritability or outbursts, difficulty with concentration, difficulty with sleep, hypervigilance, exaggerated startle response.

2. 6 months *(1 point)*.

3. Any two of the following *(1 point for each, total = 2 points)*: adjustment disorder requires a non-catastrophic event, whereas PTSD involves a traumatic event *(1 point)*. The symptoms in adjustment disorder must occur within 3 months of the event whereas PTSD can occur at any time but symptoms must persist at least 1 month *(1 point)*. The symptoms in adjustment disorder must be present for less than 6 months. In PTSD, these symptoms may last longer *(1 point)*.

4. CBT *(1 point)*, eye movement desensitization and reprocessing *(1 point)*.

5. Any two of the following *(1 point for each, total = 2 points)*: Any SSRI (most commonly paroxetine), mirtazapine, duloxetine, venlafaxine.

7 Obsessive–compulsive and related disorders

1. Obsessive–compulsive disorder/OCD *(1 point)*.

2. Illness anxiety disorder *(1 point)*, obsessive personality disorder *(1 point)*, schizophrenia *(1 point)*, depression *(1 point)*, generalized anxiety disorder *(1 point)*.

3. 'Are these thoughts that you are getting repetitive and distressing?' *(1 point)*; 'Are you aware that these thoughts are in your mind?' *(1 point)*; 'Do you feel anxious if you do not wash your hands and feet?' *(1 point)*

4. In schizophrenia, patients often believe that the thoughts and hallucinations that they develop are real, whereas patients with OCD are aware that their obsessions are coming from their own mind *(1 point)*.

5. SSRIs are the drug of choice in OCD *(1 point)*. Any of the following would be appropriate *(any two, 1 point for each = 2 points)*: fluoxetine, fluvoxamine, paroxetine, sertraline or citalopram.

6. Cognitive behavioral therapy *(1 point)*. Exposure and response prevention *(1 point)*.

8 Somatic symptom disorders

1. Somatoform disorder *(1/2 point)*, dissociative (conversion) disorder *(1/2 point)*, factitious disorder *(1/2 point)*, malingering *(1/2 point)*.

2. Somatic symptom disorder *(1 point)* since she has had multiple and recurrent physical symptoms not explained by a physical illness *(1 point)*.

3. Illness anxiety disorder *(1 point)*, conversion disorder *(1 point)* and unspecified somatic symptoms disorder *(1 point)*.

4. In both malingering and factitious disorder (also known as Munchausen's syndrome) physical or psychological symptoms are intentionally produced, i.e. faked *(1 point)*. In malingering, the patient seeks advantageous consequences of being diagnosed with a medical condition, e.g. financial gain *(1 point)*. In factitious disorder, the individual wishes to adopt the 'sick role' in order to receive the care of a patient, for internal emotional gain (i.e. primary gain) *(1 point)*.

9.1 Anorexia nervosa

1. BMI = weight (kg)/[height (m)]^2 = 42/(1.6^2) *(1 point)* = 16.4 *(1 point)*.

2. Anorexia nervosa *(1 point)*. Any two of the following: bulimia nervosa *(1/2 point)*, OCD *(1/2 point)*, depression *(1/2 point)*, hyperthyroidism *(1/2 point)*.

3. Any four of the following *(1 point for each)*: Intense fear of weight gain, restricted food intake relative to needs, deliberate weight loss, distorted body image.

4. Any four of the following *(1 point for each, total = 4 points)*: hypokalemia, hypotension, hypothermia, anemia, cardiac failure, hypoglycemia, osteoporosis, acute renal failure.

5. A bio-psychosocial approach should be adopted. The patient should be assessed medically to see whether she has any complications of AN, and this should be treated accordingly, ideally as an inpatient *(1 point)*. The patient should be educated about her condition and need for nutrition *(1 point)* and be offered long-term psychotherapy *(1 point for any of the following)*: CBT, interpersonal therapy or family therapy. Access to voluntary organizations and self-help groups should also be offered *(1 point)*. If she refuses treatment, the need for a psychiatric hold as DS or gravely disabled may be considered *(1 point)*.

9.2 Bulimia nervosa

1. Bulimia nervosa *(1 point)*. Anorexia nervosa *(1 point)* and any of the following: binge eating disorder *(1 point)*, depression *(1 point)*, OCD *(1 point)*.

2. Compensatory weight gain prevention (purging) behavior *(1 point)*, issues with body image *(1 point)*, lack of control *(1 point)* and binge eating *(1 point)*.

3. Hypokalemia *(1 point)*. Can be tested quickly via a venous blood gas (although this can be inaccurate by up to 1 mmol/L) *(1 point)*. Accurate testing would require a set of electrolytes. *(1 point)*

4. Any two of the following: pitted teeth *(1 point)*, Russell's sign *(1 point)*, enlargement of salivary glands *(1 point)*, esophageal (Mallory–Weiss) tears *(1 point)*.

5. The management of BN is based on the bio-psychosocial model. A trial of an SSRI can be offered and can ↓ frequency of binge eating/purging *(1 point)*. CBT for bulimia nervosa can also be offered *(1 point)*; interpersonal psychotherapy is an alternative *(1 point)*. Simple measures can be employed, such as a food diary to monitor eating/purging patterns, techniques to avoid bingeing (eating in company, distractions), small, regular meals *(1 point)*.

10.1 Substance use disorders

1. An opiate *(1 point)* such as heroin.

2. Schedule 1 *(1 point)*.

3. Naloxone *(1 point)* Intravenous *(1 point)*.
4. Any four of the following *(1 point for each, total = 4 points)*: compulsive need to consume drug, preoccupation with substance use, withdrawal state when substance ingestion is reduced or stopped, impaired ability to control substance-taking behavior, increased tolerance to substance, persisting despite clear evidence to harmful effects.
5. Motivational interviewing *(1 point)*, CBT *(1 point)*, contingency management *(1 point)*.

10.2 Alcohol abuse

1. Any four of the following *(1 point for each, total = 4 points)*: subjective awareness of compulsion to drink, avoidance or relief of withdrawal symptoms by further drinking, withdrawal symptoms, drink-seeking behavior predominates, reinstatement after abstinence, narrowing of drinking repertoire.
2. Any of the two medical complications *(1/2 point each)*: hepatitis, cirrhosis, hepatocellular carcinoma, peptic ulcer, esophageal varices, esophageal carcinoma, pancreatitis, hypertension, cardiomyopathy, arrhythmias, anemia, thrombocytopenia, seizures, peripheral neuropathy, cerebellar degeneration, Wernicke's encephalopathy, Korsakoff's psychosis, head injury (secondary to falls). Any two of the following psychiatric complications *(1/2 point each)*: morbid jealousy, self-harm and suicide, mood disorder, anxiety disorders, alcohol dementia, alcoholic hallucinosis, delirium tremens. Any two of the following social complications *(1/2 point each)*: domestic violence, drink driving, employment difficulties, financial problems, homelessness, accidents, relationship problems.
3. Delirium tremens is a complication of alcohol withdrawal which usually develops between 24 hours to one week after alcohol cessation *(1 point)*. It is characterized by perceptual abnormalities (hallucinations and/or illusions) *(1 point)*, cognitive impairment *(1 point)*, paranoid delusions *(1 point)*, autonomic arousal *(1 point)* (e.g. tachycardia, fever and increased sweating) and marked tremor *(1 point)*.
4. High dose benzodiazepines (commonly chlordiazepoxide) are given initially *(1 point)*, and the dose is then tapered down over roughly a one-week period *(1 point)*.

11 Personality disorders

1. Borderline personality disorder *(1 point)*.
2. Any six of the following *(1/2 point for each, total = 3 points)*: paranoid personality disorder, schizoid personality disorder, schizotypal, antisocial personality disorder, histrionic personality disorder, obsessive compulsive personality disorder, histrionic, narcissistic, avoidant personality disorder.
3. Any three of the following *(1 point for each, total = 3 points)*: callous, blame others, disregard for safety, remorseless, deceitful, impulsive tendency to violence.
4. CBT *(1 point)*, psychodynamic therapy *(1 point)*, dialectical behavioral therapy (DBT) *(1 point)*.

12.1 Deliberate self-harm

1. Any three of the following *(1 point for each, total = 3 points)*: divorced/single/living alone, severe life stressors, harmful drug/alcohol use, less than 35 (age), chronic physical health problems, domestic violence, sexual abuse or childhood maltreatment, socioeconomic disadvantage, psychiatric illness (e.g. borderline personality disorder, OCD, psychosis).
2. Any three of the following *(1 point for each, total = 3 points)*: genuine wish to die, seeking unconsciousness or pain as a means of temporary relief and escape from problems, trying to influence another person to change their views or behavior, to punish oneself, to seek attention.
3. ABCDE approach *(1 point)*, give IV N-acetylcysteine if above treatment line *(1 point)*.
4. Acute liver failure *(1 point)*.
5. Any three of the following *(1 point for each, total = 3 points)*: Was it planned? What method did they use? Was a suicide note left? Was the patient intoxicated with drugs or alcohol? Was the patient alone?

Were there any efforts to avoid discovery (e.g. waited until house empty)? Did the patient seek help after the attempt or were they found and brought in by someone else? How does the patient feel about the episode now? (regret? do they wish that they had succeeded?) How did they feel when they were found?

12.2 Suicide and risk assessment

1. Male *(1 point)*, stress *(1 point)*, medical conditions *(1 point)*, depression *(1 point)*.

2. Any four of the following risk factors *(1/2 point for each, total = 2 points)*: history of DSH, previous attempted suicide, psychiatric illness, family history of suicide, childhood abuse, age (middle aged or older), unemployed, low socioeconomic status, certain occupations, access to lethal means, low social support, living alone, institutionalized, single, widowed, divorced, recent life crisis.

3. Responsibility for someone else *(1 point)*.

4. If high risk there is a possibility for him to be hospitalized informally or via a psychiatric hold as danger to self *(1 point)*. He should first be assessed by the Crisis team to see if he could be safely managed in the community with intensive input *(1 point)*. He may need to be started on a safer antidepressant (e.g. SSRI), and consider CBT, and other support that may be available to him as a care giver *(1 point)*.

5. Any two of the following *(1 point for each, total = 2 points)*: Public education and discussion *(1 point)*, reducing access to means of suicide *(1 point)*, easy, rapid access to psychiatric care or support groups *(1 point)*, 24 hour suicide hotlines *(1 point)*.

13.1 Delirium

1.

	Delirium	Dementia	
Sleep-wake cycle	Disrupted	Usually normal	*(1 point)*
Attention	Markedly reduced	Normal/reduced	*(1 point)*
Arousal	Increased/decreased	Usually normal	*(1 point)*
Autonomic features	Abnormal	Normal	*(1 point)*
Duration	Hours to weeks	Months to years	*(1 point)*
Delusions	Fleeting	Complex	*(1 point)*
Course	Fluctuating	Stable/slowly progressive	*(1 point)*
Consciousness level	Impaired	No impairment	*(1 point)*
Hallucinations	Common (especially visual)	Less common	*(1 point)*
Onset	Acute/subacute	Chronic	*(1 point)*
Psychomotor activity	Usually abnormal	Usually normal	*(1 point)*

2. Any six of the following *(1/2 point for each, total = 3 points)*: infection, hypoxia, electrolyte disturbances, hypoglycemia, nutritional deficiencies, stroke, MI, drugs (e.g. opioids, benzodiazepines, anticholinergics), alcohol withdrawal, head trauma, epilepsy, constipation, urinary retention, bladder catheterization, hyperthyroidism, hypothyroidism, hyperglycemia, severe pain, sensory deprivation (for example leaving the person without spectacles or hearing aids), relocation (such as moving people with impaired cognition to unfamiliar environments), sleep deprivation.

3. Any of the following *(1/2 point for each, total = 5 points)*: urinalysis, CBC, BUN/Cr electrolytes, LFTs, calcium, glucose, CRP, TFTs, ECG, CXR, blood culture and urine culture.

4. The Abbreviated Mental Test *(1 point)* and Confusion Assessment Method tools *(1 point)*, Mini-Mental State Examination *(1 point)*.

5. Treat the underlying cause – in this case it is most likely to be infection and/or anesthesia-related *(1 point)*. Reassure and orientate patient *(1 point)*. The patient should be provided with the appropriate environment, e.g. a quiet well-lit side room if practical *(1 point)*, consistency in care and staff *(1 point)*, encourage presence of friend/family member, optimize sensory acuity, e.g. glasses *(1 point)*, well-lit room *(1 point)*, orientation aids (clock, calendar) *(1 point)*. Low dose sedatives should be used as a last resort, and may make the situation worse *(1 point)*. **NOTE:** The presence of friend/family member will not be practical in the middle of the night.

13.2 Dementia

1. Alzheimer's disease *(1 point)*.

2. Microscopic: neurofibrillary tangles *(1 point)* and β-amyloid plaque formation *(1 point)*. Macroscopic: cortical atrophy (commonly hippocampal) *(1 point)* with widened sulci *(1 point)* and enlarged ventricles *(1 point)*.

3. Any five of the following *(1 point for each, total = 5 points)*: CBC, BUN/Cr, electrolytes, calcium, LFTs, glucose, lipids, vitamin B_{12} and folate, TFTs, VDRL.

4. Moderate *(1 point)*.

5. Any six of the following *(1/2 point for each, total = 3 points)*: Normal pressure hydrocephalus, intracranial tumors, chronic subdural hematoma, vitamin B_{12} deficiency, folic acid deficiency, thiamine deficiency, pellagra (niacin deficiency), Cushing's syndrome, hypothyroidism.

6. Any four of the following *(1 point for each, total = 4 points)*: Social support, increasing assistance with day-to-day activities, information and education, carer support groups, community dementia teams, home nursing and personal care, community services such as meals-on-wheels, befriending services, day centers, respite care and care homes. For non-cognitive and behavioral challenges – aromatherapy, massage, therapeutic use of music or animal-assisted therapy may be considered.

7. Any two of the following *(1 point for each, total = 2 points)*: donepezil, galantamine and rivastigmine. **NOTE:** Memantine should generally be given to those with moderate Alzheimer's disease who are intolerant of or have a contraindication to acetylcholinesterase inhibitors, or those with severe Alzheimer's disease and therefore this is NOT a correct answer.

14.1 Autism

1. Autism/autism spectrum disorder *(1 point)*.

2. Have they reached all their other milestones accordingly, e.g. 'Can he walk?' *(1 point)*; 'Is there any family history of autism?' *(1 point)*; 'Does he have any other medical conditions, e.g. visual or hearing impairment?' *(1 point)*; 'Have you noticed him making any abnormal movements such as flapping his hands or walking on tiptoes?' or 'Does your child insist on the same toys, activities or foods?' *(1 point)*

3. Impairment in social interaction *(1 point)*, impairment of communication *(1 point)* and restricted, stereotyped interests and behaviors *(1 point)*.

4. Any three of the following *(1 point for each, total = 3 points)*: visual impairment, hearing impairment, sensory issues, infections, epileptic seizures, hyperkinetic disorder, pica, sleep disorders, constipation, PKU, fragile X, tuberous sclerosis, congenital rubella, CMV, toxoplasmosis.

5. Any four of the following *(1/2 point for each, total = 4 points)*: CBT, family support, access to self-help groups such as the National Autism Association, special schooling, social-communication intervention (e.g. play-based strategies), modification of environmental factors which initiate or maintain challenging behavior.

14.2 Attention deficit hyperactivity disorder

1. Attention deficit hyperactivity disorder *(1 point)*.

2. Inattention *(1 point)*, hyperactivity *(1 point)* and impulsivity *(1 point)*.

3. Any three types of questions that cover the three core features of ADHD (see *History box* in *Section 14.2*).

4. In severe ADHD in school-aged children, drug treatment is first-line with methylphenidate (Ritalin) being the usual choice *(1 point)*. Atomoxetine is second-line *(1 point)*. If this fails, dexamfetamine is the alternative when methylphenidate has been ineffective; clonidine and guanfacine may also be used *(1 point)*.

14.3 Learning disability

1. Any three of the following *(1 point for each, total = 3 points)*: palpebral fissure (up slanting), round face, occipital + nasal flattening, Brushfield spots (pigmented spots on iris), brachycephaly, epicanthic folds, mouth open + protruding tongue, strabismus (squint), sandal gap deformity.

2. Any five from *Table 14.3.1 (1 point for each, total = 5 points)*.

3. Mild: IQ = 50–70 *(1 point)*; moderate: IQ = 35–49 *(1 point)*; severe: IQ = 20–34 *(1 point)*.

4. Any four of the following *(1 point for each, total = 4 points)*: psychiatrist, speech and language therapist, specialist nurses, psychologist, occupational therapist, educational support, social worker, and pediatrician.

Appendix C

Figure acknowledgements

Fig. 2.2.4
Reproduced from http://gpuzzles.com/optical-illusion/sleeping-baby-cloud/

Fig. 8.5
Reproduced from http://theprivatetherapyclinic.co.uk/understanding-body-dysmorphic-disorder-bdd/

Fig. 9.1.2
Reproduced from www.health.com/health/gallery/0,,20665980_5,00.html

Fig. 9.2.2(a)
Reproduced from *Journal of Clinical Pediatric Dentistry* (2011) **36(2):** 155–160, P.R. Kavitha, P. Vivek, A.M. Hegde, 'Eating Disorders and their Implications on Oral Health – Role of Dentists'.

Fig. 9.2.2(b)
Reproduced courtesy of Dr Alfredo Aguirre (School of Dental Medicine, University at Buffalo, The State University of New York).

Fig. 9.2.2(c)
Loss of enamel from the inside of the upper teeth as a result of bulimia.
Licensed under the Creative Commons Attribution-Share Alike 4.0 International license.
Additional attribution: James Heilman, MD
Available at: https://commons.wikimedia.org/wiki/File:BulemiaEnamalLoss.JPG

Fig. 10.2.2(a)
Reproduced with permission from http://thehappyhospitalist.blogspot.co.uk

Fig. 10.2.2(b)
Reproduced with permission from http://blog.mmenterprises.co.uk

Fig. 10.2.2(c)
Reproduced from www.kingstonlaser.co.uk/index.php?page=acp

Fig. 10.2.2(d)
Reproduced from www.plasticsurgeryhub.com.au/plastic-surgery-before-and-after-photos/gynaecomastia-male-breast-reduction-photo-gallery/

Fig. 12.1.2
Self-injury in the form of cutting.
Licensed under the Creative Commons Attribution-Share Alike 3.0 Unported license.
Additional attribution: Hendrike
Available at: https://commons.wikimedia.org/wiki/File:Schnittwunden.JPG

Fig. 13.2.1
Reproduced from http://coloradodementia.org/2011/12/28/the-plaques-and-tangles-of-alzheimers/

Fig. 13.2.5
Reproduced with kind permission of Dr Julio Acosta-Cabronero, German Center for Neurodegenerative Diseases (DZNE).

Appendix C Figure acknowledgements

Index

abbreviated mental test (AMT), 146, 156
acalculia, 153
acamprosate, 122–3
acetaldehyde, 117, 123
acetylcholine, 149, 159
acetylcholinesterase (AChE) inhibitors, 159
activated charcoal, 136
acute and transient psychotic disorder,
    5, 194
acute intoxication, 109, 256
acute liver failure, 134
acute manic episode, 40, 202
acute stress reaction, 77
ADHD, 60, 162, 163, 167, 169–74, 178
adjustment disorder, 32, 56, 65, 69, 72,
    76–7, 184
advance care planning, 218
advance directive, 218–9
advance statement, 158, 218–9
affect, 16, 25, 47, 50, 73, 256
affective disorder, see mood disorder
agnosia, 153, 256
agoraphobia, 55–6, 62–6
agranulocytosis, 192, 197
agraphia, 153
akathisia, 197, 256, 258
alcohol
    abuse, 5, 6, 39, 102, 116–24, 136, 221–2
    detoxification, 123, 207
    withdrawal, 117–19, 123, 147, 204, 214
alcoholic hallucinosis, 118
Alcoholics Anonymous (AA), 122, 124
alexia, 153
all or nothing thinking, 182
alogia, 47
Alzheimer's disease (AD), 3, 149–59, 178
amitriptyline, 136, 189, 191–2, 207
amenorrhea, 97, 99, 105, 106, 256

amnesia, 74, 110, 207, 212, 256
amnesic syndrome, 122, 156
amphetamine, 39, 45, 113
amyloid precursor protein, 151
anabolic steroids, 111–13
anergia, 10, 29, 32, 256
Angelman syndrome, 175
anhedonia, 10, 14, 29, 31, 47, 137, 256
anorexia nervosa, 58, 69, 80, 95–100,
    104, 106
antenatal, 162
anti-adrenergic, 196
anticipatory anxiety, 63, 65, 256
antidepressants, 27, 33, 40, 91, 100, 129, 130,
    134, 158, 187–93, 207–9, 211
antidote, 114, 136, 208
antiepileptics, 208
anti-histaminergic, 190, 196
anti-muscarinic, 196
antipsychotics, 15, 33, 39–40, 44, 50–2, 100,
    129–30, 134, 147, 158–9, 167, 178,
    194–201, 202, 205, 207, 209, 211
anxiety, see anxiety disorders
anxiety disorders, 4, 5, 32, 35, 55–70, 77, 83,
    87, 89, 114, 118, 121, 173, 181, 183,
    185, 190–1, 207–8, 215
anxiolytics, 66, 207–9
apathy, 41, 50, 110, 111, 142, 152–4, 256
aphasia, 150, 153
ApoE-2, 151
ApoE-4, 151
apraxia, 150, 152–3, 256
arbitrary inference, 182
aripiprazole, 167, 194, 199–201
art therapy, 51
asocial behavior, 47, 163
Asperger's syndrome, 166
atomoxetine, 174

atropine, 136
atypical eating disorder, *see* eating disorder
    not otherwise specified (EDNOS)
auditory hallucinations, 10, 11, 18, 19, 20, 21,
    36, 38, 213
    running commentary, 10, 49
    second person, 10, 21, 30, 31, 49
    third person, 10, 19, 21, 30, 47, 49
autism spectrum disorders, 5, 162–167
autonomic nervous system, 57
avolition, 45, 47

baby blues, 32
barbiturates, 60, 110, 113, 149, 207, 208, 211
Beck, Aaron, 3, 181
Beck's cognitive triad, 30, 137, 256
Beck's anxiety inventory, 60
behavioral activation, 34, 183, 185
behavioral syndromes, 5
behavioral therapies, 183, 185
benzodiazepines, 40, 60, 66, 69, 78, 109–13,
    119, 123, 136, 143, 147, 149, 197, 202,
    207–9, 211
bereavement, 28, 34, 136, 185, 186, 256
    abnormal, 76
    normal, 32, 76–7
beta-blockers, 136, 207, 208
binge drinking, 121
binge eating disorder, 95, 99
bipolar affective disorder, 4, 25, 26, 31, 32,
    35–41, 69, 163, 181, 186, 187, 202,
    204, 212
body dysmorphic disorder,
    see dysmorphophobia
brexanolone, 188
Briquet's syndrome, *see* somatization
    disorder
bulimia nervosa, 95, 97–9, 102–7, 188
buprenorphine, 114
buspirone, 207, 208

CAGE questionnaire, 13, 120
cannabinoids, 110, 112
cannabis, 143, 169
capacity, 134, 174, 218–9

Capgras' syndrome, 256
caput medusa, 120
carbamazepine, 202, 204
catastrophic thinking, 182
catatonia, 48, 165, 211, 256
cerebrovascular disease, 121, 150–1
childhood disintegrative disorder, 165–6
chlordiazepoxide, 207
chlorpromazine, 19, 194, 199–200
circumstantiality, 17, 19, 39, 50, 256
citalopram, 66, 84, 134, 188
clang association, 16, 256
clomipramine, 69
clozapine, 194
cocaine, 55, 60, 111
cognition, 120, 144, 145
cognitive analytic therapy (CAT), 185
cognitive behavioral therapy (CBT), 181
command hallucinations, 133, 138, 223
compulsions, 80, 256
conduct disorder, 82, 173
confabulation, 256, 258
Confusion Assessment Method (CAM), 146
continuous anxiety, 56
conversion disorder, 86, 87
Cotard's syndrome, 257
counseling, 22, 34
counter-transference, 184
couples therapy, 184, 186
crack cocaine, 111, 113
Creutzfeldt–Jakob disease (CJD), 154
cyclothymia, 21, 25, 26, 39

De Clérambault's syndrome, 257
deep brain stimulation, 84, 214
deliberate self-harm (DSH), 132–4, 139
delirium, 142–5
delirium tremens, 117, 207, 257
delusion, 128, 138, 142–4, 158, 194, 223
    bizarre, 18
    grandiose, 18, 36, 38, 49, 258
    hypochondriacal, 18, 30, 44
    infestation, 18
    mood congruent, 18
    nihilistic, *see* Cotard's syndrome

paranoid, 65, 119, 120, 222, 223
persecutory, 18, 36, 38, 50
primary, 18
reference, 18
secondary, 18
delusional disorder, 43, 44
induced, 44
persistent, 44
delusional memory, 19
delusional perception, 19
dementia, 22, 26, 27, 32, 43, 83, 118, 149–60
alcohol-related, 118
fronto-temporal, 149, 150
Lewy body (DLB), 149–50, 154–5
mixed, 150, 154
vascular, 150, 154, 156, 158
dependence syndrome, 257
depersonalization, 20, 55, 59, 68, 111
depot injection, 200, 201
depression, 4, 10, 15, 16, 23, 25, 27–41, 257
atypical, 30, 32
postpartum, 184, 223
derailment of thought, 17
derealization, 17
dialectical behavioral therapy (DBT), 134, 185
diazepam, 207
disinhibition, 15, 38–9, 110, 257
dissociation, 17, 86
disulfiram, 122, 123
diurnal variation in mood, 32, 257
donepezil, 159
Down's syndrome, 151, 175, 176
doxepin, 191, 192
DSM-V, 19, 20, 257
durable power of attorney, 218, 219
dysarthria, 150, 191, 208, 257
dysmorphophobia, 257
dysphasia, 10, 153, 257
dyspraxia, 173
dysthymia, see persistent depression disorder
dystonia, 197–8, 257

early morning wakening, 14, 30
eating disorder not otherwise
specified (EDNOS), 5

eating disorders, 95–108
echolalia, 164, 257
ecstasy, 111, 113
Edward and Gross criteria, 117
electroconvulsive therapy (ECT), 192, 210–3
electroencephalogram (EEG), 211, 258
emotional numbing, 73
epilepsy, 11, 43, 50, 83, 142, 146
erotomania, 18, 258
escitalopram, 66, 188
esketamine, 190
euthymic, 16, 258
executive functioning, 47, 151–4, 158
exposure and response prevention (ERP), 183
expressed emotion, 45–6, 51
extrapyramidal side effects (EPSE), 154, 159,
194, 196, 197

factitious disorder, 90, 91
family therapy, 100, 186
flight of ideas, 17, 19, 36–9
flooding, 183
flumazenil, 136, 208
fluoxetine, 19, 84, 107, 188, 189
fluphenazine, 194, 200
fluvoxamine, 84, 188
folie à deux, 19, 258
Folstein Mini-Mental State Examination
(MMSE), 157
forensic psychiatry, 221–3
formal thought disorder, 19, 258, 259
Freud, 3, 183
frontal lobe tests, 154, 158

galantamine, 159
generalized anxiety disorder (GAD), 57–61
graduated exposure, 66, 258
group therapy, 185, 186

hallucinations, 21–2, 23, 30, 31, 36, 38,
43, 45–8
auditory, see auditory hallucinations
gustatory, 21
somatic, 21
visual, 20, 21

haloperidol, 194, 196, 198, 200
heroin, 110, 113
HIV, 112, 114, 149, 150, 152, 156
Huntington's disease, 43, 149, 156
hyperactive delirium, 142, 145
hyperarousal, 73, 76, 258
hyperthyroidism, 56, 58, 60, 68, 69, 98, 114, 142, 146
hypervigilance, 73, 74, 76, 77
hypoactive delirium, 142, 145
hypochondriacal disorder, *see* illness anxiety disorder
hypomania, 5, 15, 25, 26, 31, 36–9, 188, 189, 191, 202
hypothyroidism, 41, 142, 146, 149, 150, 175, 176, 178, 203

ICD-10, 4, 76, 135, 258
illness anxiety disorder, 5, 58, 82, 83, 89–90, 258
illusion, 20, 77, 110, 111, 119, 120, 143, 145, 155, 257, 258
insomnia, 28, 30, 111, 117, 158, 159, 174, 188, 189, 190, 191, 192, 207
interpersonal therapy (IPT), 33, 34, 107, 185

ketamine, 43, 113, 188, 190
Kleine–Levin syndrome, 106
kleptomania, 83, 258
knight's move thinking, 19, 258
Kübler–Ross stages of grief, 77

labile mood, 16, 22, 25, 110, 111, 117, 120, 145, 165, 258
lamotrigine, 46, 202, 205–6
learning disability, 5, 19, 175–8
learning theory, 116, 183, 260
Lewy body dementia, *see* dementia, Lewy body
lithium, 2–3, 15, 33, 39–41, 202–4, 211
loosening of association, 17, 19, 38, 50, 258
lorazepam, 39–40, 207
lysergic acid diethylamide (LSD), 43, 111, 113

magnification, 182
malingering, 90–1, 258

mania, 5, 9, 15–16, 21, 25–6, 35–41, 44, 60, 129, 146, 188–9, 191–2, 194, 202, 205, 211, 214, 223
medically unexplained symptoms, 91–2
memantine, 158–9
mental state examination (MSE), 2, 6, 11, 23
methadone, 110, 113–4
methamphetamine, 43, 111
methylphenidate, 113, 167, 174
Mini-Mental State Examination (MMSE), *see* Folstein Mini-Mental State Examination
minimization, 182
mirtazapine, 33, 78, 187, 188, 189, 190
monoamine hypothesis, 27, 35, 259
monoamine oxidase inhibitor (MAOI), 33, 66, 134, 187, 189, 190–3, 205, 211
Montreal Cognitive Assessment (MOCA), 22, 156
mood, 2, 3, 5, 10, 15–18, 22–3, 25, 29, 31–2, 34–9, 41, 50, 59, 65, 74–5, 77, 89–91, 98, 102, 105, 110–1, 120, 127, 129, 138, 140, 145–6, 150, 155–6, 159, 165, 173, 177
mood stabilizers, 40–1, 129, 130, 202–5
motivational interviewing, 114, 122, 123, 185
Munchausen's syndrome, *see* factitious disorder

naloxone, 114, 136
naltrexone, 114, 122, 123
negative symptoms, 45–9, 51–2, 196, 201, 213, 259
neologism, 17, 19, 38, 259
neurofibrillary tangles, 149
neuroleptic malignant syndrome, 196–7, 199, 259
neurosis, 259
noradrenaline reuptake inhibitor (NARI), 33, 188, 190
normal pressure hydrocephalus, 149, 150

obsessions, 10, 17, 19, 22, 58, 64, 68, 80–3, 95, 97, 103, 138, 165, 259

obsessive–compulsive disorder (OCD), 5, 17, 56, 58, 60, 64, 67, 68, 80–4, 89, 98, 100, 106, 132, 133–4, 163, 187–8, 208, 213, 258
olanzapine, 40, 51–2, 147, 194, 198, 200
olfactory hallucination, 22
operant conditioning, 80, 116, 183, 259
opiates, 26, 110, 136, 142, 150, 156, 193
oppositional defiant disorder, 173
Othello syndrome, 18, 259
overgeneralization, 182
overvalued ideas, 17, 38, 89, 97, 98, 102

panic disorder, 5, 55, 56, 58, 60, 63–70, 89, 188, 207–8
paraphrenia, 259
Parkinson's disease, 26, 31, 64, 149, 152, 154, 159, 197, 198, 213
parkinsonism, 15, 26, 154, 197, 258
paroxetine, 84, 188
paroxysmal anxiety, 56
passivity phenomenon, 19–20, 22, 47, 49, 259
perseveration, 17, 19, 153, 259
persistent depression disorder, 26, 32, 257
personality disorders, 5, 26, 32, 39, 60, 66, 77, 109, 126, 171, 178, 181, 183, 223
  antisocial, 127
  anxious, 56, 65
  avoidant, 126, 128
  borderline, 103, 126, 127, 185
  dependent, 126, 127
  histrionic, 39, 126–7
  OCD, 83, 126, 128
  paranoid, 126–7
  schizoid, 126–7
pervasive developmental disorder, 162, 165–6, 259
phobic anxiety, see phobic anxiety disorders
phobic anxiety disorders, 5, 55, 56, 63, 65, 66, 69, 70, 183, 207
PHQ-9, 32
Pick's disease, 149, 150, 154
post-traumatic stress disorder (PTSD), 5, 56, 68, 72–6

poverty of speech, 16, 23, 47, 50, 259
poverty of thought, 17, 259
premorbid personality, 8, 14, 259
preoccupation, see overvalued ideas
presenilin, 151
pressure of speech, 17, 36, 38, 259
primary gain, 86, 90
primary mood disorder, 25, 26
prion disease, 152, 154, 259
pseudodementia, 149, 150, 156, 259
pseudohallucination, 20, 260
psychiatric history taking, 8, 9
psychiatrist, 2–3, 6, 139, 221
psychodynamic psychotherapy, 6, 130, 181
psychoeducation, 6, 40, 51, 53, 60, 61, 84, 107, 167, 174, 184
psychomotor retardation, 15, 29, 30, 31, 34, 110, 111, 260
psychosis, 5, 9, 10, 20, 21, 36, 43–44, 46–50, 112, 114, 118, 121–2, 132, 133, 140, 163, 190, 195, 199, 207, 220, 260
  drug-induced, 26, 49, 112
  Korsakoff's, 118, 122, 258
  overview of, 43–4
psychotherapies, 6, 33, 34, 181–5
purging, 96, 97, 103–5, 107

quetiapine, 40, 194, 200

rapid cycling, 36, 41, 204, 260
recurrent depressive disorder, 25
refeeding syndrome, 100
residual disorder, 109
Rett's syndrome, 166, 175
risk assessment, 31, 33, 39, 50, 78, 100, 107, 113, 129, 133–5, 138–9, 199, 260
risperidone, 40, 51, 52, 159, 167, 194, 200
rivastigmine, 159
rumination, 17, 28, 73, 76, 82, 95, 100, 137, 260
Russell's sign, 105, 106, 260

schizoaffective disorder, 28, 39, 43–4, 48, 129, 202, 260

schizophrenia, 3–6, 15–16, 19, 21, 26, 28, 39, 43–53, 56, 58, 65, 80, 82, 83, 84, 98, 128, 129, 133, 136, 138, 146, 151, 156, 163, 166, 171, 178, 181, 185, 186, 194, 195, 196, 211–3, 221–3, 260
schizotypal disorder, 5, 126, 127
Schneider's first rank symptoms, 19, 20, 21, 47, 52, 260
seasonal affective disorder, 32
secondary gain, 86, 90
secondary mood disorder, 25, 26
sedative hypnotics, 112
selective abstraction, 182
selective serotonin reuptake inhibitor (SSRI), 3, 33, 60, 66, 69, 84, 91, 100, 134, 187, 188–93, 207–8, 211
self-injury, 132, 257
self-poisoning, 135, 257
serotonin syndrome, 189, 260
serotonin and noradrenaline reuptake inhibitor (SNRI), 189–91, 193, 208
sertraline, 66, 84, 159, 188–9, 191
sexual dysfunction, 5, 190–1, 196
sick role, 86, 90–1, 259
sleep disorders, 5, 167
social phobia, 55, 58, 62, 64–6, 188
social skills training, 174, 178
sodium valproate, 41, 162, 163, 202
somatic symptom disorder, 5, 56, 58, 65, 86–93, 260
specific phobia, 55, 60, 62, 64, 66
stress–vulnerability model, 45
substance dependence, 109
substance misuse, 13–15, 21, 27, 38, 60, 69, 70, 77, 83, 98, 102, 107, 109, 112–14, 129, 136, 181, 184, 186, 223, 258
suicide, 20, 23, 28, 29, 33, 66, 78, 84, 99, 100, 107, 113, 118, 123, 129, 134–40, 188, 191, 211, 220, 260
    attempted, 14, 137, 138
sundowning, 260
supportive psychotherapy, 53
systemic desensitization, 183

tangential thinking, see tangentiality
tangentiality, 38, 39, 50
tardive dyskinesia, 15, 197–8, 201, 258, 260
thiamine, 122, 124, 149
thought
    acceleration, 17, 19
    blocking, 17, 19, 50, 260
    broadcast, 19, 20, 47, 50, 260
    flow, 19, 37
    form, 19
    insertion, 47, 49, 50, 82, 260
    interference, 19, 20, 22, 23, 47, 260
    retardation, 17, 19
    stream, 17, 19, 23
    withdrawal, 19, 20, 47, 49–50, 260
tolerance, 99, 109, 112–13, 116–18, 121, 124, 186, 196, 209, 257, 260
Tourette's syndrome, 15, 80, 83, 173
transcranial magnetic stimulation (TMS), 3, 6, 33, 34, 213, 214
transference, 184, 260
trazodone, 187, 190
tricyclic antidepressant (TCA), 33, 69, 134, 136, 187, 189–92, 211
tuberous sclerosis, 162–3, 175

unipolar, 194, 215

vagus nerve stimulation (VNS), 3, 6, 33, 34, 215–16
venlafaxine, 60, 66, 134, 187, 190–1

Wernicke's encephalopathy, 118, 122–3, 261
withdrawal syndrome, 109, 119, 123, 208, 209, 261
word salad, 17, 19, 50, 261

X-ray, 156

Yale–Brown obsessive–compulsive scale, 83
Yerkes–Dodson law, 55, 261

zaleplon, 207, 209
zolpidem, 113, 207, 209
zopiclone, 207, 209